Perioperative Care

Perioperative Care

Editors

Richard H. Parrish II
John Kortbeek

MDPI • Basel • Beijing • Wuhan • Barcelona • Belgrade • Manchester • Tokyo • Cluj • Tianjin

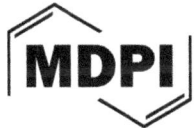

Editors
Richard H. Parrish II
Department of Biomedical
Sciences
Mercer University School of
Medicine
Columbus
United States

John Kortbeek
Departments of Surgery and
Critical Care
University of Calgary Cumming
School of Medicine
Calgary
Canada

Editorial Office
MDPI
St. Alban-Anlage 66
4052 Basel, Switzerland

This is a reprint of articles from the Special Issue published online in the open access journal *Healthcare* (ISSN 2227-9032) (available at: www.mdpi.com/journal/healthcare/special_issues/Perioperative_Care).

For citation purposes, cite each article independently as indicated on the article page online and as indicated below:

LastName, A.A.; LastName, B.B.; LastName, C.C. Article Title. *Journal Name* **Year**, *Volume Number*, Page Range.

ISBN 978-3-0365-1836-7 (Hbk)
ISBN 978-3-0365-1835-0 (PDF)

© 2021 by the authors. Articles in this book are Open Access and distributed under the Creative Commons Attribution (CC BY) license, which allows users to download, copy and build upon published articles, as long as the author and publisher are properly credited, which ensures maximum dissemination and a wider impact of our publications.

The book as a whole is distributed by MDPI under the terms and conditions of the Creative Commons license CC BY-NC-ND.

Contents

About the Editors vii

Preface to "Perioperative Care" ix

John B. Kortbeek
Peri-Operative Care
Reprinted from: *Healthcare* **2021**, *9*, 790, doi:10.3390/healthcare9070790 1

Sara J. Hyland, Kara K. Brockhaus, William R. Vincent, Nicole Z. Spence, Michelle M. Lucki, Michael J. Howkins and Robert K. Cleary
Perioperative Pain Management and Opioid Stewardship: A Practical Guide
Reprinted from: *Healthcare* **2021**, *9*, 333, doi:10.3390/healthcare9030333 5

Jenna K. Lovely and David W. Larson
Enhanced Recovery: A Decade of Experience and Future Prospects at the Mayo Clinic
Reprinted from: *Healthcare* **2021**, *9*, 549, doi:10.3390/healthcare9050549 61

Eric Johnson, Richard Parrish II, Gregg Nelson, Kevin Elias, Brian Kramer and Marian Gaviola
Expanding Pharmacotherapy Data Collection, Analysis, and Implementation in ERAS® Programs—The Methodology of an Exploratory Feasibility Study
Reprinted from: *Healthcare* **2020**, *8*, 252, doi:10.3390/healthcare8030252 73

Aysha Hasan, Remy Zimmerman, Kelly Gillock and Richard H Parrish
The Perioperative Surgical Home in Pediatrics: Improve Patient Outcomes, Decrease Cancellations, Improve HealthCare Spending and Allocation of Resources during the COVID-19 Pandemic
Reprinted from: *Healthcare* **2020**, *8*, 258, doi:10.3390/healthcare8030258 79

Kimberly Pough, Rima Bhakta, Holly Maples, Michele Honeycutt and Vini Vijayan
Evaluation of Pediatric Surgical Site Infections Associated with Colorectal Surgeries at an Academic Children's Hospital
Reprinted from: *Healthcare* **2020**, *8*, 91, doi:10.3390/healthcare8020091 85

Laura Ebbitt, Eric Johnson, Brooke Herndon, Kristina Karrick and Aric Johnson
Suspected Malignant Hyperthermia and the Application of a Multidisciplinary Response
Reprinted from: *Healthcare* **2020**, *8*, 328, doi:10.3390/healthcare8030328 95

Mariana Restrepo, Ann Marie Huffenberger, C William Hanson, Michael Draugelis and Krzysztof Laudanski
Remote Monitoring of Critically-Ill Post-Surgical Patients: Lessons from a Biosensor Implementation Trial
Reprinted from: *Healthcare* **2021**, *9*, 343, doi:10.3390/healthcare9030343 101

Alberto Emanuel Bacusca, Andrei Tarus, Alexandru Burlacu, Mihail Enache and Grigore Tinica
A Meta-Analysis on Prophylactic Donor Heart Tricuspid Annuloplasty in Orthotopic Heart Transplantation: High Hopes from a Small Intervention
Reprinted from: *Healthcare* **2021**, *9*, 306, doi:10.3390/healthcare9030306 111

Richard H. Parrish
Book Review: Cohn, S.L. (Ed.). Decision Making in Perioperative Medicine: Clinical Pearls.
(New York: McGraw-Hill), 2021. ISBN: 978-1-260-46810-6
Reprinted from: *Healthcare* **2021**, *9*, 687, doi:10.3390/healthcare9060687 . . . . **125**

About the Editors

Richard H. Parrish II

Dr. Richard Parrish is a PhD-trained, board certified clinical pharmacist with over 40 years of experience in clinical practice, administration, and academia. Currently, he is professor of pharmacology and founding faculty at Mercer University School of Medicine in Columbus, GA. Prior to this appointment, he was a director and chief pharmacist at St. Christopher's Hospital for Children in Philadelphia, and a clinical associate professor at Virginia Commonwealth University School of Pharmacy. Other career assignments include being a clinical practice leader for Alberta Health Services in Edmonton, Alberta, Canada; being a director of clinical pharmacy and residency programs at the Children's National Health System, Washington, DC; and being a professor of pharmacy practice at Shenandoah University School of Pharmacy in Winchester, VA. He has published 2 books and over 70 manuscripts in peer-reviewed pharmacy and non-pharmacy journals and has presented numerous podium and posters at national and international meetings.

John Kortbeek

Dr. John B. Kortbeek is professor of surgery, critical care, and anesthesia at the University of Calgary Cumming School of Medicine and serves as active medical staff for the Calgary Zone of Alberta Health Services (AHS) in Calgary, Alberta. He received his MD degree from the University of Alberta. Dr. Kortbeek was the head of surgery for ten years (2006–2016) at Calgary and was a co-chair of AHS's Surgery Strategic Clinical Network (2012–2016), which sponsored the province-wide implementation of the Enhanced Recovery After Surgery program in Alberta hospitals.

Preface to "Perioperative Care"

Perioperative care practices worldwide are in the midst of a seeing change with the implementation of multidisciplinary processes that improve surgical outcomes through (1) better patient education, engagement, and participation; (2) enhanced pre-operative, intra-operative, and post-operative care bundles; and (3) interactive audit programs that provide feedback to the surgical team. These improved outcomes include reductions in the frequency and severity of complications and improved throughput, which ultimately reduce operative stress. Practices in theatre as well as ward are becoming more collaborative and evidence-driven.

All professions involved in periprocedural areas were encouraged to "tell their stories"through practice-based research activities, descriptions of changes in resource utilization, and lessons learned in programmatic change management and implementation science. In addition, reports that demonstrate the impact of innovations in surgical procedures, application of new technologies and materials, and multidisciplinary collaboration in sustaining perioperative performance measures were welcome.

We dedicate this book to our patients who have taught us to be better and safer by including them in their perioperative care decision-making.

Richard H. Parrish II, John Kortbeek
Editors

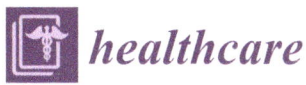

Editorial

Peri-Operative Care

John B. Kortbeek

Departments of Surgery, Anaesthesia and Critical Care Cumming School of Medicine, South Health Campus, University of Calgary, 4448 Front ST SE, Calgary, AB T3M1M4, Canada; kortbeek@ucalgary.ca

In the history of surgery, 1911 was a sentinel year. In that year, Ernest Codman resigned his staff position at the Massachusetts General Hospital to found the "End Result Hospital". He was committed to improving the quality of care of his surgical patients through careful observation and measurement. Codman was a founding member of the American College of Surgeons [1]. He understood that even the very best can err. His goal of revolutionizing surgical care through a better appreciation of patient outcomes and applying this knowledge to improve the delivery of surgical care was prescient. Unfortunately for Codman, he was a century ahead of his time and his ideas were met with ridicule and derision. I suspect that Codman would be both gratified and impressed to see the transformation that has occurred over the past several decades and the excellent work being presented in this Special Issue on perioperative care.

Olle Ljungqvist, a Swedish surgeon, and a group of like-minded surgeons from Denmark, the UK, and the Netherlands, founded the enhanced recovery after surgery study group in 2001. They were convinced, based on published studies of fast-track surgery and enhanced recovery programs, that there was a tremendous opportunity to improve outcomes in surgery through standardization, measurement, and feedback. The enhanced recovery after surgery (ERAS) era was born [2]. Studies incorporating these systems have demonstrated improvements in the length of stay and reductions in morbidity of 20–50%.

In this issue, Pough and colleagues explore variations in antibiotic administration and compliance with prophylaxis standards and identify opportunities for further reductions in surgical site infection in pediatric colorectal surgery populations [3]. They identify an approach to address these consistent with ERAS® protocols. Johnson and associates describe the methodology they will employ to harness the power of the ERAS databases from two large ERAS programs. They will expand the pharmacologic data retrieval to propose further enhancements that may reduce the important morbidities of SSI, thromboembolism, and postoperative nausea and vomiting [4]. Finally, Hasan et al. take the ERAS concept one step further in describing a Peri-operative Surgical Home in pediatrics [5]. The proposed concept was conceived during the current COVID-19 pandemic, with its devastating impact on scheduled surgeries and the need for greater coordination to mitigate the impact of COVID-19, and to streamline recovery as we emerge from the pandemic. The study outlines the potential benefits of enhanced perioperative multidisciplinary coordination.

Crisis resource management (CRM) grew from its origins in aviation, following major airline disasters, and the development of crew resource management. Anaesthesiologists were the early adopters in medicine, but CRM subsequently spread to surgery, trauma, critical care, emergency medicine, and other disciplines. The important and central role of both planning and simulation to successfully implement CRM strategies have come to be generally accepted and described [6]. Ebbitt et al. describe the development of a CRM for the rare but challenging critical event of malignant hyperthermia [7]. The essential elements of the planned response, team leadership, roles, and equipment are described in detail. An illustrative case report allows readers to live the experience.

What operation and when to perform it are questions as old as surgery. One of the fathers of surgery, Theodor Billroth, was both an exemplary teacher and a scholar, who sought to record his outcomes. His goal was to have a basis for recommending the correct surgery for his patients [8]. His legacy lives on in many ways, but perhaps none are more iconic than the classic Billroth 1 and Billroth 2 operations of upper gastro-intestinal surgery. This sentinel dilemma, what is the right procedure, has only grown with the burgeoning number of possible operations supported by modern medical science. In this issue, Bacusca et al. perform a meta-analysis on the choice between performing or not performing a prophylactic donor heart tricuspid annuloplasty in an orthotopic heart transplantation [9]. Their results are suggestive, but a definitive answer, once again, awaits a properly performed randomized clinical trial.

Charles Wilson wrote a wonderful opinion piece on the future of sensors in medicine in 1999 [10]. He predicted many of the forthcoming advances in closed loop devices, biosensors, and smart drugs. He noted that significant improvements in the quality of care will accompany these technologies and surmised that the organization and delivery of healthcare will evolve and change as a result. He had an uncanny ability to foresee coming events, illustrated by the article's closing quote advocating for, "New and better vaccines for preventing common conditions afflicting many millions throughout the world . . . ". In this issue, Restrepo and colleagues present us with a 2021 update on the status of biosensor development, with early experimental application in a critical care unit [11].

Hyland and associates include a wonderful, thorough, and comprehensive review of the use and stewardship of opiates and perioperative pain management in the 21st century [12]. The article should be required reading for surgical trainees as they navigate the changing landscape of managing pain in surgical patients. The paper summarizes approaches that employ all of the available strategies when navigating the complex waters posed by patients with opiate exposure or dependency. Patients with co morbidities, and the increasing number of patients regularly using cannabis or opioid agonists and antagonists are also addressed. Ensuring the best peri-operative experience while mitigating the risks of chronic opioid dependence are quality expectations of modern surgery programs.

The ERAS and strategies to standardize and inform surgical care have become expected norms. This does not make them easy to adopt and implement. Fortunately, Lovely and Larson have provided a road map for success and describe the dos and do not learned from many of our colleagues along the way [13].

I hope that you enjoy this Special Issue of *Healthcare* focusing on peri-operative quality and safety. Ernest Codman would have been pleased.

Funding: This research received no external funding.

Institutional Review Board Statement: Not applicable.

Informed Consent Statement: Not applicable.

Data Availability Statement: Not applicable.

Conflicts of Interest: The authors declare no conflict of interest.

References

1. Neuhauser, D. Ernest Amory Codman MD. *Qual. Saf. Health Care* **2002**, *11*, 104–105. [CrossRef] [PubMed]
2. Ljungqvist, O. ERAS—enhanced recovery after surgery: Moving evidence-based perioperative care to practice. *JPEN J. Parenter. Enteral Nutr.* **2014**, *38*, 559–566. [CrossRef] [PubMed]
3. Pough, K.; Bhakta, R.; Maples, H.; Honeycutt, M.; Vijayan, V. Evaluation of Pediatric Surgical Site Infections Associated with Colorectal Surgeries at an Academic Children's Hospital. *Healthcare* **2020**, *8*, 91. [CrossRef]
4. Johnson, E.; Parrish II, R.; Nelson, G.; Elias, K.; Kramer, B.; Gaviola, M. Expanding Pharmacotherapy Data Collection, Analysis, and Implementation in ERAS®Programs-The Methodology of an Exploratory Feasibility Study. *Healthcare* **2020**, *8*, 252. [CrossRef] [PubMed]
5. Hasan, A.; Zimmerman, R.; Gillock, K.; Parrish, R.H., II. The Perioperative Surgical Home in Pediatrics: Improve Patient Outcomes, Decrease Cancellations, Improve HealthCare Spending and Allocation of Resources during the COVID-19 Pandemic. *Healthcare* **2020**, *8*, 258. [CrossRef] [PubMed]

6. Moorthy, K.; Munz, Y.; Forrest, D.; Pandey, V.; Undre, S.; Vincent, C.; Darzi, A. Surgical crisis management skills training and assessment: A simulation [corrected]-based approach to enhancing operating room performance. *Ann. Surg.* **2006**, *244*, 139–147. [CrossRef] [PubMed]
7. Ebbitt, L.; Johnson, E.; Herndon, B.; Karrick, K.; Johnson, A. Suspected Malignant Hyperthermia and the Application of a Multidisciplinary Response. *Healthcare* **2020**, *8*, 328. [CrossRef]
8. Kazi, R.A.; Peter, R.E. Christian Albert Theodor Billroth: Master of surgery. *J. Postgrad. Med.* **2004**, *50*, 82–83. [PubMed]
9. Bacusca, A.E.; Tarus, A.; Burlacu, A.; Enache, M.; Tinica, G. A Meta-Analysis on Prophylactic Donor Heart Tricuspid Annuloplasty in Orthotopic Heart Transplantation: High Hopes from a Small Intervention. *Healthcare* **2021**, *9*, 306. [CrossRef]
10. Wilson, C.B. Sensors in medicine. *West J. Med.* **1999**, *171*, 322–325. [CrossRef] [PubMed]
11. Restrepo, M.; Huffenberger, A.M.; Hanson, C.W., III; Draugelis, M.; Laudanski, K. Remote Monitoring of Critically-Ill Post-Surgical Patients: Lessons from a Biosensor Implementation Trial. *Healthcare* **2021**, *9*, 343. [CrossRef] [PubMed]
12. Hyland, S.J.; Brockhaus, K.K.; Vincent, W.R.; Spence, N.Z.; Lucki, M.M.; Howkins, M.J.; Cleary, R.K. Perioperative Pain Management and Opioid Stewardship: A Practical Guide. *Healthcare* **2021**, *9*, 333. [CrossRef]
13. Lovely, J.K.; Larson, D.W. Enhanced Recovery: A Decade of Experience and Future Prospects at the Mayo Clinic. *Healthcare* **2021**, *9*, 549. [CrossRef] [PubMed]

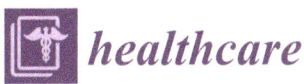

Review

Perioperative Pain Management and Opioid Stewardship: A Practical Guide

Sara J. Hyland [1,*], Kara K. Brockhaus [2], William R. Vincent [3], Nicole Z. Spence [4], Michelle M. Lucki [5], Michael J. Howkins [6] and Robert K. Cleary [7]

1. Department of Pharmacy, Grant Medical Center (OhioHealth), Columbus, OH 43215, USA
2. Department of Pharmacy, St. Joseph Mercy Hospital Ann Arbor, Ypsilanti, MI 48197, USA; kara.brockhaus@stjoeshealth.org
3. Department of Pharmacy, Boston Medical Center, Boston, MA 02118, USA; william.vincent@bmc.org
4. Department of Anesthesiology, Boston University School of Medicine, Boston Medical Center, Boston, MA 02118, USA; nicole.spence@bmc.org
5. Department of Orthopedics, Grant Medical Center (OhioHealth), Columbus, OH 43215, USA; michelle.lucki@ohiohealth.com
6. Department of Addiction Medicine, Grant Medical Center (OhioHealth), Columbus, OH 43215, USA; michael.howkins@ohiohealth.com
7. Department of Surgery, St. Joseph Mercy Hospital Ann Arbor, Ypsilanti, MI 48197, USA; robert.cleary@stjoeshealth.org
* Correspondence: sara.jordan@ohiohealth.com

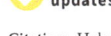

Citation: Hyland, S.J.; Brockhaus, K.K.; Vincent, W.R.; Spence, N.Z.; Lucki, M.M.; Howkins, M.J.; Cleary, R.K. Perioperative Pain Management and Opioid Stewardship: A Practical Guide. *Healthcare* 2021, 9, 333. https://doi.org/10.3390/healthcare9030333

Academic Editor: H. Michael Marsh

Received: 1 February 2021
Accepted: 10 March 2021
Published: 16 March 2021

Publisher's Note: MDPI stays neutral with regard to jurisdictional claims in published maps and institutional affiliations.

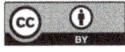

Copyright: © 2021 by the authors. Licensee MDPI, Basel, Switzerland. This article is an open access article distributed under the terms and conditions of the Creative Commons Attribution (CC BY) license (https://creativecommons.org/licenses/by/4.0/).

Abstract: Surgical procedures are key drivers of pain development and opioid utilization globally. Various organizations have generated guidance on postoperative pain management, enhanced recovery strategies, multimodal analgesic and anesthetic techniques, and postoperative opioid prescribing. Still, comprehensive integration of these recommendations into standard practice at the institutional level remains elusive, and persistent postoperative pain and opioid use pose significant societal burdens. The multitude of guidance publications, many different healthcare providers involved in executing them, evolution of surgical technique, and complexities of perioperative care transitions all represent challenges to process improvement. This review seeks to summarize and integrate key recommendations into a "roadmap" for institutional adoption of perioperative analgesic and opioid optimization strategies. We present a brief review of applicable statistics and definitions as impetus for prioritizing both analgesia and opioid exposure in surgical quality improvement. We then review recommended modalities at each phase of perioperative care. We showcase the value of interprofessional collaboration in implementing and sustaining perioperative performance measures related to pain management and analgesic exposure, including those from the patient perspective. Surgery centers across the globe should adopt an integrated, collaborative approach to the twin goals of optimal pain management and opioid stewardship across the care continuum.

Keywords: pain management; opioid stewardship; perioperative care; postoperative pain; multimodal analgesia; regional anesthesia; preemptive analgesia; perioperative medication management; transitions of care; opioid-related adverse effects

1. Introduction

Surgery is an indispensable part of healthcare, and over 300 million surgical procedures are performed around the world annually [1]. Despite tremendous benefits to survival and quality of life, surgical procedures frequently result in acute pain, among other risks. Suboptimal postoperative pain management is associated with worsened humanistic and economic outcomes, including the development of chronic pain and opioid dependence [2]. In the U.S., opioid analgesics have been the cornerstone of postoperative pain management, driven by earlier efforts to improve treatment of pain and societal expectations for surgical recovery [3–5]. The significant risks and costs associated with opioid overuse are now better understood: opioid-related adverse events frequently potentiate complications in postoperative populations and postsurgical opioid prescribing patterns have contributed to the modern U.S. opioid epidemic [6–11]. Postoperative opioid prescribing in the U.S. remains alarmingly high and in stark contrast to that of non-U.S. countries, underscoring the need for more widespread adoption of multimodal analgesia and enhanced recovery strategies by American centers [4,12–14].

Perioperative pain management and opioid stewardship are therefore comparable in necessity and interrelated in execution. To this end, many organizations have offered guidance on components of their application. This has included general postoperative pain management [15–17], perioperative management of patients on preoperative opioids [18], surgery-specific guidelines [19–24], medication-specific recommendations [25,26], conceptual frameworks for opioid stewardship [27–29], collaborative postoperative opioid prescribing guidelines [30–32], statements on perioperative opioid use [33,34], legal opioid prescribing limits [35], and various quality measures for healthcare institutions [36–38]. Despite the multitude of recommendations available, a large proportion of surgical patients report inadequately treated pain and high rates of adverse events, alongside many institutions exhibiting overreliance on opioids and underutilization of multimodal strategies [2,39,40]. This narrative review enhances awareness and adoption of perioperative pain management and opioid stewardship strategies by integrating available guidance into a single "roadmap" for interprofessional stakeholders across the surgical care continuum.

2. Statistics and Definitions

2.1. The Burdens of Perioperative Opioid Overuse and of Uncontrolled Postoperative Pain

Approximately one out of every ten opioid-exposed postoperative patients will experience at least one opioid-related adverse event (ORAE), conferring significant morbidity and economic burden [7,41]. Many postoperative complications may be appropriately classified as ORAEs, including nausea and vomiting, ileus, urinary retention, delirium, and respiratory depression, underscoring the interrelatedness of perioperative opioid use and surgical outcomes [6,41]. Despite their toxicities, opioids appear to be overprescribed for postoperative pain [42–47]. Available data suggest 42–71% of prescribed opioid pills go unused after surgery, with 73% of postoperative orthopedic patients reporting unused opioid pills at one month post-procedure [42,46]. This reservoir of unused prescription opioids in community settings has been identified as a potential contributor to the U.S. opioid epidemic. Over 80% of modern heroin users report nonmedical prescription opioid use prior to heroin initiation, and two-thirds of prescription opioids used for nonmedical purposes are obtained from a friend or relative [11,48,49].

Despite an apparent overreliance on opioids by prescribers, less than half of postoperative patients endorse adequate pain relief, with 75–88% reporting a pain severity of moderate, severe, or extreme [2,15]. Short-term morbidities related to uncontrolled acute postoperative pain span nearly every organ system, including increased risks for thrombotic events, pneumonia, ileus, oliguria, and impaired wound healing. Furthermore, inadequate acute pain control negatively impacts long-term functional recovery, mental health, and quality of life. Collectively, the economic burden of uncontrolled acute postoperative pain is vast, driven by significantly longer surgery center stays and higher rates of unplanned admissions and readmissions to emergency departments and hospitals [2].

An additional risk of poorly managed acute postoperative pain is the development of persistent postoperative pain, frequently defined as new and enduring pain of the operative or related area without other evident causes lasting more than 2 months after surgery. While prevalence of such "chronic" postsurgical pain (CPSP) varies by surgery type and generally decreases with time, it may occur in 10–60% of patients after common procedures [2,50–53]. The physical and mental consequences of persistent postoperative pain are frequently complicated by the development of persistent opioid use, which is also variably defined but largely refers to ongoing opioid use for postoperative pain in the timeframe of 90 days to 1 year after surgery [2,34]. The incidence of persistent postoperative opioid use appears highest after spine surgery and not uncommon (i.e., 5–30%) after arthroplasty and thoracic procedures. Patients on opioids prior to surgery demonstrate a 10-fold increase in the development of persistent postoperative opioid use. Still, previously opioid-naïve patients are converted to persistent opioid users by the surgical process at an alarming 6–10% rate [10,34]. Considering that 1 in 4 chronic opioid users may develop an opioid use disorder, the mitigation of persistent postoperative pain and opioid use should be a priority to healthcare providers and systems [10,54].

2.2. Opioid Stewardship, Multimodal Analgesia, and Equianalgesic Opioid Dosing

"Perioperative opioid stewardship" may be defined as the judicious use of opioids to treat surgical pain and optimize postoperative patient outcomes. The paradigm is not simply "opioid avoidance," and requires balancing the risks of both over- and under-utilization of these high-risk agents. To this end, postoperative opioid minimization should be pursued only in the greater context of optimizing acute pain management, reducing adverse events, and preventing persistent postoperative pain through comprehensive multimodal analgesia [19,33,55–61]. Multimodal analgesia, or the use of multiple modalities of differing mechanisms of action, is key to decreasing surgical recovery times and complications, and so is also a fundamental component of the enhanced recovery paradigm promoted by the international Enhanced Recovery After Surgery (ERAS®) Society [19,24,62–65]. Dedicated resources and care coordination are often required for institutions to align analgesic use with best practices, so Opioid Stewardship Programs (OSPs) are taking hold, modeled after antimicrobial stewardship practices [29,38,66–68].

Quantifying opioid exposure for patient care, process improvement, or research purposes requires the use of a standardized assessment. Opioid doses can be normalized to their equianalgesic oral morphine amounts, i.e., Oral Morphine Equivalent (OME), oral Morphine Milligram Equivalent (MME), or oral Morphine Equivalent Dose (MED) [69–71]. Current evidence-based recommendations for equianalgesic dosing of opioids commonly encountered in perioperative settings are summarized in Table 1 [71]. Guidelines on the use of opioids for chronic pain are also available and provide slightly different conversions for MME doses, citing earlier literature [54,72]. All opioid conversions for patient care purposes should include careful consideration of the limitations of these factors, including extremely wide ranges for ratios found in clinical trials, clinical inter-patient variability, incomplete cross-tolerance between opioids, and other patient-specific factors (e.g., renal impairment or genetic variants in metabolism, see Section 3.5). The newly calculated opioid dose should therefore be reduced by 25–50% when changing between opioids or routes of administration, as discussed in detail elsewhere [71].

Table 1. Current Recommendations for Equianalgesic Dosing of Opioids Commonly Encountered in Perioperative Settings.

Drug	Equianalgesic Doses (mg)	
	IV/IM/SC [1] Dose	PO/SL Dose
Oxycodone [2]	10	20
Hydrocodone [3]	N/A	25
Hydromorphone [4]	2	5
Morphine [3]	10	25
Fentanyl	0.15	N/A
Oxymorphone	1	10
Tapentadol	N/A	100
Tramadol [2]	100	120

[1] The IM route of administration is not recommended. [2] IV formulation not available in the U.S. at the time of this writing. [3] Oral equianalgesic dose equivalent of 30 mg has been used and is also reasonable, given variations in bioavailability between morphine/hydrocodone and oxycodone (equianalgesic ratio ranges from 1:1 to 2:1 morphine:oxycodone based on individual patient absorption). [4] Previous resources have used a 1:5 ratio for parenteral:oral hydromorphone, but newer data suggest a ratio 1:2.5 is more appropriate. IM = intramuscular, IV = intravenous, mg = milligrams, N/A = not applicable, PO = oral, SC = subcutaneous, SL = sublingual. Adapted from *Demystifying Opioid Conversion Calculations: A Guide for Effective Dosing, 2nd Edition, 2019* [71].

3. Pain Management and Opioid Stewardship across the Perioperative Continuum of Care

Perioperative care consists of a complex orchestra of medical professionals, physical locations, processes, and temporal phases. This continuum begins prior to the day of surgery (DOS), continues across inpatient or ambulatory stay, and extends through recovery and follow-up phases of care. A maximally effective institutional strategy for perioperative pain management and opioid stewardship includes all phases and providers across this continuum. Though there is no definitive evidence-based regimen, effective multimodal analgesia requires institutional culture and protocols for pre-admission optimization, consistent use of regional anesthesia, routine scheduled administration of nonopioid analgesics and nonpharmacologic therapies, and reservation of systemic opioids to an "as needed" basis at doses tailored to expected pain and preexisting tolerance [15,18,33]. Figure 1 summarizes the recommended strategies at each phase of care, which will be discussed in greater detail.

3.1. Pre-Admission Phase

The pre-admission phase of care occurs prior to the day of surgery (DOS) and represents the ideal opportunity for patient optimization. Safe and effective interventions exist during the pre-admission phase to improve pain control and decrease opioid requirements in the subsequent perioperative period. Recommended pre-admission interventions include evaluation of patient pain and pain history, education to patients and caregivers, assessment of patient risk for perioperative opioid-related adverse events (ORAEs) and implementation of mitigation strategies, optimization of preoperative opioid and multimodal therapies, and advance planning for perioperative management of chronic therapies for chronic pain and medication-assisted therapy for substance use disorders.

3.1.1. Patient Pain History, Evaluation and Education

Perioperative pain management planning should be pursued through a shared decision-making approach and necessitates an accurate pre-admission history and evaluation. Pain assessment should include classification of pain type(s) (e.g., neuropathic, visceral, somatic, or spastic), duration, impact on physical function and quality of life, and current therapies. Other key patient evaluation components include past medical and psychiatric comorbidities, concomitant medications, medication allergies and intolerances, assessment of chronic pain and/or substance use histories, and previous experiences with surgery and analgesic therapies [15]. Barriers to the safe use of regional anesthetic and analgesic strategies can be identified and considered, such as certain anatomic abnormalities, prior medication reactions, a history of bleeding disorders, or need for anticoagulant use [73]. Likewise, chronic medications that synergize postoperative risks for ORAEs and complications can be managed expectantly, such as benzodiazepines (e.g., respiratory depression, delirium). While such medications may not be avoided feasibly due to the risk of withdrawal syndromes, consideration could be given to preoperative tapering and/or increased education and monitoring for adverse effects in the perioperative period [15,74].

Psychosocial comorbidities and behaviors that could negatively affect the patient's perioperative pain management and general recovery include anxiety, depression, frailty, and maladaptive coping strategies such as pain catastrophizing [15,18,52,75–78]. Additionally, patients with chronic pain and/or history of a substance use disorder frequently experience anxiety regarding their perioperative pain management and/or risk of relapse [18]. While high-quality data is currently lacking to support specific pre-admission strategies for decreasing postoperative adverse events associated with mental health comorbidities, pilot studies and expert opinion support the integration of psychosocial optimization into the "prehabilitation" paradigm for surgical readiness [18,52,75,79]. Cognitive function, language barriers, health literacy, and other social determinants of health also significantly influence postoperative pain management and recovery [51,80–82]. Validated health literacy assessments have been applied to surgical populations [83–87]. Prospective identification of these challenges, including the application of standardized cognitive and psychosocial assessments, can allow for appropriate preoperative referral, patient optimization, and future study of risk mitigation strategies [15,18,52,75,78,80,88]. To this end, various predictive tools for postoperative pain are being explored [88–91].

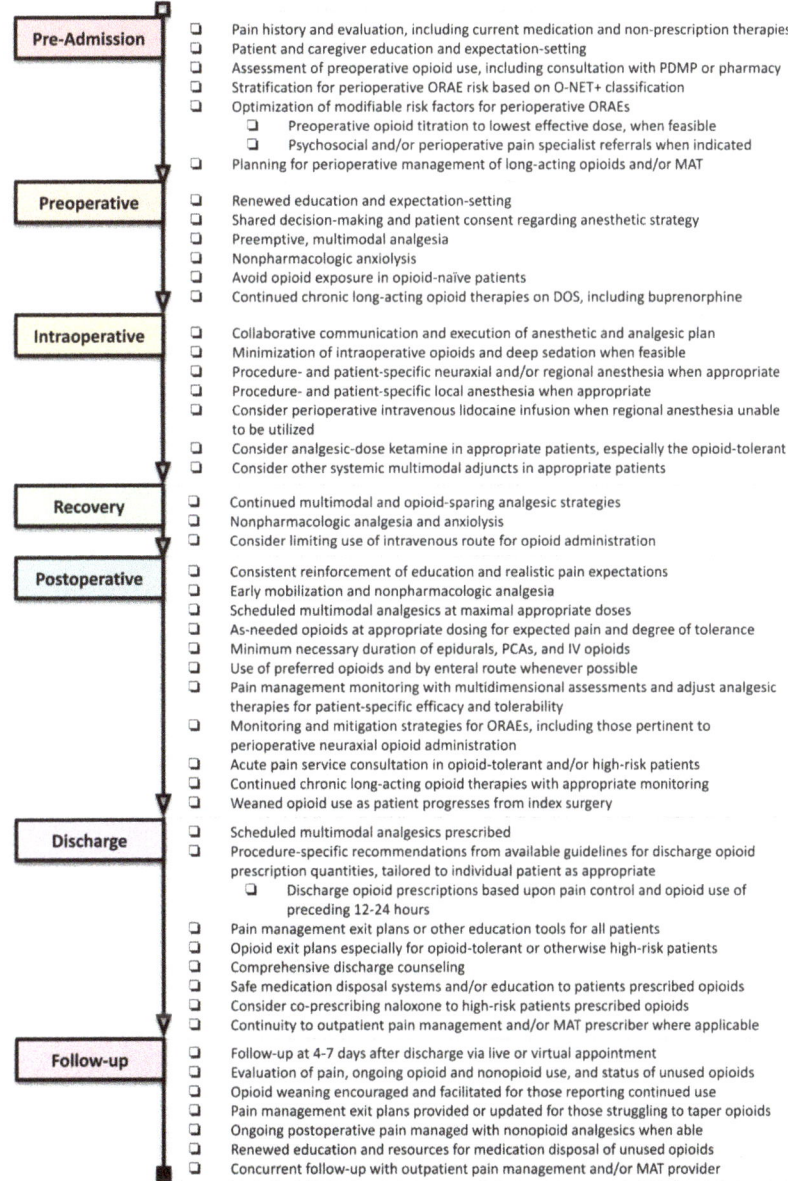

Figure 1. Perioperative Pain Management and Opioid Stewardship Interventions across the Continuum of Care. Legend: DOS = day of surgery, IV = intravenous, MAT = medication-assisted treatment (i.e., for substance use disorders), O-NET+ = opioid-naïve, -exposed or -tolerant, plus modifiers classification system, ORAE = opioid-related adverse event, PCA = patient-controlled (intravenous) analgesia, PDMP = prescription drug monitoring program.

Patient-centered education and expectation management during the pre-admission phase of care are effective strategies for improving postoperative pain control, limiting postoperative opioid use, decreasing complications and readmissions, and increasing postoperative function and quality of life [15,18,92–98]. Insufficient evidence exists to support specific educational strategies or components, but current guidelines recommend an individualized discussion about expected severity and duration of postoperative pain to generate realistic goals about pain management, a description of how pain will be assessed, and an overview of available analgesic options, including the judicious use of opioids and their associated risks, multimodal therapies in the form of nonopioid medications, local anesthetic or regional (central and peripheral) techniques, and nonpharmacologic modalities [15]. Patients with chronic pain or substance use disorders should especially be introduced to the concepts of multimodal analgesia and educated on the risks of perioperative opioids, beginning at the pre-admission phase of care [18]. Education should be provided in an effective manner considering the patient's age, health literacy, language, and cognitive ability [15,99]. The patient's prior experiences, preferences, and expectations should then be integrated into a collaborative, documented, goal-based plan [15].

Provider education, resources, and time constraints in pre-admission clinics currently limit the widespread uptake of these best practices into routine care. The pre-admission phase therefore represents an important target for process improvement related to perioperative pain management and opioid stewardship [94]. To support such efforts, some organizations have made patient education materials publicly available [100–103].

3.1.2. Pre-Admission Opioid Use Assessment, Risk Stratification for Perioperative ORAEs, and Optimization

Recent guidelines have provided an updated tool recommended for preoperative opioid assessment, termed the Opioid-Naïve, -Exposed, or -Tolerant plus Modifiers (O-NET+) classification system (Table 2) [18]. Patients are deemed opioid-naïve if they have had no opioid exposure in the 90 days prior to surgery, opioid-exposed if they have taken any amount less than 60 milligram (mg) oral morphine equivalents per day (MED) in the same time period, or opioid-tolerant if they have taken 60 MED or more in the seven days before surgery. Risk modifiers are then utilized to stratify the patient's risk for perioperative ORAEs, such as uncontrolled psychiatric disorders, any substance use disorder history, maladaptive behavioral tendencies that could impact pain management, and the surgical risk for persistent pain. These categories can then be used to guide perioperative risk mitigation strategies and optimization goals. Patients at every risk level benefit from preoperative education and expectation management in addition to multimodal analgesia throughout the perioperative care continuum. Additionally, patients at moderate risk for perioperative ORAEs should be referred for optimization of psychobehavioral comorbidities, and high risk patients should also be referred to a pain management specialist prior to surgery (Table 2). While not all identified risk factors may be modifiable in time for surgery, the O-NET+ classification system affords the ability to identify higher risk patients proactively to inform perioperative planning and support future practice research [18].

Patients using opioids prior to surgery should also receive a customized evaluation of their current analgesic regimen for optimization opportunities, which may include maximizing pre-admission multimodal therapies and/or tapering of opioid therapies. Conversely, certain pain medications may need to be interrupted for surgery (e.g., aspirin or other anti-inflammatory agents), in which case clinicians should provide clear rationale and education on safe resumption after surgery. Patients on long-term opioid therapies prior to surgery experience increased rates of postoperative complications in addition to higher rates of persistent postsurgical pain and prolonged opioid use, so preoperative opioid minimization has emerged as a potentially modifiable risk factor. To this end, current consensus statements and expert opinion suggest titrating preoperative opioid therapies to the lowest effective dose, depending on the patient's underlying condition [18,104–106]. Patients currently taking more than 60 mg MED may be evaluated for a goal of tapering to less than this threshold by one week prior to surgery as a possible mechanism for reducing risk of perioperative ORAEs, since this should theoretically reduce postoperative opioid requirements. One study found similar postoperative outcomes between opioid-naïve patients and chronic opioid users who successfully reduced their preoperative opioid dose by at least 50% before surgery, and both of these cohorts experienced significantly improved outcomes compared to chronic opioid users who were unable to wean to this threshold [107]. Some experts have proposed delaying elective surgery in chronic pain patients for a structured 12-week prehabilitation program focused on opioid reduction (general goal of ~10% per week) and increasing psychological reserve ahead of painful procedures [108]. The ultimate goals of preoperative opioid minimization include improving postoperative pain control, limiting perioperative opioid exposure and associated ORAEs, and avoiding persistent dose escalations of chronic opioid therapies [18].

Table 2. O-NET+ Classification System and Recommended Optimization for Patients on Preoperative Opioids.

Step 1: Classify Preoperative Opioid Exposure and Presence of Risk Modifiers		
Opioid-Naïve	No opioid exposure	In the 90 days prior to DOS
Opioid-Exposed	Any opioid exposure <60 MED	In the 90 days prior to DOS
Opioid-Tolerant	Any opioid exposure ≥60 MED	In the 7 days prior to DOS
+ Modifiers	+ Uncontrolled psychiatric conditions (e.g., depression, anxiety) + Behavioral tendencies likely to impact pain control (e.g., pain catastrophizing, low self-efficacy) + History of SUD (e.g., substance dependency, alcohol or opioid use disorders) + Surgical procedure associated with persistent postop pain (e.g., thoracotomy, spinal fusion)	
Step 2: Stratify Risk for Perioperative ORAEs		
Opioid-Naïve	+ No modifiers	→ Low Risk
	+ 1 modifier	→ Moderate Risk
	+ ≥2 modifiers	→ High Risk
Opioid-Exposed	+ No modifiers	→ Moderate Risk
	+ ≥1 modifier(s)	→ High Risk
Opioid-Tolerant	+ No or any modifiers	→ High Risk
Step 3: Recommend Risk-Stratified Pre-Admission Optimization		
Low Risk	Preoperative education and perioperative multimodal analgesia	
Moderate Risk	Preoperative education and perioperative multimodal analgesia + Preoperative psychological optimization	
High Risk	Preoperative education and perioperative multimodal analgesia + Preoperative psychological optimization + Preoperative referral to perioperative pain specialist	

Abbreviations: DOS = day of surgery, MED = oral morphine equivalents per day, O-NET+ = opioid-naïve, -exposed, or -tolerant plus modifiers, ORAE = opioid-related adverse event, SUD = substance use disorder. Adapted from [18].

High-quality data does not exist at this time to support strong recommendations regarding preoperative opioid reduction strategies, so a patient-specific, collaborative approach informed by appropriate expertise is vital. General guidance exists for opioid tapering in patients on chronic opioid therapy, but application to the preoperative setting is not discussed [109,110]. Opioid tapering must always be accompanied by patient education and respectful support from the healthcare team [104,109]. Transitional pain services or other perioperative pain management specialist consultation is recommended for opioid-tolerant or otherwise high-risk patients by current guidelines and is supported by implementation reports [15,18,111–114]. Current institutional expertise and resources limit availability of such services at many centers, representing an important area for future investment by health-systems and institutions.

3.1.3. Planning for Perioperative Management of Chronic Long-Acting Opioids and/or Medication Assisted Treatment (MAT)

Patients with chronic pain and/or substance use disorders pose significant challenges to perioperative pain management and opioid stewardship. These complex surgical populations are expected to continue growing, necessitating increased clinical knowledge and creativity from perioperative providers [115]. It is imperative that surgery centers create mechanisms for identifying these high-risk patients prior to surgery to allow for preoperative optimization and coordination of perioperative care. Pre-admission expert consultation is recommended, as is coordination with the patient's chronic therapy prescriber, to allow for optimal perioperative care and safe transitions throughout the recovery period [15,18].

Perioperative management of chronic long-acting opioid receptor therapies, including those used as medication-assisted treatment (MAT) for substance use disorders, should be planned during the pre-admission phase of care. These high-risk medications include long-acting pure mu-opioid receptor agonists (e.g., OxyContin®), methadone, a multitude of buprenorphine products, and the pure opioid antagonist naltrexone (Table 3). A thorough pre-admission medication reconciliation is imperative, including the assessment of available prescription drug monitoring program (PDMP) data, since the use of these products span many formulations and therapeutic indications that may not be evident upon history and physical alone. For example, buccal, transdermal, and implanted formulations of buprenorphine are increasingly used for chronic pain indications. Additionally, naltrexone is used off-label for self-mutilation behavior, and is also available in a combination oral product labeled for weight management (Contrave®). Table 3 summarizes current general recommendations for perioperative management of chronic opioid receptor therapies.

Chronic pain and opioid tolerance are frequently complicated by opioid-induced hyperalgesia, physical dependence, psychological comorbidities, and/or substance use disorders, making postoperative pain more difficult to manage in this population [104,116–118]. These factors contribute to current expert recommendations to continue chronic long-acting opioid agonists throughout the perioperative period, including methadone and buprenorphine [18,115,116,119–122]. Methadone and buprenorphine can be prescribed for either chronic pain treatment or as medication-assisted treatment for opioid use disorder (OUD) in the outpatient setting.

Table 3. Recommendations for Perioperative Management of Long-Acting Opioids and Medication Assisted Therapy (MAT).

Medication	Perioperative Plan [1]	Postoperative Plan [1]
Long-acting pure mu-opioid agonists for chronic pain (e.g., OxyContin®), including continuous transdermal use (e.g., Duragesic®) or intrathecal infusions	Continue typical dose throughout periop period including on DOS, in addition to sufficient intraop analgesia	Continue typical dose and provide opioid-tolerant dosing for PRN opioid orders, consider PCA if expect significant pain
Methadone	Continue typical dose throughout periop period including on DOS, in addition to sufficient intraop analgesia	Continue typical dose, may divide into q6-8hr dosing to maximize analgesic benefit Provide opioid-tolerant dosing for PRN opioid orders
Buprenorphine oral, sublingual, and buccal formulations (e.g., Suboxone®, Subutex®, Belbuca®), including combination products with naloxone	Option 1: Continue typical dose [2] throughout periop period including on DOS, in addition to sufficient intraop analgesia	Continue typical dose and provide opioid-tolerant dosing for PRN opioid orders
	Option 2 (*consider if high risk for relapse and/or very painful procedure*): Continue typical dose through day prior to surgery; temporarily increase and/or divide dosing into shorter intervals starting DOS, in addition to sufficient intraop analgesia	Continue increased and/or divided buprenorphine regimen and use opioid-tolerant dosing for PRN opioid orders Discharge on original/typical buprenorphine regimen with sufficient opioid-tolerant PRN opioid supply
Buprenorphine transdermal patch, subdermal implant, or subcutaneous implant (e.g., Butrans®, Probuphine®)	Continue typical dose throughout periop period including on DOS, in addition to sufficient intraop analgesia	Continue typical dose and provide opioid-tolerant dosing for PRN opioid orders

Table 3. Cont.

Medication	Perioperative Plan [1]	Postoperative Plan [1]
Naltrexone oral formulations (e.g., ReVia®, Contrave®)	Discontinue 3 days prior to surgery and hold on DOS, provide usual intraop analgesia	Continue to hold therapy postop, provide opioid-naïve dosing for PRN opioid orders with close monitoring [3]
Naltrexone extended-release IM injection (e.g., Vivitrol®)	Ideally schedule surgery for ≥4 weeks after last injection and hold throughout periop period, provide usual intraop analgesia	Discontinue naltrexone at discharge and reinitiate with outpatient prescriber after pain recovery complete

[1] All patients should receive maximal multimodal pharmacologic and nonpharmacologic adjuncts across their care continuum as discussed in other sections, and all changes to chronic therapies should be made in concert with the managing prescriber. [2] Some have advocated for preoperative dose reduction in patients on total daily doses ≥12–16 mg; see discussion. [3] Patients on chronic naltrexone therapy may exhibit increased sensitivity to opioids after naltrexone discontinuation due to opioid receptor up-regulation; increased monitoring for adverse events is warranted. Abbreviations: DOS = day of surgery, IM = intramuscular, intraop = intraoperative, periop = perioperative, PCA = patient-controlled analgesia, PRN = as needed. References: [18,116,117,119–128].

Conventional belief has been to discontinue buprenorphine therapy prior to surgery to allow for unencumbered mu-opioid receptors and more effective perioperative analgesia. Current data and clinical experience have challenged this practice, and experts cite multiple reasons for supporting perioperative continuation over interruption. Firstly, buprenorphine is now better understood as an efficacious analgesic, and likely one without ceiling dose effect for analgesia. Little data exists to support better pain control with buprenorphine cessation. Ceiling effects are observed for respiratory depression and sedation, however, likely conferring a safer risk profile than pure mu-opioid agonists [104,122,129–132]. Buprenorphine has also demonstrated protective effects against opioid-induced hyperalgesia, likely improving postoperative pain responsiveness to therapy [121]. This notion is supported by retrospective evidence that chronic buprenorphine users exhibit lower postoperative opioid requirements when buprenorphine is given on day of surgery versus when it is not [133]. These unique qualities suggest buprenorphine continuation is beneficial to pain control and opioid safety in the perioperative period, and preoperative cessation of therapy removes these benefits when they may be most advantageous. A more nuanced strategy is to temporarily increase and/or divide buprenorphine or methadone dosing starting on the day of surgery to maximize pain control without increasing peak-related adverse effects. This has pharmacologic merit in that the analgesic duration of action for buprenorphine and methadone is far shorter than their active duration for reducing cravings [121,128].

For patients on buprenorphine doses exceeding 8–12 mg/day, some experts consider a preoperative reduction to 8–12 mg/day that is then continued throughout the perioperative period, in concert with the patient and buprenorphine prescriber [122,126,132] (see also Section 3.5.3). Data describing the impact of this strategy on patient-centered outcomes remains limited. An alternative option that has previously been proposed is transitioning the patient to a pure mu-opioid agonist (e.g., methadone) prior to surgery. This strategy creates challenges when converting back to buprenorphine postoperatively due to the risk of precipitous withdrawal and length of time (days) involved. Additionally, removing the protective effects of partial agonism to overdose risk likely makes this strategy less safe, and we discourage its use [123].

Preoperative discontinuation of buprenorphine is no longer recommended [18,119,120, 122,126,132]. Complete buprenorphine cessation can lead to opioid withdrawal syndrome if sufficient alternative opioid agonists are not administered, and standard perioperative protocols may not be adequate for this purpose. While not life-threatening, opioid withdrawal is physically and psychologically taxing to the patient and is likely to contribute to increased perioperative opioid exposure, postoperative complications, prolonged hospital stays, and increased healthcare costs. In addition to necessitating increased doses of less safe opioids for adequate postoperative pain control, interruption of chronic buprenorphine therapy requires a subsequent opioid-free period prior to reinitiation. This is especially problematic in a population that may be experiencing opioid-induced hyperalgesia, uncontrolled pain, unmet psychosocial needs, continuity of care gaps, and access to non-prescribed opioids in the postoperative period. While clinical data is limited, expert opinion cites this dynamic as a key driver of postoperative opioid misuse and opioid use disorder development or relapse [74,119,120,122,123,126].

In short, buprenorphine is appropriately viewed as an effective basal analgesic therapy with possible protective effects against ORAEs, psychological destabilization, and relapse. Therapy interruption at the time of painful stimulus is likely to exacerbate the underlying indication for buprenorphine, opening the door to inadequate pain control, increased postoperative complications and costs, and opioid misuse. To this effect, a recent clinical practice advisory states, "it is almost always appropriate to continue buprenorphine at the preoperative dose; furthermore, it is rarely appropriate to reduce the buprenorphine dose" [119]. This is supported by current consensus statements and expert reviews [18,120–128]. Rigorous evidence on postoperative pain management in patients on MAT remains urgently needed to quantify these anecdotal benefits and to compare the effects of available perioperative strategies on patient-centered outcomes [115]. It is also important for healthcare providers to understand the role of buprenorphine coformulation with naloxone, and that continuing combination products (i.e., Suboxone®) poses no risk of opioid reversal when the dosage form is taken appropriately. The naloxone is only made bioavailable when the dosage form is altered in an attempt to inject it, and was developed as an abuse deterrent [126].

Conversely, naltrexone formulations must be discontinued in sufficient time to ensure complete wash-out prior to surgery to avoid iatrogenic pain crisis, since opioids are rendered largely ineffective during therapy [123,124]. Animal data suggest opioid therapies would need to be increased 10–20 times the standard clinical dose to achieve analgesia in patients on concomitant naltrexone [134], and human data is very limited [115,135]. Chronic naltrexone therapy induces opioid receptor up-regulation, however, so patients usually on naltrexone therapy may exhibit increased sensitivity to opioids after naltrexone discontinuation for surgery [117,136]. Postoperative planning for such patients should include maximal nonopioid therapies, opioid-naïve dosing for as-needed opioids, and increased monitoring for adverse events [117,124,128,135].

3.1.4. Perioperative Planning for the Patient with Active Substance Use

A thorough social history is imperative to proactively identifying other substance use that may have significant consequences for postoperative pain management. Patients who exhibit misuse of prescription and/or illicit opioids and also require surgery pose an exceptional challenge [137]. Providers should anticipate postoperative withdrawal symptoms and increased pain sensation in patients with active opioid use disorder (OUD) and ensure postoperative monitoring using validated measures [123,128,138]. Perioperative planning should include opioid withdrawal management and maximizing multimodal agents, including ketamine [104,123,139,140]. Medication-assisted treatment (MAT) initiation and optimization of psychiatric comorbidities should be attempted in the pre-admission phase when time and patient desire allow. If MAT initiation is not possible or desirable prior to surgery, planning for postoperative inpatient MAT initiation should be pursued, with patient consent. This should involve consultation with the inpatient addiction medicine consultant, who will also arrange outpatient follow-up and post-discharge resources for continued OUD management [123].

Patients with alcohol use disorder should be managed expectantly in the postoperative period using validated assessments [141,142]. While such patients do not demonstrate cross-tolerance requiring increased opioid doses to effectively treat pain, the concomitant use of benzodiazepines will confer an increased risk of respiratory depression and increased monitoring is needed. Likewise, patients using prescribed or illicit benzodiazepines should not be prescribed higher than routine opioids for postoperative pain, but are subject to increased postoperative respiratory risk [140,143]. Increased opioid tolerance has also not been observed in postoperative patients with baseline cocaine and/or amphetamine use, but stimulant withdrawal can occur upon cessation that may add to postoperative anxiety and discomfort [140].

Recreational and medicinal cannabinoid use is expanding, including various applications to chronic pain management, and may be replacing chronic opioid and other substance use in some patients [144–146]. Providers should actively engage patients in shared decision-making and education regarding the perioperative implications of chronic cannabinoid use (discussed comprehensively elsewhere [147,148]), including how postoperative pain is affected. Cannabinoid use is associated with significantly increased anesthetic requirements during surgery, higher postoperative pain scores, higher perioperative opioid consumption, and poorer postoperative sleep quality [149–152]. This may be due to cannabinoid receptor downregulation and the complex interactions of the endocannabinoid system with various neurotransmitters and pain modulation pathways [153,154]. Cannabinoids may also increase risks for perioperative medical complications and drug interactions, and so many practitioners are advising perioperative cessation [148]. Chronic cannabinoid users will experience an uncomfortable withdrawal syndrome after abrupt cessation, however, so preoperative down-titration and close postoperative monitoring may be considered [104,140,155]. High-quality evidence to guide perioperative management of active substance use remains elusive.

3.2. Preoperative Phase

The preoperative phase of surgical care begins at patient presentation to the preoperative area on the day of procedure ("postoperative day zero" or POD0). This onsite period, prior to the administration of sedatives or anxiolytics, is ideal to renew education and expectation-setting regarding perioperative analgesia. The patient and caregiver(s) should be engaged in shared decision-making to finalize the anesthetic plan and complete consent documentation.

Preoperative anxiety is common among patients and caregivers. Patient education is associated with decreased anxiety, and nonpharmacologic modalities improve relaxation and positive thinking as part of a multimodal approach to postoperative pain management [15]. While evidence is insufficient to strongly recommend specific strategies, perioperative cognitive-behavioral therapies including guided imagery and music therapy are noninvasive and unlikely to cause harm. Their positive effects on reducing anxiety may provide downstream benefits to narcotic avoidance and analgesia, but further study is needed [15,55,156–160]. Massage and physiotherapy have contributed to improved pain control in other settings and are being explored for perioperative applications [55]. Preoperative virtual reality technology has also been successfully employed to reduce perioperative anxiety and pain [161–163].

Most notably, the preoperative phase of care should be employed to administer preemptive analgesia. Preemptive analgesia refers to the administration of analgesics *prior* to a painful stimulus (i.e., surgical incision) to decrease subsequent pain response. A complex interplay between surgical incision and preexisting factors drives a cascade of central and peripheral sensitization, inflammation, and neuromodulation that intensifies and prolongs postoperative pain beyond the point of physical healing. Preemptive analgesia attenuates these processes to confer reduced postoperative pain, decreased opioid requirements, and potentially less-frequent development of persistent postsurgical pain across diverse procedures [15,53,164–172]. Preemptive analgesics can generally be administered orally with sips of water one to two hours prior to operating time. This strategy is expected to maximize efficacy by aligning pharmacokinetics with therapeutic goals and avoids the risks and costs of unnecessary intravenous agents, which are unlikely to confer meaningful benefit over their enteral counterparts [15,169,173–176]. Intravenous agents should be employed in patients with true contraindications to enteral administration or in those with significantly impaired enteral drug absorption.

While every surgical patient should be offered multimodal preemptive analgesia as a component of comprehensive perioperative analgesia and opioid stewardship, not every patient is an ideal candidate for each medication. Table 4 contains a sample preemptive analgesia protocol with applicable patient-specific exclusion criteria. The optimal pharmacologic agents and doses for preemptive analgesia are undetermined. Acetaminophen is frequently used alongside anti-inflammatory and neuropathic agents, and the combination of these three classes appears to provide the greatest opioid-sparing benefit [177]. Preemptive acetaminophen should be employed widely due to its favorable safety profile, including in patients with cirrhosis [178]. Preemptive opioids may be counterproductive, however, even in opioid-tolerant patients, and are not recommended preoperatively [15,18,106,179]. Preemptive opioids should be especially avoided in opioid-naïve patients due to the risk of increasing postoperative pain perception and opioid use [180].

Table 4. Example Preemptive Analgesia Protocol.

Drug [1]	Dose	Exclusions [2] and Comments
Acetaminophen	975 mg	Exclude in patients with acute decompensated liver failure Do not exclude in patients with chronic liver disease
Celecoxib [3]	400 mg if <65 years old, 200 mg if ≥65 years old	Exclude in patients with any current or preexisting renal impairment and in those undergoing cardiac surgery Do not exclude due to sulfa allergies
Gabapentin	300 mg if <65 years old, 100–300 mg if ≥65 years old or if any renal impairment	May consider avoiding in patients at high risk of respiratory depression, delirium, or dizziness, if risks outweigh opioid-sparing benefits

[1] All to be given as one-time medication orders by mouth in preoperative holding area within 2 h of incision, unless exclusion is met.
[2] These in addition to patients with true significant allergy to drug. [3] Additionally, reduce dose by 25–50% if known CYP2C9 poor metabolizer. References: [15,60,165,166,168,170,180–184].

The use of perioperative gabapentinoids has been increasingly controversial owing to conflicting evidence of analgesic benefit and risks of adverse effects, including dizziness and synergistic sedation with concomitant opioids [61,185–190]. The U.S. FDA has issued additional warnings regarding the risk of respiratory depression with gabapentinoids in patients who have respiratory risk factors, including the elderly, the renally impaired, those with chronic lung diseases, and those on concomitant sedatives [191]. This warning cited predominantly observational data and emphasized the need for patient-specific risk assessments. One of the reviewed studies suggested increased risk with preoperative gabapentin doses over 300 mg [61], while another did not identify any significantly increased risk when exposure was limited to a single preoperative dose [189]. A third retrospective analysis found preoperative gabapentin exposure was associated with a 47% increase in odds of experiencing a postoperative respiratory event, though the vast majority of the studied population were administered doses exceeding 300 mg [190,191]. Gabapentinoids exhibit dose-dependent propensity to increase postoperative pulmonary complications, though combination with other multimodal agents may negate this risk, and the absolute risk of adverse events with perioperative gabapentinoids appears low [177,192,193]. Hence, adverse event risks of gabapentinoids can be substantially mitigated by using conservative doses (i.e., 300 mg gabapentin preoperatively), avoiding postoperative use in patients experiencing or at risk for sedation or dizziness, and/or avoiding entirely in high-risk patients.

Despite these limitations, gabapentinoids have consistently demonstrated significant opioid-sparing benefits and reduced postoperative nausea [15,60,185,194–199]. A recent meta-analysis suggested minimal analgesic benefit to perioperative gabapentinoids in terms of patient-reported pain scores, yet found a significant opioid reduction of approximately 90 mg oral morphine over the first seventy-two postoperative hours [185]. Additionally, gabapentinoids may mitigate central sensitization and decrease the risk of persistent surgical pain, though further research is needed [53,172,200]. Opioid-tolerant patients may especially benefit [117]. Hence, gabapentinoids remain a valuable tool in the perioperative opioid stewardship arsenal for appropriate patients and are supported by multiple guidelines [15,18,197,201]. Ongoing controlled trials may further delineate the effectiveness, safety, and cost-effectiveness of perioperative gabapentinoids [202].

Some pharmacokinetic differences exist between gabapentin and pregabalin, though both are heavily renally eliminated. Pharmacokinetic profiling suggests an equipotent ratio of 6:1 for gabapentin:pregabalin doses [203]. Some have suggested that switching to pregabalin from gabapentin may reduce adverse events in the chronic neuropathic pain setting, but these benefits were not sustained or significantly different from patients who remained on gabapentin [204]. The relative safety profiles of the gabapentinoids in perioperative settings are therefore unlikely to differ when use is limited to short-term, low doses. Duloxetine, a serotonin- and norepinephrine-reuptake inhibitor with analgesic properties, has also been effective in perioperative multimodal regimens, representing a potential alternative to gabapentinoids [205–210].

Nonsteroidal anti-inflammatory drugs (NSAIDs) have long been shrouded in safety concerns of variable validity [183]. Bleeding risk has been of primary concern with perioperative NSAID exposure given the anti-platelet effects of cyclooxygenase-1 (COX-1) inhibition. Bleeding times and postoperative bleeding events do not appear significantly affected by NSAIDs at usual doses, and this risk may be further mitigated by using COX-2 selective agents [211–216]. Traditional dogma has suggested avoiding NSAIDs in spinal/orthopedic fusion surgeries because of the risk of nonunion. More recent and higher quality data suggests short-term NSAID use at normal doses does not affect spinal fusion rates and is valuable for postoperative analgesia and opioid minimization [60,167,217]. High-quality prospective studies are needed to definitively assess this risk. In gastrointestinal surgery, NSAID use has been associated with increased risk of anastomotic leak, but recent meta-analyses suggest this concern may be limited to non-selective NSAIDs [218–220].

Available literature suggests celecoxib, a selective COX-2 inhibitor, is not associated with the aforementioned concerns with NSAID use in spine and gastrointestinal surgery [60,218–220]. Celecoxib is the only NSAID specifically recommended for preoperative use in clinical practice guidelines for postoperative pain management, likely owing to the significant evidence in this setting and lower rates of some adverse effects [15,212]. While celecoxib could be viewed as the NSAID of choice for perioperative use in many surgical populations, it must be avoided in cardiac surgery, where selective COX-2 inhibitors have been associated with increased rates of major adverse cardiac events [201,221]. Increased rates of adverse cardiac events have not been demonstrated with nonselective NSAIDs in cardiac surgery, nor with selective COX-2 inhibitors in noncardiac surgery [183,222]. Caution may still be warranted with selective COX-2 inhibitors in noncardiac surgery patients with significant cardiovascular disease, but these risks may not be significant when exposure is limited to short-term perioperative use [183,212,223–225]. Patient-specific risk-benefit assessments regarding perioperative NSAID use are warranted and should include consideration of the risks of increased pain and opioid use in each given patient [183]. All perioperative NSAIDs are inadvisable in patients with preexisting renal disease or otherwise at high risk of postoperative acute kidney injury [226–230]. NSAIDs, including celecoxib, should not be withheld in patients with sulfa allergies, however [231–233]. Although chronic NSAID should be avoided in bariatric surgery patients, short-term perioperative use is considered safe and beneficial, and is recommended in this population per current guidelines [234–236]. Concomitant, temporary proton pump inhibitor therapy could be considered in patients with high gastrointestinal risk.

3.3. Intraoperative Phase

Anesthetists are crucial team members in optimizing perioperative pain management and opioid stewardship since these aspects, alongside many postoperative outcomes, hinge upon effective anesthesia. Anesthetic strategies include general, regional, and local modalities, as reviewed comprehensively elsewhere [237–241]. General anesthesia has progressed from its origins in deep, long-acting sedative-hypnotics to a more "balanced" strategy employing a combination of agents to create the anesthetized state while facilitating quicker recovery. Balanced general anesthesia now includes broader multimodal agents to mitigate surgical stress and decrease reliance on systemic opioids [242]. Regional anesthesia is divided into neuraxial and peripheral strategies, and various techniques within these strata are reviewed (Table 5). These ever-expanding anesthetic options have rendered controlled comparative efficacy studies challenging, limiting available guidance on optimal techniques for perioperative analgesia and opioid stewardship. Furthermore, the feasibility of anesthetic strategies varies widely by procedure type, anesthetist training, institutional capabilities, and patient-specific factors. Multiple professional collaboratives have generated quality procedure-specific reviews and recommendations to which perioperative teams should refer when developing anesthetic pathways at the institutional level [20,22].

3.3.1. Regional and Local Anesthesia

Regional anesthesia is a cornerstone of multimodal analgesia and opioid minimization, in addition to reducing perioperative morbidity and mortality. General anesthetics can be reduced or sometimes avoided with regional anesthesia, resulting in shorter recovery times and less adverse drug effects such as postoperative nausea and vomiting. Hence, regional anesthesia is integral to the enhanced recovery paradigm [23,62,63,243–245]. The benefits of regional anesthesia continue to be explored and include reduced cancer recurrence when used in oncologic surgeries, likely owing to the mitigation of inflammatory marker surges and other immunomodulatory effects [246,247]. While regional anesthesia is a foundational modality for perioperative analgesia and opioid stewardship, it requires input from patients, expertise from clinicians, and careful procedural assessment and institution-specific tailoring of anesthetic options [15,62,63,248]. Key components and considerations for regional and local anesthetic strategies are summarized in Table 5.

The main limitation of local anesthetics is their duration of action, which diminishes their ability to provide opioid-sparing analgesia for multiple postoperative days [249]. One strategy for extending clinical duration of regional anesthesia is the addition of pharmacologic adjuvants such as dexamethasone, clonidine or dexmedetomidine, and/or epinephrine [249–254]. While additives to local anesthetics may extend duration of peripheral nerve blockade by as much as 6–10 h and are supported by clinical practice guidelines, total duration of action for single-shot injections will still be limited to less than 24 h [15,249,252]. Additionally, despite considerable research, data remains of low quality and with conflicting results for common pharmacologic adjuvants to peripheral nerve blocks, and they may confer additional risks. These dynamics preclude strong recommendations or expert consensus regarding their use [251,252]. Alternatively, continuous catheters are effective strategies for extending local anesthetic analgesia, and are supported by clinical practice guidelines when the duration of analgesia is expected to exceed the capacity of single-injection nerve blocks [15,255,256]. Continuous catheters are not without limitations, however, including increased complexity to perform and maintain, catheter-related complications, and additional monitoring and follow-up requirements [249]. As such, controlled-release local anesthetic formulations have also been developed [257–259]. Liposomal bupivacaine has not demonstrated clinically meaningful benefits to postoperative pain control or opioid reduction when compared to conventional local anesthetics in local wound infiltration, periarticular injection, or peripheral nerve blockade [249,260–275]. Potential benefits and cost-effectiveness of extended-release local anesthetic formulations are likely to vary significantly depending on injection technique, site, and type of surgical procedure, so institutions should consider surgery- and patient-specific use of these agents.

To ensure patient safety, it is imperative to have a standardized, collaborative assessment of the total local anesthetic exposure from all sources. Clinicians must remain vigilant to ensure toxic doses are not reached inadvertently when using multiple local anesthetics across anesthesia and surgical applications (i.e., peripheral nerve block in addition to periarticular injection in total knee arthroplasty). Furthermore, local anesthetic toxicity may be masked while a patient is under general anesthesia. To avoid cardiovascular collapse and death, local anesthetic systemic toxicity must be recognized and treated early [276,277]. Accordingly, current guidelines recommend against intravenous lidocaine within four hours of most local anesthetic-containing regional anesthesia strategies, though local anesthetic infusions through wound or epidural catheters may be started without boluses at thirty minutes after IV lidocaine has been stopped [26]. Additionally, local anesthetics must be used extremely carefully in patients with Brugada Syndrome due to potential arrhythmic effect [278].

Table 5. Selected Attributes of Regional and Local Anesthetic Strategies for Pain Management and/or Opioid Stewardship.

Category, General Considerations	Anesthetic Strategy	Application	Specific Clinical Considerations
Neuraxial Regional Anesthesia Provides motor, sensory, and sympathetic blockade Includes local anesthetics +/− opioids May serve as primary or adjunctive anesthetic or analgesic strategy Significantly improves pain control and decreases use of systemic narcotics May decrease postop morbidity and mortality Increases risks of urinary retention, hypotension Rare catastrophic complications Requires interruption and careful management of antithrombotics	Spinal (intrathecal) injections	Single injection of local anesthetic +/− opioid [1] into subarachnoid space; for surgeries below umbilicus	Hypotension, pruritus (if opioid used); Requires careful assessment and monitoring of postop narcotics if opioid used
	Epidural infusions	Continuous infusion +/− PCEA or PIEB of local anesthetic +/− opioid into posterior epidural space; wide range of procedures (thoracic, abdominal, lower extremity)	Infusion pumps and catheters require special monitoring; may complicate or delay postop mobility or pose other logistical challenges; require careful postop narcotic management if opioid used
	Para-vertebral blocks	Single/multiple injections or catheter placement for continuous local anesthetic infusion along vertebra near spinal nerve emergence; for thoracic or abdominal procedures	Effective blockade of complete hemithorax or hemiabdomen but technically difficult; modern practice generally favors fascial plane blocks or alternative neuraxial modalities
Peripheral Regional Anesthesia Includes local anesthetic injections or infusions (CRA), +/− pharmacologic adjuvants Can limit/avoid need for general anesthesia for some procedures, or can be combined with anesthesia as analgesic strategy Fewer risks and contraindications than neuraxial techniques as most are IM injections Most do not provide sympathetic block Significantly improves analgesia, decreases narcotic requirements May decrease morbidity Rare risks of nerve injury, bleeding, infection, LAST Use of ultrasound guidance has increased safety and consistency	Plexus blocks	Brachial plexus blocks for unilateral upper extremity procedures; lumbar plexus blocks for hip or lower extremity	Requires significant clinician expertise of anatomy; proximal brachial plexus blockade risks hemidiaphragmatic paresis
	Peripheral nerve blocks	Provide targeted anesthesia and/or analgesia of specific nerve or nerve bundles for extremity procedures	Numb limb or distribution must be protected from inadvertent injury, such as thermal injuries, hyperextension, or falls
	Fascial plane blocks (e.g., TAP, ESPB, FIB, PECS-2)	Use higher volumes of dilute local anesthetics to target dermatomes/nerve planes; for thoracic, abdominal, spinal or extremity procedures	Provide unilateral, dermatomal, or regional analgesia; increasing use in modern practice due to safety, ease of administration and broad applications
	Intravenous blocks (IVRA)	Use high doses of short-acting local anesthetic injected into venous system of an exsanguinated distal extremity to provide anesthesia and analgesia	High doses of local anesthetic are used so dual tourniquets must be used and their release carefully timed to prevent LAST; use limited to procedures less than 1 h
Local Anesthesia Mild sensory blockade of superficial/cutaneous nerves Minimal side effects Caution with type of local anesthetic, total exposure, and comorbid conditions (e.g., Reynaud) Avoid open wounds and compromised dermis with some techniques/products	Wound infiltration	SC and/or intradermal injection(s) by surgeon for incisional pain	Less effective if injected into areas of tissue infection
	Periarticular injections	Generally injected by surgeon without use of ultrasound guidance, such as in TKA	Provides effective postop analgesia, in some cases minimizing the need for peripheral nerve blockade
	Topical	Applied as sprays, creams, gels, patches, or oral rinses for superficial pain	Some can be safely self-administered by patient

[1] Routine intrathecal opioids are not recommended by some guidelines [188]. Abbreviations: CRA = continuous regional anesthesia, ESPB = erector spinae plane block, FIB = fascia iliaca block, IM = intramuscular, IV = intravenous, IVRA = intravenous regional anesthesia (e.g., Bier block), LAST = local anesthetic systemic toxicity, PECS-2 = pectoralis nerve block (2 injections), PCEA = patient-controlled epidural analgesia, PIEB = programmed intermittent epidural bolus, SC = subcutaneous, TAP = transversus abdominis plane block, TKA = total knee arthroplasty. References: [15,18,23,170,188,237,240,242,249,250,255,279–287].

3.3.2. Systemic Multimodal Adjuncts

Limitations to regional anesthesia include patient and systems factors. As such, systemic multimodal adjuncts should be implemented or used concurrently with regional anesthesia. These systemic therapies are usually started perioperatively and limited to the intraoperative phase of care or continued into the short-term recovery or postoperative phases. Table 6 summarizes dosing and clinical considerations for common intraoperative multimodal analgesics administered systemically.

Lidocaine infusions are one adjunct that may be applied in the perioperative period. Data exist for lidocaine infusions as opioid-sparing modalities across multiple procedure types, though most literature is for intra-abdominal procedures. Multiple studies have suggested decreased pain scores, decreased 24-h postoperative opioid usage, possible decreased length of stay, and minimal adverse effects [15,18,26,281,288–291]. Studies vary widely regarding the dosing of lidocaine infusions, whether or not boluses are administered, and infusion duration [291–294]. Although lidocaine infusions are frequently started intraoperatively, some centers may instate or continue therapy in the postoperative period where supported by institutional protocols [290]. Lidocaine infusions have been used to provide analgesia outside of the surgical arena, such as in patients with traumatic rib fractures [295]. Current guidelines generally recommend a loading dose of no more than 1.5 mg/kg be given as an infusion over 10 min, followed by an infusion of no more than 1.5 mg/kg/h for no longer than 24 h [26]. All doses must be calculated based upon ideal body weight and should not exceed 120 mg/h in any patient. Doses should be substantially reduced in patients with mild renal or hepatic dysfunction, and avoided entirely in patients with moderate or significant end organ dysfunction and in those weighing less than 40 kg. Other relative contraindications should be evaluated prior to use, including cardiac disease, electrolyte disorders, seizure and other neurologic disorders, and pregnancy or breastfeeding. Serum lidocaine level monitoring is not generally warranted with short-term perioperative use but could be considered if toxicity concerns emerge. Extensive monitoring recommendations should be reviewed and standardized institutional protocols put in place for this modality [26,296].

Similarly, sub-anesthetic ketamine by bolus or infusion has been applied to perioperative and inpatient settings for nonopioid analgesia. Ketamine's ability to improve analgesia and mitigate opioid tolerance and hyperalgesia stems from its antagonism at the NMDA receptor; however, ketamine has a complex receptor profile that likely informs multiple acute and chronic pain pathways. While ketamine may be appropriately considered for opioid-naïve patients undergoing painful procedures, it is especially beneficial to the opioid-tolerant population [15,18,25,117]. Professional consensus statements exist for both intravenous lidocaine and ketamine use for postoperative analgesia and should be consulted. Patient selection, monitoring, and systems implementation are imperative for safety and success with these agents [25,26].

Magnesium has been investigated for its role in attenuating acute and chronic pain. Proposed mechanisms include magnesium's antagonism of the NMDA-receptor, similar to that of ketamine. NMDA-receptor antagonism may interrupt central sensitization of pain, therefore allaying the pathologic transition from acute to chronic pain. An additional potential mechanism is magnesium's antagonistic effects on calcium, as elevated levels of calcium are involved in central sensitization [297–300].

Table 6. Clinical Considerations for Intraoperative Systemic Multimodal Analgesics.

Drug [Refs]	Dosing [1]	Potential Benefits	Monitoring and Cautions [2]
Lidocaine [15,18,26,33,57,261,288–292,301–307]	0.5–1.5 mg/kg loading dose over 10 min then 1–1.5 mg/kg/h infusion through end of procedure Infusions continued or instated postop at 0.5–1 mg/min in some protocols with appropriate monitoring, though some recommend limiting to ≤24 h Always dose based on IBW and do not exceed max exposure of 120 mg/h	Provides improved pain control, decreased opioid use May decrease risk of persistent postop pain, increase functional recovery, decrease ORAEs, and hasten bowel recovery May decrease cancer recurrence, though further study is needed	Avoid in patients with significant end organ dysfunction, certain cardiac abnormalities [3], uncontrolled seizure disorders, electrolyte imbalances, during pregnancy, and in those weighing <40 kg Unsafe to combine with most local anesthetic-based regional anesthesia techniques or topical patches (see discussion) Monitoring protocols for cardiac function and LAST prevention
Ketamine [15,18,25,33,217,261,308–310]	0.1–0.35 mg/kg bolus followed by intraop infusion at 0.1–1 mg/kg/h, and/or postop infusion at 0.1–0.5 mg/kg/h Alternatively, consider 5–10 mg boluses q1hr prn	May decrease risk of persistent postop pain and hasten recovery times Improved pain control and decreased opioid use Evidence of benefits in opioid-tolerant patients Can be given intranasally	Avoid in patients with severe or uncontrolled psychiatric, cardiovascular, or hepatic disease, and in pregnancy Avoid in acute hypertension or tachyarrhythmia and in decompensated patients with high shock index

Table 6. Cont.

Drug [Refs]	Dosing [1]	Potential Benefits	Monitoring and Cautions [2]
Magnesium [33,297,298,309,311–314]	1–3 g loading dose over 15 min then 0.5–1 g/h during procedure	May improve antinociception and reduce sedative and opioid requirements similarly to ketamine	Important to monitor BP, HR, RR, and muscle relaxation Caution or avoid in renal insufficiency, neuromuscular disorders, electrolyte imbalances, bradyarrhythmias, hypotension or at high risk for hemodynamic compromise
Dexmed-etomidine [33,250,261,315–322]	0.3–1 MCG/kg/h, with or without 0.5–0.6 MCG/kg loading dose over 10 min	May improve pain control, decrease opioid requirements, decrease delirium risk, and inhibit catecholamine surges to mitigate surgical stress and end organ damage, but data is limited	Dose- and rate-dependent bradycardia and hypotension: monitor and titrate carefully or avoid if susceptible May be comparable to IV when added to perineural or neuraxial injections instead, but safety unclear
Esmolol [323–325]	500 MCG/kg bolus followed by 5–50 MCG/kg/min infusion	May reduce postop pain scores, opioid use, and ORAEs, but evidence is currently limited	Patient selection and monitoring related to systemic beta blocker therapy should apply, including consideration of concomitant beta blocker/AV-nodal blocking therapies
Dexamethasone [33,250,254,259,309,326–333]	1–10 mg once at beginning of procedure	May prolong duration of regional anesthesia, reduce pain and opioid use	Systemic corticosteroid administration can contribute to postop hyperglycemia and demargination; comparable efficacy between IV and perineural administration
Methadone [334–340]	0.1–0.3 mg/kg (max 30 mg) once at beginning of procedure	May have additional analgesic benefits similar to ketamine or neuropathic agents May be preferable to high-dose fentanyl or preemptive opioids	Duration of plasma half-life can exceed 24 h—monitor for ORAEs Caution in patients at risk for ventricular dysrhythmias given QTc-prolonging risk

[1] All agents given intravenously. [2] These in addition to patients with true significant allergy to drug. [3] Includes second or third degree sinoatrial, atrioventricular, or intraventricular heart block without a functioning artificial pacemaker, Adam-Stokes syndrome, Wolff-Parkinson-White syndrome, or other active dysrhythmia, severe cardiac failure (ejection failure <20%), or concomitant Class I antiarrhythmic. Abbreviations: AV = atrioventricular, BP = blood pressure, HR = heart rate, IBW = ideal body weight, ICP = intracranial pressure, IOP = intraocular pressure, LAST = local anesthetic systemic toxicity, MCG = microgram, mg = milligram, ORAE-opioid-related adverse event, RR = respiratory rate.

Other systemic medications studied for nonopioid perioperative analgesia include the α_2-adrenergic receptor agonists dexmedetomidine and clonidine. These medications provide central analgesia and decrease agitation and sympathetic tone without significant inhibition of respiratory drive. Dexmedetomidine is a highly selective agonist at the α_2-2A receptor subtype, which mediates analgesia and sedation from multiple locations within the central nervous system. This central sympatholysis blunts surgical stress and decreases kidney injury, though evidence is limited [261,317,320,321]. Similarly, esmolol has been investigated as a synergistic analgesic intraoperatively. Esmolol may contribute to antinociception by blunting sympathetic arousal transmission through β-adrenergic receptor antagonism, but mechanisms and benefits are still being elucidated [324,325].

Systemic multimodal analgesics have been studied as additives to peripheral and/or neuraxial regional anesthetic strategies, including magnesium, α_2-agonists, dexamethasone, and methadone. Limited comparative efficacy among routes of administration has emerged. This appears most true for dexamethasone, which confers similar benefits to pain control and opioid use when administered via either modality [259,327–330,333]. Although administering dexamethasone as a component of peripheral nerve blockade may avoid systemic side effects, perineural dexamethasone may have a local effect on nerve tissues that may be undesirable in some patient populations. While literature exists for individual additives to various regional anesthetic techniques, there is no widely accepted consensus regarding ideal drug selection and dosing and if/when systemic administration is preferred [15,250,254,259,300,331,332,341].

Methadone is a systemic multimodal agent explored with increasing interest. A unique opioid in kinetic and mechanistic properties, methadone can be administered once intravenously at procedure commencement to provide prolonged analgesia into the postoperative period. In addition to mu-opioid receptor agonism, methadone's complex mechanism includes NMDA-receptor antagonism and inhibition of serotonin and norepinephrine uptake in the central nervous system. These actions confer benefit in the treatment of chronic neuropathic pain and may also inhibit surgical stress and central sensitization, thus reducing the risks of opioid-related hyperalgesia, tolerance, and persistent postoperative pain [335–337,339,342,343]. Appropriate monitoring and communication across transitions of care is important when the anesthetist administers methadone intraoperatively. Education and processes should be implemented to ensure reduced subsequent opioid use and minimization of ORAEs, especially the risk of respiratory depression with concomitant narcotics given during methadone's prolonged and variable half-life. Alerts embedded in the medication administration record may be ideal, since a "once" dose of intraoperative methadone is likely to be missed by providers in subsequent phases of care, despite its ongoing medication effects in the patient. Still, methadone appears a viable option in the multimodal arsenal and likely a preferable alternative to some clinicians' use of long-acting pure opioids (e.g., OxyContin®) in preemptive protocols.

Systemic multimodal agents available to the intraoperative phase of care are plentiful but remain underutilized. This phenomenon results from the lack of high-quality data to guide many patient care decisions, especially comparative efficacy to inform agent selection, dosing, combination, and contraindications. Institutions are encouraged to generate collaborative protocols and processes that support the safe use of these agents in appropriate patients, including pre-built order sets with recommended patient selection, drug dosing, and monitoring. Deciding and designing an institution-specific "menu" of supported intraoperative options with appropriate safeguards should increase practice utilization and research opportunities.

3.4. Recovery Phase

Ample research supports preoperative nerve blocks to facilitate quicker discharge from post-anesthesia care units (PACUs), owing to their opioid-sparing properties and associated reductions in ORAEs, especially postoperative nausea and vomiting. Patients who undergo surgical procedures with nerve blocks as their primary anesthetic may bypass PACU Phase I with a quicker discharge, enabling increased throughput and efficiency of care while maintaining patient safety and opioid stewardship [63,255,261,344,345].

Multimodal and opioid-sparing strategies should be continued while a patient is in the recovery phase. However, when continuing multimodal strategies, clinicians must be mindful of prior doses of similar agents administered in prior phases of care. When patients are sufficiently awake, providers should limit the intravenous route of opioid administration per current guidelines [15]. Oral administration facilitates longer analgesia with fewer peak-related adverse effects and risks as compared to intravenous routes. Sublingual administration of concentrated oral opioid preparations may be an advantageous strategy for increasing onset of analgesic action with fewer risks than the intravenous route, but this warrants additional study [346]. Additionally, nonpharmacologic analgesic and anxiolytic strategies should be reintroduced in the recovery phase to facilitate patient comfort without reliance on narcotics [158–160,347–352].

Deliberate opioid stewardship, avoidance of the IV route of administration, and maximal multimodal analgesics are also crucial for facilitating timely discharge from PACU for same-day surgical patients. Regional anesthesia and lighter levels of intraoperative sedation, combined with more minimally invasive surgical techniques, are allowing many previously inpatient procedures to be pursued in the ambulatory setting [353–355].

3.5. Postoperative Phase

Postoperative pain management should be individualized to the needs of each patient, noting goals and response to the prescribed approach. This requires the use of a validated pain assessment tool (e.g., numerical, verbal, or faces rating scales, or visual analog score) to assess pain intensity on a recurring basis in addition to functional assessments and evaluation for adverse events [15]. Additionally, pain assessment tools should be appropriate for the patient's age, language, and cognitive ability [15]. The pain assessment should be made during movement as well as at rest, and must include location, onset and pattern, quality or type of pain (i.e., nociceptive, visceral, neuropathic, or inflammatory), aggravating factors, and response to treatment. Typically, assessments should be performed 15–30 min and 1–2 h after administration of parenteral and oral analgesics, respectively, and less frequently for patients with stable pain control. However, analgesic regimens should not be adjusted based on pain ratings alone, given their inherent limitations for predicting analgesic requirements and the increased risk for opioid overexposure [356–359]. Functional assessment of how pain is influencing the patient's ability to achieve postoperative recovery goals should be integrated into a multidimensional approach to adjusting therapeutic regimens [360,361]. Providers should also use pain assessment interactions to reinforce realistic expectations and include the patient in treatment plans throughout the hospital stay. Providers should also be mindful of implicit bias risks when assessing and treating pain. Multiple analyses have found that lower amounts of analgesics are routinely prescribed to Black and other patients of color despite higher degrees of self-reported pain, and that race influences prescriber perceptions of risk for opioid misuse [362–364].

Many of the strategies discussed herein for inpatient postoperative patients may also be applied to various special populations, including trauma/emergent surgical patients, the elderly, the obese, obstetric populations, and pediatrics, as discussed in more detail elsewhere [293,300,365–377].

3.5.1. Postoperative Nonopioid Considerations

Postoperative pain management should continue to incorporate multiple treatment modalities to maximize therapeutic benefits and minimize complications, including nonpharmacologic strategies (Table 7) [15,55]. Physical modalities, including transcutaneous electrical nerve stimulation (TENS), acupuncture, massage, or cold therapy, alone or in combination with medications, may offer pain relief and reduce opioid use, though evidence is variable [15,55,158,160,347,350,378]. Preliminary evidence also suggests cognitive behavioral therapy (CBT), acceptance and commitment therapy (ACT), other mindfulness-based psychotherapy and music may reduce postoperative pain intensity and disability [15,79,379–381]. Surgery centers should devote due resources to making a variety of nonpharmacologic therapies standardly available to postoperative patients, as strongly supported by current guidelines and regulatory requirements [15,18,36].

To provide effective multimodal and opioid-sparing analgesia, clinicians should standardly provide around-the-clock nonopioid medications after surgery [15,18,33]. Acetaminophen, NSAIDs, and gabapentinoids are commonly prescribed nonopioids in postoperative settings. When used in combination, they are more effective in reducing pain and minimizing opioids compared with monotherapy [177,382–384]. Around-the-clock oral acetaminophen should be the backbone of postoperative pain regimens because of its safety and low cost, in the absence of acute decompensated liver disease [178,385]. Compared with the oral route, intravenous acetaminophen administration may offer faster onset and better analgesia thirty minutes after administration, but overall drug exposure after repeated doses and general clinical benefits are not significantly different [176,386–388]. Additionally, the intravenous formulation may impose financial toxicity without additional benefit in patients with functional gastrointestinal tracts as discussed previously [389–391].

Table 7. Nonpharmacologic Interventions for Postoperative Analgesia and Comfort.

Category	Examples
Behavioral/cognitive	Progressive muscle relaxation, mindfulness meditation, art therapy, guided imagery/audio-visual distraction
Psychological	Cognitive behavioral therapy (CBT), acceptance and commitment therapy (ACT), locus of control assessment

Table 7. Cont.

Category	Examples
Environmental	Music, lighting, comfort items, sleep hygiene (e.g., ear plugs, eye shield), personal hygiene (e.g., shower, hair or nail care)
Physical	Heat, ice/cooling, physical therapy, repositioning, acupuncture, massage, osteopathic manipulation, tai chi, yoga, nutrition counseling, healing touch therapy, reiki
Activities	Hobbies/leisure (e.g., playing cards, magazines/books, puzzles, games, journaling, knitting), relaxation (e.g., stress ball, television), pet visitation
Spiritual	Religious literature & services, onsite spiritual counseling

References: [55,163,347,378,380,392].

Selective COX-2 inhibitors or other NSAIDs should be incorporated into most postoperative pain regimens with consideration of the type of surgery, renal function, and cardiovascular risk factors (see Section 3.2). Since inflammation is a key driver of pain after surgery, early anti-inflammatories may be the most effective postoperative analgesic strategies, as evidenced by their superior performance over opioids in analyses of randomized controlled studies [164,393–396]. Novel intravenous formulations of ibuprofen and diclofenac currently have limited roles in therapy due to a lack of demonstrated superiority to ketorolac and significantly higher cost [214,215]. Escalating doses of ketorolac greater than 10–15 mg per dose and ibuprofen greater than 400 mg per dose may offer additional analgesic benefit, and the duration of ketorolac therapy should generally be limited to no more than 5 days [212,397–400]. Gabapentin or pregabalin should be considered for patients with neuropathic pain and may help reduce postoperative opioid use in select patients (see Section 3.2). If initiating postoperative gabapentinoids, dose reductions and close monitoring should be provided for the elderly, those with impaired renal or lung function, and those on multiple narcotic medications [191]. Genetic phenotypes at multiple metabolic enzymes contribute to variation in patient response to NSAID and other nonopioid analgesics, and emerging guidelines provide therapeutic recommendations [184,401].

Other nonopioid agents including cannabinoids, muscle relaxants, and tricyclic antidepressants cannot be recommended for routine postoperative use based on available data but may have roles in select surgical populations (e.g., chronic pain, spinal surgery) [144,217,402,403]. Analyses of the endocannabinoid system suggest certain cannabinoid receptors mediate pain sensitization and hyperalgesia, possibly increasing risk of acute pain conversion to chronic pain. Cannabinoids may therefore be detrimental in the acute pain setting despite being beneficial in chronic pain management [150,153,154,404].

3.5.2. Postoperative Opioid Considerations

In addition to nonopioid analgesia, many patients undergoing major painful procedures may benefit from short-term postoperative opioid therapy. Table 8 provides a comprehensive example of postoperative opioid and nonopioid medication orders. As with nonopioid agents, oral opioids should be used preferentially over intravenous agents for patients who can utilize oral administration. The intravenous route does not confer superior efficacy and carries greater risk for adverse events, and should therefore be reserved for patients unable to use the oral route or patients with severe pain that is refractory to increased doses of oral agents [15,38,405]. When the intravenous route is intermittently warranted for severe breakthrough pain, healthcare provider administration of opioid doses according to patient-reported and functional pain assessments is typically adequate, especially for opioid-naïve inpatients. The sublingual and subcutaneous routes are also reasonable, but the intramuscular route should be avoided due to delayed and erratic absorption [15]. One single-center retrospective cohort study suggests sublingual opioids can be utilized for postoperative breakthrough pain with comparable efficacy as the intravenous route, and the sublingual route was associated with reduced opioid-related respiratory depression [346].

Table 8. Example of Postoperative Inpatient Pain Management Orders.

Medication (Route [1])	Application	Dose Range [2]	Comments
Acetaminophen (PO)	All patients without contraindication	650 mg PO q4h while awake or 975 mg PO q6h [2]	Selective use of the IV & PR routes may be appropriate, see discussion
Anti-inflammatory—Choose one in all patients without contraindication (see Section 3.2)			
Celecoxib (PO)		100–200 mg PO q12–24h [2]	May be preferred to ibuprofen
Ketorolac (IV)		15 mg IV q6h × 24h, max duration 5 days [2]	Limit use to first 24–48 h, change to alternative when can take PO
Ibuprofen (PO)		400 mg PO TID with meals or q6h [2]	
Neuropathic Agent—Choose one in patients with significant pain or high opioid use, weighing patient-specific risks and benefits (see Section 3.2)			
Gabapentin (PO)		100 mg PO TID, or 100 mg with breakfast and lunch plus 300 mg qHS dose [2]	Opioid-sparing benefits must be weighed against patient-specific risks for sedation, respiratory depression, and dizziness
Pregabalin (PO)		25–50 mg PO BID [2]	
Oral As-needed Opioid—Choose one in patients undergoing painful procedures for duration of expected moderate-to-severe surgical pain, gradually decreasing dose during recovery period			
Oxycodone (PO)		Opioid-naïve: 5 mg PO q4 h PRN moderate-to-severe pain, may repeat 5 mg dose within 1 hr if ineffective (total available range 5–10 mg q4h PRN)	Initial dosing for opioid-tolerant patients should be based upon baseline opioid use, usually allowing for 25–100% increase from baseline exposure in immediate postop period [4]
Hydrocodone (PO)		Dosing as above, recognizing this is slightly lower analgesic potency (see Table 1)	Decrease or discontinue scheduled acetaminophen to avoid overexposure if using combination products
As-needed Opioid for Breakthrough pain—Choose one for first 24 h postop; if used frequently and/or needed beyond immediate recovery phase then assess for other causes of pain and/or increase primary as-needed opioid			
Oxycodone (SL)		5 mg PO/SL q4 h PRN moderate-to-severe breakthrough pain	Consider "may repeat" dose and/or initial 10 mg dose for breakthrough pain in opioid-tolerant patients [4]
Hydromorphone (IV)		0.2–0.5 mg IV/SC q3 h PRN moderate-to-severe breakthrough pain [3]	Only order IV opioids for severe breakthrough pain or absolute contraindications to oral analgesia. Consider "may repeat" dose and/or initial 0.8–1 mg dose for breakthrough pain in opioid-tolerant patients
NMDA Antagonist—Consider in severely painful procedures, in opioid-tolerant patients, or in cases of pain-sedation mismatch in appropriate patients			
Ketamine (IV)		0.1–0.35 mg/kg or 5–10 mg IVP once or q2 h PRN for refractory pain, or in cases of pain-sedation mismatch precluding opioid use	Continuous infusion of 0.05–0.35 mg/kg/h may be considered postoperatively where supported by institutional protocol

[1] All represented oral formulations are short-acting/immediate release dosage forms. [2] For medications with dosing ranges provided, consider using lower doses within the suggested range for patients with advanced age and/or chronic kidney and liver disease. Patients with chronic pain and and/or opioid use disorders may benefit from higher doses. [3] Available concentrations of hydromorphone injectable should determine the measurable dose, within this range, in order to ensure practical drug administration (e.g., rounded doses to the nearest 0.1 mL or 0.25 mL). [4] A number of practical strategies exist to accomplish this—see Section 3.5.3). Abbreviations: IV = intravenous, IVP = intravenous push, PO = oral or by mouth, SC = subcutaneous, SL = sublingual.

When complete reliance on the intravenous route is considered necessary due to severe gastrointestinal dysfunction or surgical need for strict bowel rest, patient-controlled analgesia (PCA) is recommended over intermittent bolus by healthcare providers by some guidelines [24,403]. This notion is increasingly challenged by enhanced recovery practice, however, especially in minimally invasive colorectal surgery [24,406,407]. Providers may consider reserving use of PCA for patients with acute on chronic pain or otherwise requiring significant amounts of intermittent IV opioids, and only until other routes can be used. Maximizing multimodal therapies in earlier phases of care, especially regional anesthesia or lidocaine infusions, may allow for avoidance of PCA in routine patients undergoing colorectal surgery [24]. The use of intraoperative methadone (see Section 3.3.2) or the sublingual route of administration for postoperative opioids are also promising modalities that could be explored for reducing reliance on PCAs. Medication and patient safety issues abound with PCAs [408,409]. Accordingly, average duration of PCA use has been discussed as a quality indicator of hospital opioid stewardship practices [38]. Use of PCAs should be guided by institutional order sets with pre-built doses stratified for opioid-naïvety and risk for opioid-related respiratory depression, and continuous infusions should generally be avoided in opioid-naïve patients [15,71,408,409].

Empiric opioid selection should align with generally preferred agents, patient-specific pharmacologic needs, and the oral route of administration. Oxycodone, hydrocodone, and hydromorphone should be used preferentially due to their decreased propensities for active metabolites, accumulation in end organ dysfunction, drug-drug interactions, and histamine release (Table 9) [410–414]. Morphine, tramadol, and codeine are significantly metabolized to active metabolites and heavily renally eliminated, increasing the risk of adverse effects in some patient populations [410,415]. Codeine and tramadol have limited roles in postoperative pain management due to well-documented interindividual variability in efficacy and safety [416,417]. Polymorphisms at CYP2D6 and drug-drug interactions significantly affect codeine bioactivation to morphine, the pathway most responsible for analgesic efficacy. Likewise, tramadol is metabolized by CYP2D6 into an active metabolite more potent than the parent drug. Patients possessing increased metabolic variants at CYP2D6 (1.5–9.5% of the worldwide population) are at heightened risk of adverse effects from these agents due to greater conversion to active metabolites, and patients with poor metabolizer phenotypes (25.3–70.3% of the worldwide population) may report decreased efficacy from reduced bioactivation [410–412,417,418]. These medications should be avoided in most patients since phenotype testing is not routinely performed before prescribing and since multiple agents with more favorable safety and efficacy profiles exist.

Individual patient response to preferred opioids still varies substantially. Genetic polymorphisms affecting opioid metabolism are not uncommon, so rotation to an agent utilizing an alternative metabolic pathway should be considered in patients with unexplained lack of response and/or significant intolerance (e.g., extreme nausea and vomiting with or without insufficient analgesia from oxycodone may be remedied by change to hydrocodone or hydromorphone) (Table 9) [414,418,419]. Newer opioid agonists can also be considered. Oxymorphone may be advantageous in cases of persistent opioid overexposure related to altered metabolism from phase I enzymatic alterations and/or significant renal impairment. Tapentadol is unique in pharmacologic and pharmacokinetic profiles and can be a valuable option in cases of significant widespread opioid intolerance, but is completely reliant on renal function for excretion. While tramadol is also sometimes considered in patients with intolerance to preferred opioids, its diverse receptor profile confers increased adverse event risks that are especially undesirable in the postoperative period, in addition to previously discussed risks related to its metabolic pathways [417,420–428]. Pharmacists can also assess medication regimens for clinically significant drug-drug pharmacokinetic interactions, especially in patients on antiepileptic medications, azole antifungals, or rifampin [413,429,430]. The interprofessional team should also evaluate for pharmacodynamic interactions affecting the patient's response, such as additive toxicity risk with concomitant sedatives or anticholinergics.

While allergic reactions to opioids are frequently reported, true IgE-mediated hypersensitivity is rare. Only 15% of patients referred for drug provocation testing due to concern with anaphylactic opioid reactions were diagnosed with opioid allergy in one analysis, and opioids are believed to be implicated in less than 2% of all cases of intraoperative anaphylaxis [431,432]. Angioedema and hemodynamic instability are more likely to indicate true hypersensitivity than other reactions [431,433]. In cases of true opioid hypersensitivity, opioids of different structural classes are unlikely to demonstrate cross-allergenicity, though this risk remains uncertain. The majority of opioid reactions are not mediated by IgE but by mast cell degranulation, however, and may present as hives, hypotension, urticaria, pruritus, and/or severe anaphylactoid responses. More synthetic opioids exhibit decreasing rates of opioid-mediated histamine release, so should be considered in cases of pseudoallergy [431–434].

Clinicians should adjust the empiric postoperative pain management plan in cases for efficacy and tolerability, taking into account the duration and intensity of expected pain for the specific surgical procedure [15]. The use of "may repeat" doses and separate orders only for breakthrough pain can usually allow for a workable escalation pathway for uncontrolled pain within standardized postoperative order sets, as displayed in Table 8. Incomplete analgesic response precluding usual postoperative functional progress despite these orders should prompt a 25–50% increase to the first-line opioid order dose, based on severity of ongoing pain and in the absence of dose-limiting adverse effects. Breakthrough pain regimens should generally be limited to the first 24 postoperative hours, with acceptable pain control maintained by adjusting oral doses if needed. Adjusting opioid regimens in longer-term pain and in cancer-related pain is discussed extensively elsewhere [71,435]. Patients with adequate analgesia but experiencing ORAEs should be assessed for opioid dose reductions, and all opioids should be tapered after surgery as acute postoperative pain improves. If usual surgical recovery is inhibited by unsuccessful functional pain management and/or unacceptable adverse effects despite appropriate multimodal therapies and patient-specific opioid optimization, postoperative pain management specialty consultation is advised. Acute and transitional pain services for surgical patients are evolving, and have been associated with reduced opioid use and length of stay [113,436–441].

Table 9. Opioid Properties to Consider When Selecting or Modifying Postoperative Regimens.

Opioid (Structural Class)	Major Metabolic Pathways	Active Metabolites	Effects of End Organ Function [1]
Phenanthrene opium alkaloids–highest rate of histamine release			
Morphine, Codeine (after bioactivation) [2]	UGT2B7 (phase II metabolism)	Extensive production of active metabolites	Renal impairment significantly increases exposure
Semisynthetic phenanthrene derivatives of opium alkaloids–cross-reactivity possible between agents			
Oxycodone	CYP3A4 (primary), CYP2D6 (minor)	Produces small amounts of oxymorphone and other active metabolites	Renal impairment mildly increases exposure
Hydrocodone	CYP3A4 (primary), CYP2D6 (minor)	Produces small amount of hydromorphone and other active metabolites	Not significantly altered by renal impairment
Hydromorphone	UGT2B7 (phase II metabolism)	Multiple active metabolites but clinically unimportant	Not significantly altered by renal impairment
Oxymorphone	UGT2B7 (phase II metabolism)	Metabolites have little activity	Not significantly altered by renal impairment
Synthetic phenylpropylamine derivatives of opioid alkaloids–cross-reactivity with phenanthrenes unlikely			
Tapentadol	Unspecified glucuronidation	No active metabolites	Renal impairment significantly increases exposure
Tramadol	CYP2D6, CYP3A4	Extensive production of active metabolites by CYP2D6	Renal impairment increases exposure

[1] All listed opioids should be reduced in cases of significant hepatic impairment. [2] Codeine is a prodrug of morphine (activated by CYP2D6) and is not recommended for postoperative pain management; see text. Abbreviations: CYP = cytochrome P450 enzyme superfamily, i.e., hepatic enzymes responsible for phase I metabolism. References: [178,410–412,414,415,423,425,426,429,430].

Despite employing opioid minimization and evidence-based opioid selection when treating postoperative pain, the interprofessional team should actively anticipate and mitigate opioid-related adverse events (ORAEs, Table 10). Nausea/vomiting, constipation, pruritus, respiratory depression, sedation, and delirium continue to be common adverse effects negatively affecting postoperative outcomes and costs of care [6–8]. Sedation and respiratory depression are the most concerning ORAEs and should be actively mitigated through institutional monitoring protocols based on current practice guidelines and published literature. Protocols should include the use of the Pasero Opioid-Induced Sedation Scale (POSS) and capnography monitoring in addition to conventional respiratory parameters and nursing assessments [15,442–446]. Avoiding concomitant sedatives, especially benzodiazepines, to all feasible extent is also an important modifiable risk for postoperative respiratory depression, sedation, and delirium. This is crucial in patients with higher baseline risks for this complications, including the elderly, obese, and those with preexisting lung disease [38,143,190,447–452]. Specialized monitoring for patients receiving perioperative neuraxial opioids must be standardly executed and supported by institutional order sets as outlined elsewhere [15,453]. Some enhanced recovery guidelines recommend against routine intrathecal opioids as this strategy may not have a positive benefit-risk profile in this setting [188].

Patients prescribed opioids should also receive scheduled stimulant bowel regimens to avoid opioid-induced constipation and progression to ileus, a risk that is heightened in the postoperative period (Table 10). Standard preventative use of a stimulant laxative such as senna or bisacodyl is generally effective in preventing opioid-induced constipation in opioid-naive patients, and available evidence does not suggest a superior agent [454–458]. The addition of stool softeners (i.e., docusate) and/or laxatives of alternative classes (e.g., osmotic agents like polyethylene glycol or magnesium oxide) may be added if needed postoperatively, but sugar-based strategies such as lactulose or sorbitol should be avoided due to adverse event risks [454,455]. Unique considerations exist in major colorectal surgery and are discussed in enhanced recovery guidelines [281]. Peripherally acting opioid antagonists have been developed to combat opioid-induced constipation with mixed results for clinical outcomes and cost-effectiveness related to postoperative ileus [459–462]. Naloxegol and alvimopan may have comparable efficacy in the postoperative period [463]. An alternative agent used in chronic constipation, lubiprostone, does not appear to have superior efficacy over senna in the postoperative setting [464].

Table 10. Recommended Monitoring and Mitigation Strategies for Postoperative ORAEs.

ORAE	Monitoring and Mitigation Strategies
Sedation, Respiratory, Depression, Delirium	Vigilant monitoring of respiratory and mental status by validated scales (e.g., POSS) and respiratory function data, especially EtCO2, per standardized institutional protocols based on available guidelines Evaluate for opioid dose reduction and/or rotation Avoid concomitant sedatives, especially benzodiazepines Standard opioid antagonist protocols for urgent/emergent reversal Optimize physical and environmental contributing factors (e.g., allow sunlight in room during daytime hours, limit interruptions to sleep)
Constipation, Ileus	Early ambulation, diet advancement as tolerated, and goal-directed hydration as per surgery-specific enhanced recovery protocol Standard postoperative scheduled bowel regimen started on DOS continued for duration of opioid therapy, including stimulant laxative and stool softener (e.g., senna-docusate 8.6–100 mg PO BID), reduced as opioid requirements decrease and bowel function returns to normal Standard additional PRN laxative for constipation (e.g., polyethylene glycol 17 g daily PRN), escalation to PR suppository in refractory cases
Nausea, Vomiting	Standard postoperative PRN antiemetic orders (e.g., ondansetron 4 mg PO q6hr PRN or droperidol 1.25 mg IV q6h PRN nausea/vomiting) Assess for opioid reduction and/or rotation (see text) Optimize physical and environmental contributing factors (e.g., nutrition, noxious stimuli)
Urinary Retention	Monitor per standard institutional protocol Decrease anticholinergic burden (e.g., remove scopolamine patches, avoid antihistamines) Hold chronic anticholinergic therapies in the immediate postoperative period where possible (e.g., oxybutynin) Avoid neuraxial opioids, consider avoiding neuraxial anesthesia entirely in patients at high risk (e.g., older males with prostate disease)
Pruritus	Low-dose nalbuphine PRN is likely most efficacious and safe strategy and may be warranted for duration of neuraxial opioids in some cases May consider age-appropriate, low-dose antihistamines where needed (e.g., diphenhydramine 12.5–25 mg PO q6hr PRN), but this is less efficacious than nalbuphine and may increase risk for other ORAEs Avoid neuraxial opioids in susceptible patients

Abbreviations: BID = twice daily; DOS = day of surgery; EtCO2 = end-tidal carbon dioxide; ORAE = opioid-related adverse drug event; PO = by mouth/oral; POSS = Pasero Opioid-Induced Sedation Scale; PR = per rectum. References: [15,442–444,453–456,465–467].

3.5.3. Postoperative Considerations in the Opioid-Tolerant and/or Substance Use Disorder Populations

Postoperative pain management in patients with preexisting opioid tolerance and/or substance use disorders is more complicated and high-risk than that of opioid-naïve counterparts, and specialist consultation is strongly advised [15,18,36]. Nonopioid medications and nonpharmacologic options are especially important in this population due to significant opioid receptor up-regulation. In the opioid-tolerant surgical patient, multimodal analgesia may help limit opioid dose escalation, reduce the incidence of adverse events, and facilitate faster postoperative opioid weaning. Stronger consideration should be given to postoperative use of gabapentinoids, ketamine, and regional anesthesia than what may be used in opioid-naïve patients.

Empiric as-needed opioid regimens should be dosed with consideration to baseline opioid use and closely monitored, recognizing that higher doses and/or longer tapers may be warranted. Patients on preoperative opioids have increased risk for suffering if undertreated and increased rates of ORAEs if overexposed. Still, opioids should be utilized only after first-line administration of nonopioids and used at the lowest effective dose, avoiding persistent dose escalations in the postoperative period [18]. To this end, opioid-exposed patients (i.e., those with preoperative opioid use below 60 MED) can usually be prescribed routine postoperative opioid orders as for opioid-naïve patients, with increased monitoring and adjustment for efficacy as needed. Truly opioid-tolerant patients (i.e., those with preoperative opioid use $\geq$60 MED) should be interviewed to discern their precise preoperative daily utilization to inform a patient-specific postoperative opioid regimen. Postoperative opioids should not be dosed solely upon prescription drug monitoring program (PDMP) data to avoid unnecessary narcotic exposure in patients taking less than maximum quantities prescribed. Opioid-tolerant patients undergoing minor procedures may only warrant routine as-needed opioid dose orders (e.g., oxycodone 5 mg q4h PRN, may repeat within 1 h if ineffective) in addition to their baseline opioid exposure.

After major painful procedures, opioid-tolerant patients often warrant opioid exposure equivalent to a 50–100% increase from their baseline MED to achieve adequate analgesia and functional outcomes in the immediate postoperative period. Some literature suggests postoperative opioid requirements up to four times that of opioid-naïve patients may be necessary after the same procedure, and little published guidance exists on how best to accomplish this [18,117,128]. Chronic opioid requirements may be maintained by modestly increasing the patient's usual as-needed opioid dose at the same dosing interval, with additional orders as-needed for breakthrough pain. Alternatively, opioid doses could be scheduled throughout daytime hours to provide the patient's baseline MED, with additional as-needed doses to allow for adequate control of postoperative pain. A third option may be to order the patient's usual as-needed opioid dose at a shorter dosing interval (e.g., every 3 h as needed instead of every 4 h) with a breakthrough pain option. To illustrate, a patient regularly taking oxycodone 10 mg every 4 h throughout the day prior to admission (i.e., 60–75 MED baseline use) could be ordered one of the following sets of empiric opioid orders upon postoperative inpatient admission after a major painful procedure, assuming the oral route of administration for primary analgesia and the sublingual route for breakthrough pain:

(a) oxycodone 10 mg PO q4hr PRN moderate-to-severe pain, may repeat 5 mg dose within 1 h if pain unrelieved; oxycodone 5 mg SL q4hr PRN moderate-to-severe breakthrough pain × 24 h.
(b) oxycodone 10 mg PO q4hr scheduled while awake; oxycodone 5 mg PO q4hr PRN moderate-to-severe pain; oxycodone 5 mg SL q4hr PRN moderate-to-severe breakthrough pain × 24 h.
(c) oxycodone 10 mg q3hr PRN moderate-to-severe pain; oxycodone 5 mg SL q4hr PRN moderate-to-severe breakthrough pain × 24 h.

All initial opioid options are in addition to maximal scheduled nonopioid and nonpharmacologic orders, and accompanied by close monitoring for any appropriate adjustments. Orders for opioids as-needed for breakthrough pain should generally still be limited to the immediate postoperative period (i.e., order should automatically expire after the first 24 h of inpatient ward admission). Ongoing need for breakthrough pain opioid doses should prompt evaluation for nonsurgical causes of pain, further optimization nonopioid therapies, and an increase to the primary as-needed opioid order on a patient-specific basis.

Patients with chronic pain and/or opioid use disorders may benefit from a patient-controlled analgesia (PCA) modality when pain is very difficult to control or when the oral route cannot be used [15,117,128,468]. Empiric reliance on intravenous opioids via PCA is increasingly falling out of favor, however, and should not be viewed as routinely necessary in colorectal surgery when enhanced recovery and multimodal analgesia modalities are maximized [24,406]. Experts are increasingly finding this to be true even in opioid-tolerant patients, and opioid-free intraoperative analgesia is even being explored in this population [18]. If PCAs are employed for opioid-tolerant patients, dosing should be patient-specific after assessment of baseline opioid use, as discussed in detail elsewhere [71,117,128,469].

Continuation of chronic long-acting pain medication regimens is recommended, in consultation with the patient's outpatient prescriber (see Section 3.1.3). Chronic buprenorphine or methadone therapy should be continued either at baseline dosing regimens or by dividing the total daily dose throughout the day to maximize their analgesic activity (see Section 3.1.3). The patient's usual total daily dose, or a slightly increased total daily dose, is divided into 2 to 4 doses throughout the day starting on the day of surgery. The patient can then be discharged on their usual preoperative regimen without therapy interruption [121,125,128]. Alternatively, some have advocated for a buprenorphine dose reduction in the perioperative period if the patient is on higher chronic doses and/or is experiencing inadequate pain relief despite appropriately dosed as-needed opioids, citing the dose-dependent mu opioid receptor antagonism of buprenorphine [119,122,126,132]. Patients on maintenance buprenorphine or methadone must also be ordered as-needed opioids at tolerant doses (see examples provided earlier in this section) to effectively treat postoperative pain in addition to the continued buprenorphine/methadone regimen, regardless of the dosing strategy employed for them.

Despite available evidence and guidance, healthcare providers may carry prejudices that result in under-treatment of postoperative pain in the opioid-tolerant and/or opioid use disorder populations. Such misconceptions often include that maintenance therapy with buprenorphine or methadone alone provides sufficient postoperative analgesia, that additional opioids for analgesia may cause addiction relapse or undue respiratory depression risk, or that the use of patient-controlled analgesia (PCA) may exacerbate these risks. In actuality, receptor up-regulation and the pharmacology of these agents confer the need for additional short-acting opioids at opioid-tolerant doses in order to provide equipotent analgesia to that provided to opioid-naïve patients. Available evidence does not support that this strategy exacerbates substance use disorders or increases risk for respiratory depression when appropriate dosing and monitoring are employed. Conversely, under-treated pain is likely a more significant risk factor for opioid misuse, ORAEs, and relapse [74,128,470].

3.6. Discharge Phase

Discharge opioid prescribing following surgery has significantly contributed to the ongoing U.S. opioid epidemic [29]. Collaborative discussions surrounding discharge opioid prescribing are imperative to minimize the risks of dependency and misuse, and should include all analgesics that are to be continued after discharge. Enhanced recovery programs that integrate standardized opioid-sparing analgesic regimens have significantly reduced or eliminated opioid use in the postoperative setting [13]. Opioid-sparing analgesics should therefore be optimized during the inpatient stay and continued at discharge. Postdischarge multimodal analgesia has been associated with decreased outpatient opioid consumption after major procedures [471]. Duration of opioid-sparing analgesics after hospital discharge should be tailored to the individual needs of the patient and the anticipated length of pain expected after surgery. To mitigate adverse effects and dependence, prescriptions for NSAIDs and gabapentinoids should generally be limited to 1–2 weeks postdischarge. If refills are to be prescribed, an evaluation from a prescriber should be conducted to assess etiology of ongoing pain and appropriateness of continued therapies [472].

Until recently, evidence-based guidelines on postoperative opioid prescribing were not readily available. Variable and often excessive opioid quantities have been prescribed after surgery, especially in the U.S. [4,473]. In 2016, the Michigan Opioid Prescribing Engagement Network (OPEN) released procedure-specific guidelines to help reduce overprescribing of opioids after surgery. These guidelines are adjusted regularly using expert opinion, patient claims data, and evidence-based literature, and are only intended for patients who are considered opioid-naïve [32]. Since implementation at 43 hospitals, there has been a significant reduction in the quantity of opioids prescribed after surgery and a corresponding reduction in opioid consumption by patients [474]. Subsequently, multiple other collaboratives have also published postoperative opioid prescribing guidelines for adults [30,31,475,476] and for children [477].

These guidelines should be used as a foundation to inform procedure-specific institutional practices for opioid prescribing at the point of hospital discharge after surgery. However, opioid prescribing must be individualized within this framework. The patient's pain control and opioid use in the 12–24 h preceding discharge should be evaluated before prescribing discharge analgesics [478]. Patients undergoing minor procedures, those experiencing minimal pain, or patients who are opioid-naïve may not require opioid prescriptions at discharge. When opioids are prescribed to the opioid-naïve patient population, it is best practice to minimize the duration of supply to three days or less for procedures associated with rapid recovery from severe pain, seven days or less for medium term recovery procedures, and fourteen days or less for expected longer term recovery procedures [31]. Long-acting opioids should not be prescribed for the management of acute postoperative pain after discharge and should be especially avoided in patients who were previously opioid-naïve [15,32]. Opioid-tolerant patients generally have higher opioid requirements than opioid-naïve patients and prescribing a postdischarge opioid taper for this patient population is recommended. Typically, tapering the opioid dose by 20–25% every one to two days is tolerated by most patients as their pain is improving [15]. Detailed postoperative opioid taper examples are presented elsewhere [478]. Additionally, prescription drug monitoring programs (PDMPs) should be reviewed prior to prescribing opioids at discharge to chronic opioid users. This allows for review of the patient's current home supply and prevents overprescribing of unnecessary opioids at discharge [478].

Despite successful institutional efforts to decrease inpatient opioid prescribing, this has not necessarily translated into reduced opioid quantities prescribed at hospital discharge [479]. Discharge analgesic prescriptions are therefore unlikely to correlate with inpatient orders unless enhanced recovery pathways also have effective transitions of care procedures in place. This should include multidisciplinary communication informing patient-specific prescriptions as opposed to "per protocol" discharge opioid prescriptions for a given procedure. Additionally, data is emerging that shared decision-making, where patients are able to play a role in the amount of opioids they are prescribed at discharge, in conjunction with patient discharge education, can reduce the number of pills prescribed [480]. When considering reduced opioid quantities at discharge, a common concern among surgeons is an increase in office calls from patients requesting opioid prescription refills. Ample evidence supports that a large portion of opioids prescribed at discharge after surgery go unused, however, and initiatives to limit discharge opioid prescription quantities have successfully reduced opioid exposure without adversely affecting pain management or refill requests [42,44–46,93,473,476,481–490]. Maximizing nonopioid therapies and developing patient-specific plans are essential to the success and safety of such practice changes.

Pain management exit plans (PMEP) are an excellent resource for all postoperative patients, especially those with high opioid requirements [478]. Exit plans provide a detailed summary of the analgesics prescribed at discharge, including how each medication should be taken, common side effects, and appropriate disposal techniques (Figure 2). Exit plans focus on multimodal analgesia with an emphasis on nonopioids as the mainstay of therapy. If opioids are prescribed, a taper is developed and outlined in the PMEP using the lowest effective dose. Attention to tablet size and formulation should be considered for those given a taper in order to improve patient compliance. Note that splitting tablets can be challenging for some and use of whole tablets may be preferred for those undergoing a taper. Combination opioid products (e.g., oxycodone/acetaminophen) should be avoided in discharge opioid prescriptions since they limit the ability to safely maximize opioid-sparing analgesia throughout the recovery phase.

Postoperative Medication Home Management

Pt Name/ Surgeon:

PAIN MEDICATIONS AND BOWEL MANAGEMENT
Please bring pain medications to your first follow-up appointment

Class of Medication Generic (Brand) Name	Why am I taking this medication?	Common Possible Side Effects	Helpful Hints
Non-Opioid Pain Medications Acetaminophen (Tylenol®) Gabapentin (Neurontin®) Ibuprofen (Motrin®) OR Celecoxib (Celebrex®)	To treat mild to moderate pain in addition to or in place of your opioid medication.	Gabapentin may cause dizziness and sedation. Ibuprofen may cause upset stomach. It is important to take with food.	While using opioid pain medications please take the following medications as outlined below. ♯ Take acetaminophen (APAP) _____mg ____ tablets every ____ hours. Other over the counter medications may contain acetaminophen. *Do not exceed 4000mg of APAP in a day.* You may continue this for up to two weeks after surgery. ♯ Take gabapentin _____mg ____ tablets every ____ hours for 1-2 weeks after surgery. ♯ Take ibuprofen/celecoxib _____mg ____ tablets every ___ hours with food for one week after surgery.
Opioid Pain Medications _____	To treat moderate to severe postoperative pain	Constipation, tiredness, upset stomach, vomiting, itching. *If extreme drowsiness or difficulty breathing occurs, get emergency medical help.	• Take with food to prevent upset stomach • Avoid driving and alcohol while taking this medication • Use enough to control pain to allow to keep up activity at home • Information regarding proper medication disposal can be found at: https://michigan-open.org/safe-opioid-disposal/ Suggested goals to slowly come off this medication: _____: Take _____ tablets, _____ times a day _____: Take _____ tablets, _____ times a day _____: Take _____ tablets, _____ times a day
You may have constipation after your surgery. This can be caused by the surgery or the opioids you are taking. To help manage constipation, use BOTH a stool softener and laxative agent until you are not taking opioid pain medication and you have normal bowel movements without straining.			
Stool Softener Docusate sodium (Colace®)	Softens the stool to avoid straining during a bowel movement	Diarrhea, rash	• Docusate 100mg: Take 1 tablet 1 – 2 times per day with a full glass of water

Contact Information for the Surgery Clinic: (xxx) xxx-xxxx

Figure 2. Example of a Pain Management Exit Plan (PMEP) to be used at postoperative hospital Discharge.

Discharge counseling, with an emphasis on nonopioid analgesics as first line therapy, is essential for safe and successful postoperative pain control [15,101,478]. Discharge counseling should be pursued in conjunction with a PMEP or other standardized educational tool and may be completed by a pharmacist, pharmacy or medical student, advanced practice provider, or physician. Patients being discharged with opioid prescriptions should be educated about proper opioid storage and disposal. Opioids should be kept in a locked cabinet, away from children, pets and friends or family. Storing opioids appropriately can reduce accidental overdoses and decrease opioid diversion, since a majority of people who misuse opioids obtain them from a friend or family member [491]. Providers may consider involving a family member to secure and administer the medication to provide accountability and reduce temptation for opioid misuse or diversion in at-risk patients. If able, facilities dispensing opioid prescriptions should provide safe, at-home medication disposal systems to encourage appropriate and prompt disposal of unused opioids [480,492–494]. Other disposal methods include medication collecting bins, often found in hospitals, pharmacies, or police stations, and community medication take back events. As a last resort, patients may consider mixing unused medications in a plastic bag with coffee grounds or cat litter and disposing of them in the household trash. Flushing unwanted medications down the toilet should be discouraged as this leads to pharmaceutical contamination of the water supply [27,100,478,495,496].

Careful attention to the quantity of opioids prescribed at discharge to patients planning to resume medical marijuana or other illicit substances, such as heroin, is vital. In 2018,

67,367 drug overdoses were reported in the U.S., with 69.5% involving opioids [497]. Incidence of opioid overdose after postoperative discharge is greatest in the early period, and estimated to be 26.3 events per person-year during the first thirty postoperative days [498]. Co-prescribing of naloxone, a rapid-acting opioid antagonist, should therefore be considered at the point of postoperative discharge for patients at risk of opioid overdose. These patients may include those prescribed more than 50 MED per day, patients prescribed concomitant benzodiazepines, and patients with a history of respiratory disease, substance use disorder, or mental health disorders [54,499,500]. Naloxone may also be prescribed to patients if they are concerned about opioid misuse in their household.

While acute pain management prescribing is the responsibility of the surgical team, collaboration with chronic pain prescribers and/or addiction medicine specialists is crucial for successful postoperative pain control and mitigation of adverse events in these high-risk populations. This communication can help prevent relapse in those with a history of substance use disorder and promote a smooth transition to maintenance medication regimens; hence, the outpatient provider should be engaged before surgery and as soon as feasible after discharge [104,119]. For patients on chronic buprenorphine, therapy should almost always be continued perioperatively, including at the point of hospital discharge, in addition to a short-acting full mu-opioid agonist prescription for acute pain management where usually indicated [119,126,132]. Surgical providers should ensure the patient has enough buprenorphine to last until they can see their buprenorphine prescriber, contacting the prescriber to troubleshoot any foreseeable gaps. Ideally, this appointment should be within 3 days of discharge. As an alternative to the "bridge prescription," patients can return to the emergency department for administration of buprenorphine for up to 72 h after discharge. For methadone, if the patient's home dose was decreased or split during the perioperative period, the dose should generally be returned to home dosing at discharge. Arrangements must be made for the patient on methadone to go to their clinic the following day to receive their medication. It is imperative to discontinue chronic naltrexone products at discharge and to defer their reinitiation to the outpatient prescriber after the patient has been off of opioids (see also Section 3.1.3) [117,124].

3.7. Follow-Up Phase

Development of persistent opioid use is a risk when prescribing opioids for the treatment of acute pain. This risk is amplified by increased doses, additional days supplied, and duration of use. The likelihood of long-term opioid use significantly increases after five days of opioid therapy [501]. For this reason, patient follow-up should ideally take place within five days of discharge, particularly for those who were prescribed opioids. Follow-up may be conducted in person or via telemedicine. A mobile phone app, downloaded by the patient prior to hospital admission, has been shown to effectively monitor patient pain and opioid requirements after surgery. The patient answers daily mobile phone app questions that include pain assessment. These data are reviewed and pain management revisions are implemented at an in-person or telemedicine clinic visit within 4–7 days after discharge [502].

Follow-up assessments should evaluate ongoing postoperative pain, opioid and nonopioid use, and the status of unused opioids. The pain evaluation should assess pain trajectory, which includes pain intensity as well as time to resolution of pain. Patients identified as having an abnormal pain trajectory (e.g., those experiencing numeric pain scores greater than four on postoperative days three-seven) have been found to have a higher risk of developing persistent postoperative pain and should be monitored closely [503]. Closer follow up may also be warranted in those with a history of substance use disorder or those with mental health comorbidities.

Patients identified as having difficulty with postoperative pain control should receive education about proactive pain management. By taking scheduled doses of nonopioid medications, patients are able to "stay ahead" of their pain and prevent severe pain breakthroughs. For those struggling to wean off of opioids, providers should further optimize nonopioid medications, reiterate nonpharmacologic modalities, and encourage opioid tapers whenever possible. Pain management exit plans can be employed as they are at hospital discharge or updated in the outpatient setting, and should be strongly considered in this patient population [478]. The need for additional opioid prescriptions should be limited and assessed on a case-by-case basis, e.g., in opioid-tolerant patients requiring longer tapers. Coordination with the patient's other outpatient providers is important, and opioid refills from both surgical and nonsurgical providers should be accounted for [504].

For patients with unused opioids, medication disposal education should be reiterated. Providing patients with local medication take-back locations or safe disposal devices can facilitate appropriate narcotic disposal and limit redistribution within the community [492–494].

4. Interprofessional Collaboration in Sustaining Perioperative Performance Measures Related to Pain Management and Opioid Prescribing

4.1. From the Surgical Institution Perspective

Pain assessment and management metrics have been critical focus areas for healthcare institutions in recent decades, sometimes with deleterious effects. In 2001, as part of a national effort to address the widespread underassessment and undertreatment of pain, The Joint Commission (formerly The Joint Commission on the Accreditation of Healthcare Organizations or JCAHO) introduced pain management standards for healthcare organizations [505]. While well-intended, the standards were also informed by an unfortunately misguided understanding of the addictive potential of opioids at the time [3,506]. This practice movement ultimately resulted in the elevation of pain as the "fifth vital sign", giving pain equal status with blood pressure, heart rate, respiratory rate, and temperature. Nurses were required to assess pain as an objective sign, instead of as a subjective symptom of surgical recovery [507–509]. Hospitals have also been incentivized to improve patient satisfaction with pain management via the Centers for Medicare & Medicaid Services (CMS) Value-Based Purchasing (VBP) program, which adjusts each hospital inpatient payment according to its performance on quality measures [510]. One tool used to evaluate quality measures within VBP is the Hospital Consumer Assessment of Healthcare Providers and Systems (HCAHPS) survey. This survey is administered to patients after hospital discharge and previously asked patients how often hospital providers did, "everything in their power to control your pain" [505]. By directly linking patient satisfaction with pain management to hospital compensation, the survey may have incentivized opioid overprescribing [511].

The Joint Commission and other organizations have since recognized a need to modify standards to mitigate unintended consequences in the wake of the ensuing opioid epidemic [3,359,508,509,512]. The Joint Commission revised their pain standards to include an emphasis on patient safety and the promotion of multimodal analgesia in 2018 [3,36]. Additionally, the revised pain management-related HCAHPS questions shifted from a focus on the perceived quality of pain management efforts to quality of communication about pain management [513]. Furthermore, many U.S. states have enacted opioid prescribing restrictions affecting surgical providers [35]. These revised standards and a shifting paradigm to reduce opioid prescribing are driving surgery centers to reevaluate their approach to perioperative pain management. The requirement by many states to review prescription drug monitoring programs (PDMPs) when prescribing opioids has been linked with a reduced rate of opioid prescriptions in hospitals [514]. Additionally, The Joint Commission requires hospitals to collect and analyze data to monitor their ability to safely prescribe opioids, an important step in the effort to demonstrate reductions in perioperative opioid prescribing without negatively impacting the quality of pain management [67].

In addition to reimbursement-driving quality metrics and legal pressures, healthcare institutions are motivated by increased transparency of their patients' pain management-related outcomes. Tools such as the CMS Hospital Compare websites and Leapfrog Hospital Safety Grade are available online to consumers [515–517]. These quality data are influenced by subjective patient satisfaction indicators in addition to objective outcome metrics. Evaluations of elective surgical programs, such as those providing hip and knee replacements, are therefore only an internet search away from prospective patients. Evidence suggests that an institution's reputation for postoperative pain management has an important influence on potential healthcare consumers. A recent study assessed the preferences of hip and knee arthroplasty patients regarding publicly available quality metrics. This discrete choice experiment yielded that patients are willing to accept suboptimal hospital ratings and facility cleanliness in exchange for better postoperative pain management and complication rates [518].

Some institutions have implemented opioid stewardship programs (OSPs) to achieve these goals. Core pillars of OSPs include interprofessional collaboration on protocols and services related to multimodal pain management, education on opioid prescribing and stewardship to staff and providers, education to patients, caregivers and community members on safe opioid use and disposal, opioid-related risk reduction, and data analysis and reporting of related quality metrics [38,66,68,519–522]. An expert panel has proposed quality indicators for measuring opioid stewardship interventions in hospital and emergency settings. These nineteen measures assess quality of inpatient pain management, opioid prescribing practices, ORAE prevention, and transitions of care [38,523].

Although current quality standards and market incentives better align with shared goals by patients, providers, and institutions, the cost of nonopioid medications can pose a barrier for institutions to implement multimodal analgesia throughout perioperative care. Intravenous acetaminophen (pending the widespread availability of this formulation from generic manufacturers in early 2021), intravenous NSAID formulations, and liposomal bupivacaine represent newer nonopioid interventions that drive analgesics to rank among the most expensive therapeutic drug categories [524]. The substantial cost of these agents relative to conventional generic medications may contribute to overreliance on cheap, widely available opioid medications in the perioperative setting [391]. Fortunately, collaborative investigator-initiated research has provided comparative efficacy data to inform cost–benefit comparisons between some of these high-cost agents and their conventional counterparts [176,268,270]. Interprofessional stewardship efforts have demonstrated success in mitigating the potential financial toxicity of perioperative multimodal analgesia by limiting such high-cost agents to populations unable to achieve the same degree of benefit from conventional alternatives [390,525].

It has long been recognized that successful perioperative care involves interdisciplinary collaboration among surgeons, anesthetists, medicine physicians, nurses, and physical therapy providers. Perhaps historically underrecognized has been the value of the clinical pharmacist in improving perioperative patient outcomes and efficiencies [526]. Despite well-supported benefits to diverse patient outcomes and care teams, pharmacists may be underutilized in postoperative pain management. As pharmacotherapy experts with a longitudinal view of the perioperative care continuum, pharmacists are well-poised to perform or oversee many important functions to optimize surgical patient analgesia and institutional opioid stewardship efforts [27,478,527]. These may include completing pre-admission medication reconciliation, advising on preoperative optimization and planning for perioperative management of chronic pain therapies, developing standardized preemptive analgesic protocols with appropriate patient-specific adjustments, supporting intraoperative multimodal analgesic use through protocol development, education, and operationalization, managing postoperative analgesic therapies, advising on discharge opioid and nonopioid prescribing, developing patient educational materials and providing discharge counseling, and assessing patients at follow-up to optimize opioid tapers and screen for postoperative complications [68,478,528,529]. One pre- and post-intervention study spanning 6 years evaluated the impact of a pharmacy-directed pain management service that performed both consult-based and stewardship functions at a large public hospital. The service was associated with decreased total institutional opioid use, increased nonopioid analgesic use, fewer opioid-related respiratory depression events, and ongoing improvement in pain-related HCAHPS patient survey domains [530]. Similarly, a pharmacist-led post-discharge opioid deescalation service was implemented at a major tertiary institution for orthopedic surgery patients recently discharged from the institution's acute pain service. In the published evaluation of this service, the post-intervention group realized similar pain intensity ratings with significantly lowered opioid doses and incidence of constipation [437]. Healthcare institutions may therefore consider investment in pharmacy services to help drive quality improvement and cost-savings initiatives related to postoperative pain management and opioid stewardship.

4.2. From the Surgeon Perspective

The surgeon perspective of best-practices evidence-based perioperative performance is a team approach within standardized enhanced recovery pathways. Each member of the perioperative interdisciplinary team provides valuable knowledge that contributes to opioid stewardship efforts. Where resources are available, perioperative pain management and opioid stewardship is ideally pharmacist-led, from preoperative evaluation through the inpatient stay and postdischarge follow-up [531]. Described below is an example of the teamwork required in a colorectal enhanced recovery pathway to minimize opioid use while effectively treating postoperative pain.

Nonopioid pain management options are optimized throughout the care continuum for all patients on the surgical service. Through preadmission screening, an enhanced recovery nurse navigator may identify patients with a history of chronic opioid use. This allows the pharmacist to contact the patient and develop a focused perioperative pain management plan. Anesthetists are other important enhanced recovery collaborators. Their expertise in perioperative pain management and postoperative nausea and vomiting (PONV) prevention assist with minimizing the need for opioids. Enhanced recovery patients without complications typically receive transversus abdominis plane (TAP) blocks in the preoperative suite from the anesthetist. Postoperative patients are never "nothing by mouth" after surgery when awake and alert, therefore, enhanced recovery postoperative orders should not routinely include intravenous opioids. The pharmacist leads the multimodal pain management strategy at daily inpatient interdisciplinary rounds that include surgeon, resident surgeon, physician assistant, case manager, social worker, enterostomal nursing, and patient care unit nursing staff. Knowledgeable patient care nurses, well-informed in pain management goals and providing consistent care plan messages to patients, are an integral component of standardized perioperative pain control.

Surgeon opioid and nonopioid discharge prescriptions are written in consultation with the enhanced recovery team pharmacist and are based on inpatient pain control and opioid needs in the 12–24 h leading up to discharge. Pain management exit plans are developed by the pharmacist and provided to those with high opioid requirements. Patients receiving an exit plan are seen by pharmacy and educated about the importance of multimodal analgesia and opioid tapers. One study showed that a pharmacist-led enhanced recovery pain management plan resulted in less than 50% of patients requiring opioid prescriptions at the time of discharge for patients having robotic colorectal surgery. The average number of 5 mg oxycodone tablets prescribed in those who received prescriptions was 6 to 8 while the average number used was 2.5 to 3 tablets. Only 0.5% to 0.75% of patients required opioid prescription refills [531].

Perioperative pain management and opioid stewardship continues after patient discharge in the surgeon clinic. One study showed that enhanced recovery pharmacist participation in an early post-discharge clinic where all postoperative patients are seen within 4–7 days of discharge maximized assessment of pain management and reinforcement of nonopioids as the primary pain management option. Additionally, overall readmission rates were significantly decreased, especially with postoperative pain as a readmission diagnosis [502]. In addition to improved patient outcomes, longitudinal involvement of clinical pharmacists in perioperative pain management has been associated with surgical provider satisfaction [528]. Pharmacists may therefore be valuable to optimizing patient care and in maximizing surgeon resources.

Pain management in enhanced recovery is therefore a dynamic, collaborative, interprofessional effort that requires reassessment and evidence-based changes. A prospectively maintained database allows real-time collection and evaluation of enhanced recovery data that includes opioid and nonopioid information [65]. Implementation of an opioid stewardship program is applicable to all surgical specialties and should be incorporated into enhanced recovery pathways.

4.3. From the Patient Perspective

Patient-centered outcomes and the surgical patient experience should remain the focus of collaborative care and process improvement. Clinical practice guidelines endorse an individualized approach to all aspects of postoperative pain management based on patient needs and preferences, and echo the need to engage patients in shared decision-making throughout this process [15]. Available evidence suggests clinical pharmacists can positively impact patient experience indicators related to postoperative pain management. The incorporation of clinical pharmacists into patient education prior to joint arthroplasty was associated with modest increases in pain-related domains of the HCAHPS satisfaction survey [532]. A comprehensive clinical pharmacy service in a total joint arthroplasty population at another institution included preoperative education, postoperative pain management optimization, and discharge counseling interventions. This service was associated with improved patient understanding of discharge medications and patients indicated a high degree of satisfaction with pharmacist interactions [529].

To illustrate the importance of postoperative pain management and opioid stewardship to the patient perspective, the following account was authored by a colorectal surgical patient of two of the authors and published with his permission (edited only for brevity):

4.3.1. Preparing for Surgery

"For patients, fully understanding how surgery will affect them physically and emotionally and what type of pain management practices will be employed both before and after is a critical first step if they are to take charge of their own health care. Surgery is a scary proposition for the patient. If you add in the anticipated discomfort and pain it only escalates the unknown, elevating fear and anxiety. Speaking from experience, this quickly takes center stage in a patient's mind. With my three surgeries, I found it essential to take ownership and control and learn as much as I could about these surgeries and my recovery. Fully understanding possible surgical risks and complications, as well as the overall goal and expected positive outcomes, was vital if I was going to gain mental control of a challenging health situation.

Most patients do not realize the power exists within themselves to take better control of their surgical outcomes. Deciding on my frame of mind and focusing on the positives, rather than the negatives, immediately put me in a better position to reach my recovery goals. As I saw it, I had two choices: (1) I could worry about the possible complications associated with surgery. If I took that route, I was sure to be miserable, anxious, and not fully connected with my end goal; or (2) I could prepare by becoming knowledgeable about my surgery, perceiving it as another life challenge that would enable me to continue living and to improve my quality of life. For me, surgical challenges are a lot like flying a kite. If you run your kite before the wind, you cannot take off and fly. You have to turn into the wind and face it head-on. The challenge you push against is the very force that lifts you. Therefore, it was clear to me I had to face the headwinds."

4.3.2. The Enhanced Recovery Program, Phone Applications, and Opioid Use

"My three surgeries would involve perioperative pain control, with transverse abdominis plane (TAP) or epidural pain blocks and a combination of oral pain medications including acetaminophen, ibuprofen, gabapentin, and oxycodone. Today, I'm a veteran when it comes to pain medication, but the real inspiration that empowered me and gave me reassurance that I could make a significant contribution to my recovery was the Enhanced

Recovery Program (ERP) offered by my health provider. Along with that, I was able to use a phone application when I returned home. This application allowed me to have morning check-ins with my health-care team, if needed. My health provider also offered an informative class several weeks before my surgery that gave me valuable and concise information to help me understand my upcoming procedure and how to prepare for it and my hospital stay. The class also gave me important information about my postoperative care and recovery at home.

The ERP gave me the reassurance and tools needed to control my health care, creating a solid foundation for a good outcome. After attending this class, I realized that I had the power to actively engage as a patient who can contribute, participate, and determine outcomes. I was no longer a bystander but a player in this game. This significantly reduced my anxiety, replacing it with positive energy. I honestly believe this shortened my recovery time for all three surgeries.

In the ERP class, a nurse navigator and a pharmacist addressed the most concerning aspect of my surgery: How to control pain? I realized I am afraid of pain. I honestly believe all of us are. However, getting preoperative education on pain management led to the insight that I needed to take control of my pain rather than let it control me. Understanding opioid risks and benefits gave me the confidence and courage to set a goal to get them out of my life after surgery as soon as reasonably possible. Most of us are keenly aware of the opioid crisis still raging both worldwide and in the United States. I was initially concerned that this might eventually be me.

Well, it could have been me. All of us can be throttled by addictions when we least expect it. However, the underlying key to my success was the preoperative and postoperative education I received. What I did learn, and benefit from was the powerful combination of ibuprofen and acetaminophen and how they work together very well to relieve surgical pain. After stopping opioids, I was continued on a regimen of these over-the-counter pain relievers and quickly discovered my pain was being managed without the use of narcotics. This alternate step was presented and outlined in my ERP class. This was an enabler for me, and I was able to be more mentally alert, have less constipation issues and feel comfortable enough to go home. The ERP umbrella provided an open and honest conversation through clear and straightforward directions about what must be done before and after surgery. ERP and the medical staff gave me realistic and attainable goals for my recovery. I was a partner in my own health-care decisions, and I took ownership for my successful recovery. The well-trained medical staff promptly addressed my concerns. The addition of the phone application, which I found to be an excellent communication tool, provided me much needed emotional reassurance and support before, during, and after surgery."

4.3.3. Lessons Learned

"As a frequent-flyer patient with lots of surgeries, treatments, and narcotics use, I can report that I landed safely back in my everyday life. Additionally, this was mainly because of the expert care as well as the comprehensive education I received from the medical staff, doctors, pharmacists, and nurses. In all cases, my ERP experience gave me the solid foundation I needed to empower myself and focus on the win, not the illness. I discovered journaling every day with accompanying photos, audio, and video. I now have five solid years of life experience, good and bad, that I can look back on.

All of us will eventually face fragility and mortality. However, for this patient, my medical experiences and the numerous medical staff who helped me during trying times have given me the gift of life. I am grateful that I was forced to confront an often inevitable part of being alive and to now fully understand that we as patients can take ownership of and apply direction to our recoveries."

5. Conclusions and Future Directions

While myriad multimodal strategies exist, ongoing comparative assessments of analgesic combinations and anesthetic approaches within enhanced recovery practice are warranted to further understand and optimize perioperative patient care. Novel analgesic agents and modalities continue to be developed, and their place in therapy should be thoughtfully studied [56,286,533–536]. Pharmacogenomic assessments show promise in elucidating precision pain management [537,538]. Additional evaluation of the influence of perioperative analgesic strategies on the development of persistent postoperative pain and opioid use would be an invaluable contribution to the literature [2,50,539]. Implementation studies describing successful opioid stewardship programs should be pursued to address practice challenges and increase universal adoption [38,68,540].

Effective perioperative pain management requires a multifaceted team-based approach that begins prior to admission and continues after discharge. Healthcare providers must collaborate throughout institutional practice and process improvement with the shared goals of providing optimal patient care while minimizing opioid exposure. Standardized perioperative pathways should maximize nonpharmacologic therapies and multimodal analgesics, provide decision-support for the judicious use of opioids, and include mitigation strategies for ORAEs and postsurgical opioid dependence. Collaborative practice models should ensure appropriate patient-specific application of available strategies to high-risk and/or opioid-tolerant surgical populations. Pain and addiction medicine specialist consultation, transitional pain services, and opioid stewardship programs should be appropriately resourced across healthcare systems and surgery centers. Incorporating evidence-based pain management and opioid stewardship strategies into a standardized perioperative program will support safe, high-quality, and consistent surgical patient care.

Author Contributions: Conceptualization, S.J.H.; methodology, S.J.H., K.K.B., W.R.V.; writing—original draft preparation, S.J.H., K.K.B., W.R.V., N.Z.S., M.M.L., M.J.H., R.K.C.; writing—review and editing, S.J.H., K.K.B., W.R.V., N.Z.S., M.M.L., M.J.H., R.K.C.; visualization, S.J.H.; supervision, S.J.H. All authors have read and agreed to the published version of the manuscript.

Funding: This research received no external funding.

Acknowledgments: The authors gratefully acknowledge the support and mentorship of Cheryl K. Genord, RPh, BSPharm and Richard H. Parrish II, PhD, FCCP. Additionally, we are honored to have had the support of Robert H. Miller, who lended his voice to this manuscript from the patient perspective. We appreciate his willingness to share his story with us and with the world so that providers everywhere may better understand the patient experience regarding perioperative pain management and opioid stewardship.

Conflicts of Interest: The authors declare no conflict of interest.

References

1. Meara, J.G.; Leather, A.J.M.; Hagander, L.; Alkire, B.C.; Alonso, N.; Ameh, E.A.; Bickler, S.W.; Conteh, L.; Dare, A.J.; Davies, J.; et al. Global Surgery 2030: Evidence and solutions for achieving health, welfare, and economic development. *Lancet* **2015**, *386*, 569–624. [CrossRef]
2. Gan, T.J. Poorly controlled postoperative pain: Prevalence, consequences, and prevention. *J. Pain Res.* **2017**, *10*, 2287–2298. [CrossRef]
3. Baker, D.W. History of The Joint Commission's Pain Standards. *JAMA* **2017**, *317*, 1117–1118. [CrossRef]
4. El Moheb, M.; Mokhtari, A.; Han, K.; Van Erp, I.; Kongkaewpaisan, N.; Jia, Z.; Rodriguez, G.; Kongwibulwut, M.; Kaafarani, H.M.; Sakran, J.V.; et al. Pain or No Pain, We Will Give You Opioids: Relationship Between Number of Opioid Pills Prescribed and Severity of Pain after Operation in US vs Non-US Patients. *J. Am. Coll. Surg.* **2020**, *231*, 639–648. [CrossRef]
5. Loh, F.E.; Herzig, S.J. Pain in the United States: Time for a Culture Shift in Expectations, Messaging, and Management. *J. Hosp. Med.* **2019**, *14*, 787–788. [CrossRef]
6. Oderda, G.M.; Senagore, A.J.; Morland, K.; Iqbal, S.U.; Kugel, M.; Liu, S.; Habib, A.S. Opioid-related respiratory and gastrointestinal adverse events in patients with acute postoperative pain: Prevalence, predictors, and burden. *J. Pain Palliat. Care Pharmacother.* **2019**, *33*, 82–97. [CrossRef]
7. Kane-Gill, S.L.; Rubin, E.C.; Smithburger, P.L.; Buckley, M.S.; Dasta, J.F. The Cost of Opioid-Related Adverse Drug Events. *J. Pain Palliat. Care Pharmacother.* **2014**, *28*, 282–293. [CrossRef]

8. Oderda, G.M.; Said, Q.; Evans, R.S.; Stoddard, G.J.; Lloyd, J.; Jackson, K.; Rublee, D.; Samore, M.H. Opioid-Related Adverse Drug Events in Surgical Hospitalizations: Impact on Costs and Length of Stay. *Ann. Pharmacother.* **2007**, *41*, 400–407. [CrossRef]
9. Brat, G.A.; Agniel, D.; Beam, A.; Yorkgitis, B.; Bicket, M.; Homer, M.; Fox, K.P.; Knecht, D.B.; McMahill-Walraven, C.N.; Palmer, N.; et al. Postsurgical prescriptions for opioid naive patients and association with overdose and misuse: Retrospective cohort study. *BMJ* **2018**, *360*, j5790. [CrossRef]
10. Brummett, C.M.; Waljee, J.F.; Goesling, J.; Moser, S.; Lin, P.; Englesbe, M.J.; Bohnert, A.S.B.; Kheterpal, S.; Nallamothu, B.K. New Persistent Opioid Use After Minor and Major Surgical Procedures in US Adults. *JAMA Surg.* **2017**, *152*, e170504. [CrossRef]
11. Kharasch, E.D.; Brunt, L.M. Perioperative Opioids and Public Health. *Anesthesiology* **2016**, *124*, 960–965. [CrossRef]
12. Kaafarani, H.M.A.; Han, K.; El Moheb, M.; Kongkaewpaisan, N.; Jia, Z.; El Hechi, M.W.; Van Wijck, S.; Breen, K.; Eid, A.; Rodriguez, G.; et al. Opioids after Surgery in the United States Versus the Rest of the World. *Ann. Surg.* **2020**, *272*, 879–886. [CrossRef]
13. Echeverria-Villalobos, M.; Stoicea, N.; Todeschini, A.B.; Fiorda-Diaz, J.; Uribe, A.A.; Weaver, T.; Bergese, S.D. Enhanced Recovery after Surgery (ERAS). *Clin. J. Pain* **2020**, *36*, 219–226. [CrossRef]
14. Ladha, K.S.; Neuman, M.D.; Broms, G.; Bethell, J.; Bateman, B.T.; Wijeysundera, D.N.; Bell, M.; Hallqvist, L.; Svensson, T.; Newcomb, C.W.; et al. Opioid Prescribing after Surgery in the United States, Canada, and Sweden. *JAMA Netw. Open* **2019**, *2*, e1910734. [CrossRef] [PubMed]
15. Chou, R.; Gordon, D.B.; de Leon-Casasola, O.A.; Rosenberg, J.M.; Bickler, S.; Brennan, T.; Carter, T.; Cassidy, C.L.; Chittenden, E.H.; Degenhardt, E.; et al. Management of Postoperative Pain: A Clinical Practice Guideline from the American Pain Society, the American Society of Regional Anesthesia and Pain Medicine, and the American Society of Anesthesiologists' Committee on Regional Anesthesia, Executive Committee, and Administrative Council. *J. Pain* **2016**, *17*, 131–157. [CrossRef]
16. Ansari, A.; Rizk, D.; Whinney, C. The Society of Hospital Medicine. The Society of Hospital Medicine's (SHM's) Multimodal Pain Strategies Guide for Postoperative Pain Management. 2017. Available online: https://www.hospitalmedicine.org/globalassets/clinical-topics/clinical-pdf/ctr-17-0004-multi-model-pain-project-pdf-version-m1.pdf (accessed on 14 September 2020).
17. American Society of Anesthesiologists Task Force on Acute Pain. Management Practice Guidelines for Acute Pain Management in the Perioperative Setting. *Anesthesiology* **2012**, *116*, 248–273. [CrossRef]
18. Edwards, D.A.; Hedrick, T.L.; Jayaram, J.; Argoff, C.; Gulur, P.; Holubar, S.D.; Gan, T.J.; Mythen, M.G.; Miller, T.E.; Shaw, A.D.; et al. American Society for Enhanced Recovery and Perioperative Quality Initiative Joint Consensus Statement on Perioperative Management of Patients on Preoperative Opioid Therapy. *Anesth. Analg.* **2019**, *129*, 553–566. [CrossRef]
19. McEvoy, M.D.; Scott, M.J.; Gordon, D.B.; Grant, S.A.; Thacker, J.K.; Wu, C.L.; Gan, T.J.; Mythen, M.G.; Shaw, A.D.; Miller, T.E.; et al. American Society for Enhanced Recovery (ASER) and Perioperative Quality Initiative (POQI) joint consensus statement on optimal analgesia within an enhanced recovery pathway for colorectal surgery: Part 1—From the preoperative period to PACU. *Perioper. Med.* **2017**, *6*, 1–13. [CrossRef]
20. Joshi, G.P.; Van De Velde, M.; Kehlet, H.; Pogatzki-Zahn, E.; Schug, S.; Bonnet, F.; Rawal, N.; Delbos, A.; Lavand'Homme, P.; Beloeil, H.; et al. Development of evidence-based recommendations for procedure-specific pain management: PROSPECT methodology. *Anaesthesia* **2019**, *74*, 1298–1304. [CrossRef] [PubMed]
21. European Society for Regional Anesthesia & Pain Therapy. Procedure Specific Postoperative Pain Management (PROSPECT) Guidelines. Available online: http://postoppain.org/ (accessed on 14 September 2020).
22. List of Guidelines. Enhanced Recovery After Surgery (ERAS) (R) Society. Available online: https://erassociety.org/guidelines/list-of-guidelines/ (accessed on 14 September 2020).
23. Memtsoudis, S.G.; Cozowicz, C.; Bekeris, J.; Bekere, D.; Liu, J.; Soffin, E.M.; Mariano, E.R.; Johnson, R.L.; Hargett, M.J.; Lee, B.H.; et al. Anaesthetic care of patients undergoing primary hip and knee arthroplasty: Consensus recommendations from the International Consensus on Anaesthesia-Related Outcomes after Surgery group (ICAROS) based on a systematic review and meta-analysis. *Br. J. Anaesth.* **2019**, *123*, 269–287. [CrossRef]
24. McEvoy, M.D.; Scott, M.J.; Gordon, D.B.; Grant, S.A.; Thacker, J.K.; Wu, C.L.; Gan, T.J.; Mythen, M.G.; Shaw, A.D.; Miller, T.E.; et al. American Society for Enhanced Recovery (ASER) and Perioperative Quality Initiative (POQI) Joint Consensus Statement on Optimal Analgesia within an Enhanced Recovery Pathway for Colorectal Surgery: Part 2—From PACU to the Transition Home. *Perioper. Med.* **2017**, *6*, 1–10. [CrossRef]
25. Schwenk, E.S.; Viscusi, E.R.; Buvanendran, A.; Hurley, R.W.; Wasan, A.D.; Narouze, S.; Bhatia, A.; Davis, F.N.; Hooten, W.M.; Cohen, S.P. Consensus Guidelines on the Use of Intravenous Ketamine Infusions for Acute Pain Management From the American Society of Regional Anesthesia and Pain Medicine, the American Academy of Pain Medicine, and the American Society of Anesthesiologists. *Reg. Anesth. Pain Med.* **2018**, *43*, 456–466. [CrossRef]
26. Foo, I.; Macfarlane, A.J.R.; Srivastava, D.; Bhaskar, A.; Barker, H.; Knaggs, R.; Eipe, N.; Smith, A.F. The use of intravenous lidocaine for postoperative pain and recovery: International consensus statement on efficacy and safety. *Anaesthesia* **2021**, *76*, 238–250. [CrossRef] [PubMed]
27. Bicket, M.C.; Brat, G.A.; Hutfless, S.; Wu, C.L.; Nesbit, S.A.; Alexander, G.C. Optimizing opioid prescribing and pain treatment for surgery: Review and conceptual framework. *Am. J. Health-Syst. Pharm.* **2019**, *76*, 1403–1412. [CrossRef]
28. Yorkgitis, B.K.; Brat, G.A. Postoperative opioid prescribing: Getting it RIGHTT. *Am. J. Surg.* **2018**, *215*, 707–711. [CrossRef] [PubMed]
29. Varley, P.R.; Zuckerbraun, B.S. Opioid Stewardship and the Surgeon. *JAMA Surg.* **2018**, *153*, e174875. [CrossRef]

30. Overton, H.N.; Hanna, M.N.; Bruhn, W.E.; Hutfless, S.; Bicket, M.C.; Makary, M.A.; Matlaga, B.; Johnson, C.; Sheffield, J.; Shechter, R.; et al. Opioid-Prescribing Guidelines for Common Surgical Procedures: An Expert Panel Consensus. *J. Am. Coll. Surg.* **2018**, *227*, 411–418. [CrossRef]
31. Dr. Robert Bree Collaborative and Washington State Agency Medical Directors' Group. Prescribing Opioids for Postoperative Pain—Supplemental Guidance. July 2018. Available online: http://www.agencymeddirectors.wa.gov/Files/FinalSupBreeAMDGPostopPain091318wcover.pdf (accessed on 14 September 2020).
32. Michigan OPEN. Prescribing Recommendations. Available online: https://michigan-open.org/prescribing-recommendations/ (accessed on 14 September 2020).
33. Wu, C.L.; King, A.B.; Geiger, T.M.; Grant, M.C.; Grocott, M.P.W.; Gupta, R.; Hah, J.M.; Miller, T.E.; Shaw, A.D.; Gan, T.J.; et al. American Society for Enhanced Recovery and Perioperative Quality Initiative Joint Consensus Statement on Perioperative Opioid Minimization in Opioid-Naïve Patients. *Anesth. Analg.* **2019**, *129*, 567–577. [CrossRef]
34. Kent, M.L.; Hurley, R.W.; Oderda, G.M.; Gordon, D.B.; Sun, E.; Mythen, M.; Miller, T.E.; Shaw, A.D.; Gan, T.J.; Thacker, J.K.M.; et al. American Society for Enhanced Recovery and Perioperative Quality Initiative-4 Joint Consensus Statement on Persistent Postoperative Opioid Use. *Anesth. Analg.* **2019**, *129*, 543–552. [CrossRef]
35. Pharmacy Times. Opioid Prescribing Limits Across the States. Available online: https://www.pharmacytimes.com/contributor/marilyn-bulloch-pharmd-bcps/2019/02/opioid-prescribing-limits-across-the-states (accessed on 14 September 2020).
36. The Joint Commission. R3 Report: Pain Assessment and Management Standards for Hospitals. 2017 Aug. Report No.: Issue 11. Available online: https://www.jointcommission.org/-/media/tjc/documents/standards/r3-reports/r3_report_issue_11_2_11_19_rev.pdf (accessed on 14 September 2020).
37. Meissner, W.; Huygen, F.; Neugebauer, E.A.; Osterbrink, J.; Benhamou, D.; Betteridge, N.; Coluzzi, F.; De Andres, J.; Fawcett, W.; Fletcher, D.; et al. Management of acute pain in the postoperative setting: The importance of quality indicators. *Curr. Med. Res. Opin.* **2017**, *34*, 187–196. [CrossRef]
38. Rizk, E.; Swan, J.T.; Cheon, O.; Colavecchia, A.C.; Bui, L.N.; Kash, B.A.; Chokshi, S.P.; Chen, H.; Johnson, M.L.; Liebl, M.G.; et al. Quality indicators to measure the effect of opioid stewardship interventions in hospital and emergency department settings. *Am. J. Health Pharm.* **2019**, *76*, 225–235. [CrossRef] [PubMed]
39. Gan, T.J.; Habib, A.S.; Miller, T.E.; White, W.; Apfelbaum, J.L. Incidence, patient satisfaction, and perceptions of post-surgical pain: Results from a US national survey. *Curr. Med. Res. Opin.* **2014**, *30*, 149–160. [CrossRef]
40. Ladha, M.K.S.; Patorno, M.E.; Huybrechts, M.K.F.; Liu, M.J.; Rathmell, M.J.P.; Bateman, M.B.T. Variations in the Use of Perioperative Multimodal Analgesic Therapy. *Anesthesiology* **2016**, *124*, 837–845. [CrossRef] [PubMed]
41. Shafi, S.; Collinsworth, A.W.; Copeland, L.A.; Ogola, G.O.; Qiu, T.; Kouznetsova, M.; Liao, I.-C.; Mears, N.; Pham, A.T.; Wan, G.J.; et al. Association of Opioid-Related Adverse Drug Events with Clinical and Cost Outcomes among Surgical Patients in a Large Integrated Health Care Delivery System. *JAMA Surg.* **2018**, *153*, 757–763. [CrossRef]
42. Bicket, M.C.; White, E.; Pronovost, P.J.; Wu, C.L.; Yaster, M.; Alexander, G.C. Opioid Oversupply after Joint and Spine Surgery. *Anesth. Analg.* **2019**, *128*, 358–364. [CrossRef]
43. Neuman, M.D.; Bateman, B.T.; Wunsch, H. Inappropriate opioid prescription after surgery. *Lancet* **2019**, *393*, 1547–1557. [CrossRef]
44. Huang, P.; Copp, S.N. Oral Opioids Are Overprescribed in the Opiate-Naive Patient Undergoing Total Joint Arthroplasty. *J. Am. Acad. Orthop. Surg.* **2019**, *27*, e702–e708. [CrossRef]
45. Saini, S.; McDonald, E.L.; Shakked, R.; Nicholson, K.; Rogero, R.; Chapter, M.; Winters, B.S.; Pedowitz, D.I.; Raikin, S.M.; Daniel, J.N. Prospective Evaluation of Utilization Patterns and Prescribing Guidelines of Opioid Consumption Following Orthopedic Foot and Ankle Surgery. *Foot Ankle Int.* **2018**, *39*, 1257–1265. [CrossRef]
46. Bicket, M.C.; Long, J.J.; Pronovost, P.J.; Alexander, G.C.; Wu, C.L. Prescription Opioid Analgesics Commonly Unused after Surgery. *JAMA Surg.* **2017**, *152*, 1066–1071. [CrossRef]
47. Kim, N.; Matzon, J.L.; Abboudi, J.; Jones, C.; Kirkpatrick, W.; Leinberry, C.F.; Liss, F.E.; Lutsky, K.F.; Wang, M.L.; Maltenfort, M.; et al. A Prospective Evaluation of Opioid Utilization after Upper-Extremity Surgical Procedures: Identifying Consumption Patterns and Determining Prescribing Guidelines. *J. Bone Jt. Surg. Am. Vol.* **2016**, *98*, e89. [CrossRef]
48. Jones, C.M. Heroin use and heroin use risk behaviors among nonmedical users of prescription opioid pain relievers—United States, 2002–2004 and 2008–2010. *Drug Alcohol Depend.* **2013**, *132*, 95–100. [CrossRef]
49. Lipari, R.N.; Hughes, A. How People Obtain the Prescription Pain Relievers They Misuse. The CBHSQ Report. Rockville (MD): Substance Abuse and Mental Health Services Administration (US). 2017. Available online: https://www.ncbi.nlm.nih.gov/pubmed/28252901 (accessed on 14 September 2020).
50. Glare, P.; Aubrey, K.R.; Myles, P.S. Transition from acute to chronic pain after surgery. *Lancet* **2019**, *393*, 1537–1546. [CrossRef]
51. Núñez-Cortés, R.; Chamorro, C.; Ortega-Palavecinos, M.; Mattar, G.; Paredes, O.; Besoaín-Saldaña, Á.; Cruz-Montecinos, C. Social determinants associated to chronic pain after total knee arthroplasty. *Int. Orthop.* **2019**, *43*, 2767–2771. [CrossRef]
52. Weinrib, A.Z.; Azam, M.A.; Birnie, K.A.; Burns, L.C.; Clarke, H.; Katz, J. The psychology of chronic post-surgical pain: New frontiers in risk factor identification, prevention and management. *Br. J. Pain* **2017**, *11*, 169–177. [CrossRef]
53. Ravindran, D. Chronic Postsurgical Pain: Prevention and Management. *J. Pain Palliat. Care Pharmacother.* **2014**, *28*, 51–53. [CrossRef]
54. Dowell, D.; Haegerich, T.M.; Chou, R. CDC Guideline for Prescribing Opioids for Chronic Pain—United States, 2016. *JAMA* **2016**, *315*, 1624–1645. [CrossRef]

55. Kaye, A.D.; Granier, A.L.; Garcia, A.J.; Carlson, S.F.; Fuller, M.C.; Haroldson, A.R.; White, S.W.; Krueger, O.L.; Novitch, M.B.; Cornett, E.M. Non-Opioid Perioperative Pain Strategies for the Clinician: A Narrative Review. *Pain Ther.* **2020**, *9*, 25–39. [CrossRef]
56. Ramirez, M.F.; Kamdar, B.B.; Cata, J.P. Optimizing Perioperative Use of Opioids: A Multimodal Approach. *Curr. Anesthesiol. Rep.* **2020**, *10*, 404–415. [CrossRef]
57. Wick, E.C.; Grant, M.C.; Wu, C.L. Postoperative Multimodal Analgesia Pain Management with Nonopioid Analgesics and Techniques. *JAMA Surg.* **2017**, *152*, 691–697. [CrossRef]
58. Ogura, Y.; Gum, J.L.; Steele, P.; Iii, C.H.C.; Djurasovic, M.; Ii, R.K.O.; Laratta, J.L.; Davis, E.; Brown, M.; Daniels, C.; et al. Multi-modal pain control regimen for anterior lumbar fusion drastically reduces in-hospital opioid consumption. *J. Spine Surg.* **2020**, *6*, 681–687. [CrossRef]
59. Hajewski, C.J.; Westermann, R.W.; Holte, A.; Shamrock, A.; Bollier, M.; Wolf, B.R. Impact of a Standardized Multimodal Analgesia Protocol on Opioid Prescriptions after Common Arthroscopic Procedures. *Orthop. J. Sports Med.* **2019**, *7*. [CrossRef]
60. Kurd, M.F.; Kreitz, T.; Schroeder, G.; Vaccaro, A.R. The Role of Multimodal Analgesia in Spine Surgery. *J. Am. Acad. Orthop. Surg.* **2017**, *25*, 260–268. [CrossRef]
61. Weingarten, T.N.; Jacob, A.K.; Njathi, C.W.; Wilson, G.A.; Sprung, J. Multimodal Analgesic Protocol and Postanesthesia Respiratory Depression during Phase I Recovery after Total Joint Arthroplasty. *Reg. Anesth. Pain Med.* **2015**, *40*, 330–336. [CrossRef] [PubMed]
62. Dunkman, W.J.; Manning, M.W. Enhanced Recovery after Surgery and Multimodal Strategies for Analgesia. *Surg. Clin. North Am.* **2018**, *98*, 1171–1184. [CrossRef]
63. Beverly, A.; Kaye, A.D.; Ljungqvist, O.; Urman, R.D. Essential Elements of Multimodal Analgesia in Enhanced Recovery after Surgery (ERAS) Guidelines. *Anesthesiol. Clin.* **2017**, *35*, e115–e143. [CrossRef]
64. Kaye, A.D.; Urman, R.D.; Rappaport, Y.; Siddaiah, H.; Cornett, E.M.; Belani, K.; Salinas, O.J.; Fox, C.J. Multimodal analgesia as an essential part of enhanced recovery protocols in the ambulatory settings. *J. Anaesthesiol. Clin. Pharmacol.* **2019**, *35*, S40–S45. [CrossRef]
65. Ljungqvist, O.; Scott, M.; Fearon, K.C. Enhanced Recovery After Surgery. *JAMA Surg.* **2017**, *152*, 292–298. [CrossRef] [PubMed]
66. Fawcett, W.; Levy, N.; Scott, M.; Ljunqvist, O.; Lobo, D. The ERAS® society's 2018 survey on post-operative opioid stewardship. *Clin. Nutr. ESPEN* **2019**, *31*, 122. [CrossRef]
67. Frazee, R.; Garmon, E.; Isbell, C.; Bird, E.; Papaconstantinou, H. Postoperative Opioid Prescription Reduction Strategy in a Regional Healthcare System. *J. Am. Coll. Surg.* **2020**, *230*, 631–635. [CrossRef]
68. Uritsky, T.J.; Busch, M.E.; Chae, S.G.; Genord, C. Opioid Stewardship: Building on Antibiotic Stewardship Principles. *J. Pain Palliat. Care Pharmacother.* **2020**, 1–3. [CrossRef]
69. Agency Medical Directors' Group. AMDG—Interagency Guidelines. Available online: http://www.agencymeddirectors.wa.gov/guidelines.asp (accessed on 1 December 2020).
70. CDC Guideline for Prescribing Opioids for Chronic Pain. 28 August 2019. Available online: https://www.cdc.gov/drugoverdose/prescribing/guideline.html (accessed on 1 December 2020).
71. McPherson, M.L. *Demystifying Opioid Conversion Calculations: A Guide for Effective Dosing*, 2nd ed.; American Society of Health-System Pharmacists: Bethesda, MD, USA, 2019; Available online: https://play.google.com/store/books/details?id=1g9uDwAAQBAJ (accessed on 14 September 2020).
72. Von Korff, M.; Saunders, K.; Ray, G.T.; Boudreau, D.; Campbell, C.; Merrill, J.; Sullivan, M.D.; Rutter, C.M.; Silverberg, M.J.; Banta-Green, C.; et al. De Facto Long-term Opioid Therapy for Noncancer Pain. *Clin. J. Pain* **2008**, *24*, 521–527. [CrossRef]
73. American Society of Regional Anesthesia and Pain Medicine. Advisories & Guidelines. Available online: https://www.asra.com/advisory-guidelines (accessed on 28 December 2020).
74. Huxtable, C.A.; Roberts, L.J.; Somogyi, A.A.; MacIntyre, P.E. Acute Pain Management in Opioid-Tolerant Patients: A Growing Challenge. *Anaesth. Intensiv. Care* **2011**, *39*, 804–823. [CrossRef]
75. Doan, L.V.; Blitz, J. Preoperative Assessment and Management of Patients with Pain and Anxiety Disorders. *Curr. Anesthesiol. Rep.* **2020**, *10*, 28–34. [CrossRef] [PubMed]
76. Banning, L.B.; El Moumni, M.; Visser, L.; van Leeuwen, B.L.; Zeebregts, C.J.; Pol, R.A. Frailty leads to poor long-term survival in patients undergoing elective vascular surgery. *J. Vasc. Surg.* **2020**. [CrossRef] [PubMed]
77. Shah, R.; Attwood, K.; Arya, S.; Hall, D.E.; Johanning, J.M.; Gabriel, E.; Visioni, A.; Nurkin, S.; Kukar, M.; Hochwald, S.; et al. Association of Frailty with Failure to Rescue after Low-Risk and High-Risk Inpatient Surgery. *JAMA Surg.* **2018**, *153*, e180214. [CrossRef]
78. Feldman, L.S.; Carli, F. From Preoperative Assessment to Preoperative Optimization of Frailty. *JAMA Surg.* **2018**, *153*, e180213. [CrossRef]
79. Dindo, L.; Zimmerman, M.B.; Hadlandsmyth, K.; StMarie, B.; Embree, J.; Marchman, J.; Tripp-Reimer, T.; Rakel, B. Acceptance and Commitment Therapy for Prevention of Chronic Postsurgical Pain and Opioid Use in At-Risk Veterans: A Pilot Randomized Controlled Study. *J. Pain* **2018**, *19*, 1211–1221. [CrossRef] [PubMed]
80. Kim, S.; Duncan, P.W.; Groban, L.; Segal, H.; Abbott, R.M.; Williamson, J.D. Patient-Reported Outcome Measures (PROM) as a Preoperative Assessment Tool. *J. Anesth. Perioper. Med.* **2017**, *4*, 274–281. [CrossRef]
81. Nyman, M.H.; Nilsson, U.; Dahlberg, K.; Jaensson, M. Association between Functional Health Literacy and Postoperative Recovery, Health Care Contacts, and Health-Related Quality of Life among Patients Undergoing Day Surgery. *JAMA Surg.* **2018**, *153*, 738–745. [CrossRef]

82. De Oliveira, G.S.; Errea, M.; Bialek, J.; Kendall, M.C.; McCarthy, R.J. The impact of health literacy on shared decision making before elective surgery: A propensity matched case control analysis. *BMC Health Serv. Res.* **2018**, *18*, 958. [CrossRef]
83. De Oliveira, G.S., Jr.; McCarthy, R.J.; Wolf, M.S.; Holl, J.L. The impact of health literacy in the care of surgical patients: A qualitative systematic review. *BMC Surg.* **2015**, *15*, 1–7. [CrossRef]
84. Roy, M.; Corkum, J.P.; Urbach, D.R.; Novak, C.B.; Von Schroeder, H.P.; McCabe, S.J.; Okrainec, K. Health Literacy among Surgical Patients: A Systematic Review and Meta-analysis. *World J. Surg.* **2019**, *43*, 96–106. [CrossRef]
85. Chang, M.E.; Baker, S.J.; Marques, I.C.D.S.; Liwo, A.N.; Chung, S.K.; Richman, J.S.; Knight, S.J.; Fouad, M.N.; Gakumo, C.A.; Davis, T.C.; et al. Health Literacy in Surgery. *HLRP Health Lit. Res. Prract.* **2020**, *4*, e46–e65. [CrossRef] [PubMed]
86. Weiss, B.D.; Mays, M.Z.; Martz, W.; Castro, K.M.; DeWalt, D.A.; Pignone, M.P.; Mockbee, J.; Hale, F.A. Quick Assessment of Literacy in Primary Care: The Newest Vital Sign. *Ann. Fam. Med.* **2005**, *3*, 514–522. [CrossRef] [PubMed]
87. Chew, L.D.; Bradley, K.A.; Boyko, E.J. Brief questions to identify patients with inadequate health literacy. *Health* **2004**, *11*, 12.
88. Wolmeister, A.S.; Schiavo, C.L.; Nazário, K.C.K.; Castro, S.M.D.J.; De Souza, A.; Caetani, R.P.; Caumo, W.; Stefani, L.C. The Brief Measure of Emotional Preoperative Stress (B-MEPS) as a new predictive tool for postoperative pain: A prospective observational cohort study. *PLoS ONE* **2020**, *15*, e0227441. [CrossRef] [PubMed]
89. Yang, M.M.; Riva-Cambrin, J. Prediction tools for postoperative pain. *PAIN Rep.* **2021**, *6*, e875. [CrossRef]
90. Braun, M.; Bello, C.; Riva, T.; Hönemann, C.; Doll, D.; Urman, R.D.; Luedi, M.M. Quantitative Sensory Testing to Predict Postoperative Pain. *Curr. Pain Headache Rep.* **2021**, *25*, 1–8. [CrossRef]
91. Palanisami, D.R.; Reddy, D.A.; Huggi, V.; Rajasekaran, R.B.; Natesan, R.; Shanmuganathan, R. Assessing Preoperative Pain Sensitivity Predicts the Postoperative Analgesic Requirement and Recovery after Total Knee Arthroplasty: A Prospective Study of 178 Patients. *J. Arthroplast.* **2020**, *35*, 3545–3553. [CrossRef]
92. Horn, A.; Kaneshiro, K.; Tsui, B.C.H. Preemptive and Preventive Pain Psychoeducation and Its Potential Application as a Multimodal Perioperative Pain Control Option. *Anesth. Analg.* **2020**, *130*, 559–573. [CrossRef]
93. Bohan, P.M.K.; Chick, R.C.; Wall, M.E.; Hale, D.F.; Tzeng, C.-W.D.; Peoples, G.E.; Vreeland, T.J.; Clifton, G.T. An Educational Intervention Reduces Opioids Prescribed Following General Surgery Procedures. *J. Surg. Res.* **2021**, *257*, 399–405. [CrossRef]
94. Khorfan, R.; Shallcross, M.L.; Yu, B.; Sanchez, N.; Parilla, S.; Coughlin, J.M.; Johnson, J.K.; Bilimoria, K.Y.; Stulberg, J.J. Preoperative patient education and patient preparedness are associated with less postoperative use of opioids. *Surgery* **2020**, *167*, 852–858. [CrossRef]
95. Rucinski, K.; Cook, J.L. Effects of preoperative opioid education on postoperative opioid use and pain management in orthopaedics: A systematic review. *J. Orthop.* **2020**, *20*, 154–159. [CrossRef]
96. Rief, W.; Shedden-Mora, M.C.; Laferton, J.A.C.; Auer, C.; Petrie, K.J.; Salzmann, S.; Schedlowski, M.; Moosdorf, R. Preoperative optimization of patient expectations improves long-term outcome in heart surgery patients: Results of the randomized controlled PSY-HEART trial. *BMC Med.* **2017**, *15*, 1–13. [CrossRef]
97. Martin, L.A.; Finlayson, S.R.G.; Brooke, B.S. Patient Preparation for Transitions of Surgical Care: Is Failing to Prepare Surgical Patients Preparing Them to Fail? *World J. Surg.* **2017**, *41*, 1447–1453. [CrossRef]
98. Poland, F.; Spalding, N.; Gregory, S.; McCulloch, J.; Sargen, K.; Vicary, P. Developing patient education to enhance recovery after colorectal surgery through action research: A qualitative study. *BMJ Open* **2017**, *7*, e013498. [CrossRef]
99. Liebner, L.T. I Can't Read That! Improving Perioperative Literacy for Ambulatory Surgical Patients. *AORN J.* **2015**, *101*, 416–427. [CrossRef] [PubMed]
100. Michigan OPEN. Patient Education. Available online: https://michigan-open.org/wp-content/uploads/2019/07/POP-education.7.01.19.pdf (accessed on 21 December 2020).
101. Michigan OPEN. Patient Counseling. Available online: https://michigan-open.org/prescribing-recommendations/patient-counseling/ (accessed on 22 December 2020).
102. Northwestern Medicine. Prescription Opioids—What You Need to Know. Available online: https://www.surgjournal.com/cms/10.1016/j.surg.2020.01.002/attachment/49637b3a-9996-4d9b-a612-935c44f0923f/mmc1.pdf (accessed on 22 December 2020).
103. Patient Information. Enhanced Recovery after Surgery (ERAS) (R) Society. Available online: https://erassociety.org/patient-information/ (accessed on 21 December 2020).
104. MacIntyre, P.E.; Roberts, L.J.; Huxtable, C.A. Management of Opioid-Tolerant Patients with Acute Pain: Approaching the Challenges. *Drugs* **2019**, *80*, 9–21. [CrossRef] [PubMed]
105. McAnally, H.B.; Freeman, L.W.; Darnall, B. *Preoperative Optimization of the Chronic Pain Patient: Enhanced Recovery Before Surgery*; Oxford University Press: Oxford, UK, 2019. Available online: https://play.google.com/store/books/details?id=jpCqDwAAQBAJ (accessed on 14 September 2020).
106. Hannon, C.P.; Fillingham, Y.A.; Nam, D.; Courtney, P.M.; Curtin, B.M.; Vigdorchik, J.M.; Buvanendran, A.; Hamilton, W.G.; Della Valle, C.J.; Deen, J.T.; et al. Opioids in Total Joint Arthroplasty: The Clinical Practice Guidelines of the American Association of Hip and Knee Surgeons, American Society of Regional Anesthesia and Pain Medicine, American Academy of Orthopaedic Surgeons, Hip Society, and Knee Society. *J. Arthroplast.* **2020**, *35*, 2709–2714. [CrossRef] [PubMed]
107. Nguyen, L.-C.L.; Sing, D.C.; Bozic, K.J. Preoperative Reduction of Opioid Use Before Total Joint Arthroplasty. *J. Arthroplast.* **2016**, *31*, 282–287. [CrossRef]
108. McAnally, H. Rationale for and approach to preoperative opioid weaning: A preoperative optimization protocol. *Perioper. Med.* **2017**, *6*, 19. [CrossRef]

109. Pergolizzi, J.V.; Varrassi, G.; Paladini, A.; LeQuang, J. Stopping or Decreasing Opioid Therapy in Patients on Chronic Opioid Therapy. *Pain Ther.* **2019**, *8*, 163–176. [CrossRef]
110. Opioid Taper Decision Tool. Veterans Affairs. Available online: https://www.pbm.va.gov/AcademicDetailingService/Documents/Pain_Opioid_Taper_Tool_IB_10_939_P96820.pdf (accessed on 23 December 2020).
111. Buys, M.J. Multidisciplinary Transitional Pain Service for the Veteran Population. *Fed. Pract.* **2020**, *37*, 472–478. [CrossRef]
112. Vetter, T.R.; Kain, Z.N. Role of the Perioperative Surgical Home in Optimizing the Perioperative Use of Opioids. *Anesth. Analg.* **2017**, *125*, 1653–1657. [CrossRef]
113. Katz, J.; Weinrib, A.; Fashler, S.R.; Katznelson, R.; Shah, B.R.; Ladak, S.S.; Jiang, J.; Li, Q.; McMillan, K.; Mina, D.S.; et al. The Toronto General Hospital Transitional Pain Service: Development and implementation of a multidisciplinary program to prevent chronic postsurgical pain. *J. Pain Res.* **2015**, *8*, 695–702. [CrossRef]
114. Montbriand, J.J.; Weinrib, A.Z.; Azam, M.A.; Ladak, S.S.J.; Shah, B.R.; Jiang, J.; McRae, K.; Tamir, D.; Lyn, S.; Katznelson, R.; et al. Smoking, Pain Intensity, and Opioid Consumption 1–3 Months after Major Surgery: A Retrospective Study in a Hospital-Based Transitional Pain Service. *Nicotine Tob. Res.* **2018**, *20*, 1144–1151. [CrossRef]
115. Veazie, S.; Mackey, K.; Peterson, K.; Bourne, D. Managing Acute Pain in Patients Taking Medication for Opioid Use Disorder: A Rapid Review. *J. Gen. Intern. Med.* **2020**, *35*, 945–953. [CrossRef] [PubMed]
116. Compton, P. Acute Pain Management for Patients Receiving Medication-Assisted Therapy. *AACN Adv. Crit. Care* **2019**, *30*, 335–342. [CrossRef] [PubMed]
117. Simpson, G.; Jackson, M. Perioperative management of opioid-tolerant patients. *BJA Educ.* **2016**, *17*, 124–128. [CrossRef]
118. Colvin, L.A.; Bull, F.; Hales, T.G. Perioperative opioid analgesia—When is enough too much? A review of opioid-induced tolerance and hyperalgesia. *Lancet* **2019**, *393*, 1558–1568. [CrossRef]
119. Goel, A.; Azargive, S.; Weissman, J.S.; Shanthanna, H.; Hanlon, J.G.; Samman, B.; Dominicis, M.; Ladha, K.S.; Lamba, W.; Duggan, S.; et al. Perioperative Pain and Addiction Interdisciplinary Network (PAIN) clinical practice advisory for perioperative management of buprenorphine: Results of a modified Delphi process. *Br. J. Anaesth.* **2019**, *123*, e333–e342. [CrossRef]
120. Mehta, D.; Thomas, V.; Johnson, J.; Scott, B.; Cortina, S.; Berger, L. Continuation of Buprenorphine to Facilitate Postoperative Pain Management for Patients on Buprenorphine Opioid Agonist Therapy. *Pain Physician* **2020**, *23*, E163–E174. [PubMed]
121. Buresh, M.; Ratner, J.; Zgierska, A.; Gordin, V.; Alvanzo, A. Treating Perioperative and Acute Pain in Patients on Buprenorphine: Narrative Literature Review and Practice Recommendations. *J. Gen. Intern. Med.* **2020**, *35*, 3635–3643. [CrossRef]
122. Lembke, A.; Ottestad, E.; Schmiesing, C. Patients Maintained on Buprenorphine for Opioid Use Disorder Should Continue Buprenorphine Through the Perioperative Period. *Pain Med.* **2019**, *20*, 425–428. [CrossRef]
123. Ward, E.N.; Quaye, A.N.-A.; Wilens, T.E. Opioid use disorders: Perioperative management of a special population. *Anesth. Analg.* **2018**, *127*, 539–547. [CrossRef]
124. Harrison, T.K.; Kornfeld, H.; Aggarwal, A.K.; Lembke, A. Perioperative Considerations for the Patient with Opioid Use Disorder on Buprenorphine, Methadone, or Naltrexone Maintenance Therapy. *Anesthesiol. Clin.* **2018**, *36*, 345–359. [CrossRef]
125. Sritapan, Y.; Clifford, S.; Bautista, A. Perioperative Management of Patients on Buprenorphine and Methadone: A Narrative Review. *Balk. Med. J.* **2020**, *37*, 247–252. [CrossRef]
126. Quaye, A.N.-A.; Zhang, Y. Perioperative Management of Buprenorphine: Solving the Conundrum. *Pain Med.* **2018**, *20*, 1395–1408. [CrossRef] [PubMed]
127. Jonan, A.B.; Kaye, A.D.; Urman, R.D. Buprenorphine Formulations: Clinical Best Practice Strategies Recommendations for Perioperative Management of Patients Undergoing Surgical or Interventional Pain Procedures. *Pain Physician* **2018**, *21*, e1–e12. [PubMed]
128. Coluzzi, F.; Bifulco, F.; Cuomo, A.; Dauri, M.; Leonardi, C.; Melotti, R.M.; Natoli, S.; Romualdi, P.; Savoia, G.; Corcione, A. The challenge of perioperative pain management in opioid-tolerant patients. *Ther. Clin. Risk Manag.* **2017**, *13*, 1163–1173. [CrossRef]
129. Pergolizzi, J.; Aloisi, A.M.; Dahan, A.; Filitz, J.; Langford, R.; Likar, R.; Mercadante, S.; Morlion, B.; Raffa, R.B.; Sabatowski, R.; et al. Current Knowledge of Buprenorphine and Its Unique Pharmacological Profile. *Pain Pract.* **2010**, *10*, 428–450. [CrossRef]
130. Dahan, A.; Yassen, A.; Romberg, R.; Sarton, E.; Teppema, L.; Olofsen, E.; Danhof, M. Buprenorphine induces ceiling in respiratory depression but not in analgesia. *Br. J. Anaesth.* **2006**, *96*, 627–632. [CrossRef] [PubMed]
131. Richardson, M.G.; Raymond, B.L. Lack of Evidence for Ceiling Effect for Buprenorphine Analgesia in Humans. *Anesth. Analg.* **2018**, *127*, 310–311. [CrossRef]
132. Warner, N.S.; Warner, M.A.; Cunningham, J.L.; Gazelka, H.M.; Hooten, W.M.; Kolla, B.P.; Warner, D.O. A Practical Approach for the Management of the Mixed Opioid Agonist-Antagonist Buprenorphine During Acute Pain and Surgery. *Mayo Clin. Proc.* **2020**, *95*, 1253–1267. [CrossRef]
133. MacIntyre, P.E.; Russell, R.A.; Usher, K.A.N.; Gaughwin, M.; Huxtable, C.A. Pain Relief and Opioid Requirements in the First 24 Hours after Surgery in Patients Taking Buprenorphine and Methadone Opioid Substitution Therapy. *Anaesth. Intensive Care* **2013**, *41*, 222–230. [CrossRef]
134. Dean, R.L.; Todtenkopf, M.S.; Deaver, D.R.; Arastu, M.F.; Dong, N.; Reitano, K.; O'Driscoll, K.; Kriksciukaite, K.; Gastfriend, D.R. Overriding the blockade of antinociceptive actions of opioids in rats treated with extended-release naltrexone. *Pharmacol. Biochem. Behav.* **2008**, *89*, 515–522. [CrossRef] [PubMed]
135. Petri, C.R.; Richards, J.B. Management of Sedation and Analgesia in Critically Ill Patients Receiving Long-Acting Naltrexone Therapy for Opioid Use Disorder. *Ann. Am. Thorac. Soc.* **2020**, *17*, 1352–1357. [CrossRef]

136. Yoburn, B.C.; Sierra, V.; Lutfy, K. Chronic opioid antagonist treatment: Assessment of receptor upregulation. *Eur. J. Pharmacol.* **1989**, *170*, 193–200. [CrossRef]
137. Menendez, M.E.; Ring, D.; Bateman, B.T. Preoperative Opioid Misuse is Associated with Increased Morbidity and Mortality after Elective Orthopaedic Surgery. *Clin. Orthop. Relat. Res.* **2015**, *473*, 2402–2412. [CrossRef] [PubMed]
138. Wesson, D.R.; Ling, W. The Clinical Opiate Withdrawal Scale (COWS). *J. Psychoact. Drugs* **2003**, *35*, 253–259. [CrossRef]
139. Vadivelu, N.; Kai, A.M.; Kodumudi, V.; Zhu, R.; Hines, R. Pain Management of Patients with Substance Abuse in the Ambulatory Setting. *Curr. Pain Headache Rep.* **2017**, *21*, 9. [CrossRef] [PubMed]
140. Quinlan, F.F.J.; Cox, F.F. Acute pain management in patients with drug dependence syndrome. *Pain Rep.* **2017**, *2*, e611. [CrossRef] [PubMed]
141. Makdissi, R.; Stewart, S.H. Care for hospitalized patients with unhealthy alcohol use: A narrative review. *Addict. Sci. Clin. Pract.* **2013**, *8*, 11. [CrossRef]
142. Sullivan, J.T.; Sykora, K.; Schneiderman, J.; Naranjo, C.A.; Sellers, E.M. Assessment of Alcohol Withdrawal: The revised clinical institute withdrawal assessment for alcohol scale (CIWA-Ar). *Br. J. Addict.* **1989**, *84*, 1353–1357. [CrossRef]
143. Babalonis, S.; Walsh, S.L. Warnings Unheeded: The Risks of Co-Prescribing Opioids and Benzodiazepines. *Pain Clin. Updates.* **2015**, *23*, 1–7. Available online: https://www.ncbi.nlm.nih.gov/pubmed/33343182 (accessed on 14 September 2020).
144. Aviram, J.; Samuelly-Leichtag, G. Efficacy of Cannabis-Based Medicines for Pain Management: A Systematic Review and Meta-Analysis of Randomized Controlled Trials. *Pain Physician* **2017**, *20*, E755–E796. [CrossRef] [PubMed]
145. Lucas, P.; Boyd, S.; Milloy, M.-J.; Walsh, Z. Cannabis Significantly Reduces the Use of Prescription Opioids and Improves Quality of Life in Authorized Patients: Results of a Large Prospective Study. *Pain Med.* **2020**, pnaa396. [CrossRef]
146. Lucas, P.; Baron, E.P.; Jikomes, N. Medical cannabis patterns of use and substitution for opioids & other pharmaceutical drugs, alcohol, tobacco, and illicit substances; results from a cross-sectional survey of authorized patients. *Harm Reduct. J.* **2019**, *16*, 9. [CrossRef]
147. Alexander, J.C.; Joshi, G.P. A review of the anesthetic implications of marijuana use. *Bayl. Univ. Med. Cent. Proc.* **2019**, *32*, 364–371. [CrossRef]
148. Goel, A.; McGuinness, B.; Jivraj, N.K.; Wijeysundera, D.N.; Mittleman, M.A.; Bateman, B.T.; Clarke, H.; Kotra, L.P.; Ladha, K.S. Cannabis Use Disorder and Perioperative Outcomes in Major Elective Surgeries. *Anesthesiology* **2020**, *132*, 625–635. [CrossRef] [PubMed]
149. Liu, C.W.; Bhatia, A.; Buzon-Tan, A.; Walker, S.; Ilangomaran, D.; Kara, J.; Venkatraghavan, L.; Prabhu, A.J. Weeding out the Problem. *Anesth. Analg.* **2019**, *129*, 874–881. [CrossRef]
150. Salottolo, K.; Peck, L.; Ii, A.T.; Carrick, M.M.; Madayag, R.; McGuire, E.; Bar-Or, D. The grass is not always greener: A multi-institutional pilot study of marijuana use and acute pain management following traumatic injury. *Patient Saf. Surg.* **2018**, *12*, 1–8. [CrossRef]
151. American Society of Anesthesiologists. Cannabis and Postoperative Pain. Available online: https://www.asahq.org/about-asa/newsroom/news-releases/2020/10/cannabis-and-postoperative-pain (accessed on 10 January 2021).
152. Twardowski, M.A.; Link, M.M.; Twardowski, N.M. Effects of Cannabis Use on Sedation Requirements for Endoscopic Procedures. *J. Am. Osteopat. Assoc.* **2019**, *119*, 307. [CrossRef]
153. Paulsen, R.T.; Burrell, B.D. Comparative studies of endocannabinoid modulation of pain. *Philos. Trans. R. Soc. B Biol. Sci.* **2019**, *374*, 20190279. [CrossRef]
154. Pernía-Andrade, A.J.; Kato, A.; Witschi, R.; Nyilas, R.; Katona, I.; Freund, T.F.; Watanabe, M.; Filitz, J.; Koppert, W.; Schüttler, J.; et al. Spinal Endocannabinoids and CB1 Receptors Mediate C-Fiber-Induced Heterosynaptic Pain Sensitization. *Science* **2009**, *325*, 760–764. [CrossRef] [PubMed]
155. Bonnet, U.; Preuss, U.W. The cannabis withdrawal syndrome: Current insights. *Subst. Abus. Rehabil.* **2017**, *8*, 9–37. [CrossRef] [PubMed]
156. Bradt, J.; Dileo, C.; Shim, M. Music interventions for preoperative anxiety. *Cochrane Database Syst. Rev.* **2013**, CD006908. [CrossRef] [PubMed]
157. Gasti, V.; Kurdi, M.S. Intraoperative meditation music as an adjunct to subarachnoid block for the improvement of postoperative outcomes following cesarean section: A randomized placebo-controlled comparative study. *Anesth. Essays Res.* **2018**, *12*, 618–624. [CrossRef] [PubMed]
158. Matsota, P.; Christodoulopoulou, T.; Smyrnioti, M.E.; Pandazi, A.; Kanellopoulos, I.; Koursoumi, E.; Karamanis, P.; Kostopanagiotou, G. Music's Use for Anesthesia and Analgesia. *J. Altern. Complement. Med.* **2013**, *19*, 298–307. [CrossRef] [PubMed]
159. Kühlmann, A.Y.R.; de Rooij, A.; Kroese, L.F.; van Dijk, M.; Hunink, M.G.M.; Jeekel, J. Meta-analysis evaluating music interventions for anxiety and pain in surgery. *BJS* **2018**, *105*, 773–783. [CrossRef]
160. Poulsen, M.J.; Coto, J. Nursing Music Protocol and Postoperative Pain. *Pain Manag. Nurs.* **2018**, *19*, 172–176. [CrossRef]
161. Koo, C.-H.; Park, J.-W.; Ryu, J.-H.; Han, S.-H. The Effect of Virtual Reality on Preoperative Anxiety: A Meta-Analysis of Randomized Controlled Trials. *J. Clin. Med.* **2020**, *9*, 3151. [CrossRef]
162. Eijlers, R.; Dierckx, B.; Staals, L.M.; Berghmans, J.M.; Van Der Schroeff, M.P.; Strabbing, E.M.; Wijnen, R.M.; Hillegers, M.H.; Legerstee, J.S.; Utens, E.M. Virtual reality exposure before elective day care surgery to reduce anxiety and pain in children. *Eur. J. Anaesthesiol.* **2019**, *36*, 728–737. [CrossRef]

163. Ding, L.; Hua, H.; Zhu, H.; Zhu, S.; Lu, J.; Zhao, K.; Xu, Q. Effects of virtual reality on relieving postoperative pain in surgical patients: A systematic review and meta-analysis. *Int. J. Surg.* **2020**, *82*, 87–94. [CrossRef] [PubMed]
164. Pogatzki-Zahn, E.M.; Segelcke, D.; Schug, S.A. Postoperative pain—From mechanisms to treatment. *Pain Rep.* **2017**, *2*, e588. [CrossRef] [PubMed]
165. Urman, R.D.; Vadivelu, N.; Mitra, S.; Kodumudi, V.; Kaye, A.D.; Schermer, E. Preventive analgesia for postoperative pain control: A broader concept. *Local Reg. Anesth.* **2014**, *7*, 17–22. [CrossRef] [PubMed]
166. Dilip, C.R.S.; Shetty, A.P.; Subramanian, B.; Kanna, R.M.; Rajasekaran, S. A prospective randomized study to analyze the efficacy of balanced pre-emptive analgesia in spine surgery. *Spine J.* **2019**, *19*, 569–577. [CrossRef]
167. Haffner, M.; Saiz, A.M.; Nathe, R.; Hwang, J.; Migdal, C.; Klineberg, E.; Roberto, R. Preoperative multimodal analgesia decreases 24-hour postoperative narcotic consumption in elective spinal fusion patients. *Spine J.* **2019**, *19*, 1753–1763. [CrossRef]
168. Nir, R.-R.; Nahman-Averbuch, H.; Moont, R.; Sprecher, E.; Yarnitsky, D. Preoperative preemptive drug administration for acute postoperative pain: A systematic review and meta-analysis. *Eur. J. Pain* **2016**, *20*, 1025–1043. [CrossRef]
169. Barker, J.C.; DiBartola, K.; Wee, C.; Andonian, N.; Abdel-Rasoul, M.; Lowery, D.; Janis, J.E. Preoperative Multimodal Analgesia Decreases Postanesthesia Care Unit Narcotic Use and Pain Scores in Outpatient Breast Surgery. *Plast. Reconstr. Surg.* **2018**, *142*, 443e–450e. [CrossRef]
170. Moucha, C.S.; Weiser, M.C.; Levin, E.J. Current Strategies in Anesthesia and Analgesia for Total Knee Arthroplasty. *J. Am. Acad. Orthop. Surg.* **2016**, *24*, 60–73. [CrossRef]
171. Doleman, B.; Read, D.; Lund, J.N.; Williams, J.P. Preventive Acetaminophen Reduces Postoperative Opioid Consumption, Vomiting, and Pain Scores After Surgery. *Reg. Anesth. Pain Med.* **2015**, *40*, 706–712. [CrossRef] [PubMed]
172. Clarke, H.; Bonin, R.P.; Orser, B.A.; Englesakis, M.; Wijeysundera, D.N.; Katz, J. The Prevention of Chronic Postsurgical Pain Using Gabapentin and Pregabalin. *Anesth. Analg.* **2012**, *115*, 428–442. [CrossRef]
173. Cain, K.E.; Iniesta, M.D.; Fellman, B.M.; Suki, T.S.; Siverand, A.; Corzo, C.; Lasala, J.D.; Cata, J.P.; Mena, G.E.; Meyer, L.A.; et al. Effect of preoperative intravenous vs oral acetaminophen on postoperative opioid consumption in an enhanced recovery after surgery (ERAS) program in patients undergoing open gynecologic oncology surgery. *Gynecol. Oncol.* **2021**, *160*, 464–468. [CrossRef]
174. Johnson, R.J.; Nguyen, D.K.; Acosta, J.M.; O'Brien, A.L.; Doyle, P.D.; Medina-Rivera, G. Intravenous Versus Oral Acetaminophen in Ambulatory Surgical Center Laparoscopic Cholecystectomies: A Retrospective Analysis. *PT Peer-Rev. J. Formul. Manag.* **2019**, *44*, 359–363.
175. Westrich, G.H.; Birch, G.A.; Muskat, A.R.; Padgett, D.E.; Goytizolo, E.A.; Bostrom, M.P.; Mayman, D.J.; Lin, Y.; YaDeau, J.T. Intravenous vs Oral Acetaminophen as a Component of Multimodal Analgesia after Total Hip Arthroplasty: A Randomized, Blinded Trial. *J. Arthroplast.* **2019**, *34*, S215–S220. [CrossRef] [PubMed]
176. Hickman, S.R.; Mathieson, K.M.; Bradford, L.M.; Garman, C.D.; Gregg, R.W.; Lukens, D.W. Randomized trial of oral versus intravenous acetaminophen for postoperative pain control. *Am. J. Health Pharm.* **2018**, *75*, 367–375. [CrossRef] [PubMed]
177. Ohnuma, T.; Raghunathan, K.; Ellis, A.R.; Whittle, J.; Pyati, S.; Bryan, W.E.; Pepin, M.J.; Bartz, R.R.; Krishnamoorthy, V. Effects of Acetaminophen, NSAIDs, Gabapentinoids, and Their Combinations on Postoperative Pulmonary Complications after Total Hip or Knee Arthroplasty. *Pain Med.* **2020**, *21*, 2385–2393. [CrossRef]
178. Dwyer, J.P.; Jayasekera, C.; Nicoll, A. Analgesia for the cirrhotic patient: A literature review and recommendations. *J. Gastroenterol. Hepatol.* **2014**, *29*, 1356–1360. [CrossRef]
179. Doleman, B.; Leonardi-Bee, J.; Heinink, T.P.; Bhattacharjee, D.; Lund, J.N.; Williams, J.P. Pre-emptive and preventive opioids for postoperative pain in adults undergoing all types of surgery. *Cochrane Database Syst. Rev.* **2018**, *12*, CD012624. [CrossRef]
180. Cooper, H.J.; Lakra, A.; Maniker, R.B.; Hickernell, T.R.; Shah, R.P.; Geller, J.A. Preemptive Analgesia with Oxycodone Is Associated with More Pain Following Total Joint Arthroplasty. *J. Arthroplast.* **2019**, *34*, 2878–2883. [CrossRef]
181. Ong, C.K.-S.; Lirk, P.; Seymour, R.A.; Jenkins, B.J. The Efficacy of Preemptive Analgesia for Acute Postoperative Pain Management: A Meta-Analysis. *Anesth. Analg.* **2005**, *100*, 757–773. [CrossRef]
182. Kim, M.P.; Godoy, C.; Nguyen, D.T.; Meisenbach, L.M.; Chihara, R.; Chan, E.Y.; Graviss, E.A. Preemptive pain-management program is associated with reduction of opioid prescriptions after benign minimally invasive foregut surgery. *J. Thorac. Cardiovasc. Surg.* **2020**, *159*, 734–744.e4. [CrossRef] [PubMed]
183. Chang, R.W.; Tompkins, D.M.; Cohn, S.M. Are NSAIDs Safe? Assessing the Risk-Benefit Profile of Nonsteroidal Anti-inflammatory Drug Use in Postoperative Pain Management. *Am. Surg.* **2020**. [CrossRef] [PubMed]
184. Theken, K.N.; Lee, C.R.; Gong, L.; Caudle, K.E.; Formea, C.M.; Gaedigk, A.; Klein, T.E.; Agúndez, J.A.; Grosser, T. Clinical Pharmacogenetics Implementation Consortium Guideline (CPIC) for CYP2C9 and Nonsteroidal Anti-Inflammatory Drugs. *Clin. Pharmacol. Ther.* **2020**, *108*, 191–200. [CrossRef] [PubMed]
185. Verret, M.; Lauzier, F.; Zarychanski, R.; Perron, C.; Savard, X.; Pinard, A.-M.; Leblanc, G.; Cossi, M.-J.; Neveu, X.; Turgeon, A.F.; et al. Perioperative Use of Gabapentinoids for the Management of Postoperative Acute Pain. *Anesthesiology* **2020**, *133*, 265–279. [CrossRef] [PubMed]
186. Kang, J.; Zhao, Z.; Lv, J.; Sun, L.; Lu, B.; Dong, B.; Ma, J.; Ma, X. The efficacy of perioperative gabapentin for the treatment of postoperative pain following total knee and hip arthroplasty: A meta-analysis. *J. Orthop. Surg. Res.* **2020**, *15*, 1–9. [CrossRef] [PubMed]
187. Kharasch, E.D.; Clark, J.D.; Kheterpal, S. Perioperative Gabapentinoids. *Anesthesiology* **2020**, *133*, 251–254. [CrossRef] [PubMed]

188. Wainwright, T.W.; Gill, M.; McDonald, D.A.; Middleton, R.G.; Reed, M.; Sahota, O.; Yates, P.; Ljungqvist, O. Consensus statement for perioperative care in total hip replacement and total knee replacement surgery: Enhanced Recovery after Surgery (ERAS®) Society recommendations. *Acta Orthop.* **2020**, *91*, 3–19. [CrossRef] [PubMed]
189. Deljou, A.; Hedrick, S.; Portner, E.; Schroeder, D.; Hooten, W.; Sprung, J.; Weingarten, T. Pattern of perioperative gabapentinoid use and risk for postoperative naloxone administration. *Br. J. Anaesth.* **2018**, *120*, 798–806. [CrossRef]
190. Cavalcante, A.N.; Sprung, J.; Schroeder, D.R.; Weingarten, T.N. Multimodal Analgesic Therapy with Gabapentin and Its Association with Postoperative Respiratory Depression. *Anesth. Analg.* **2017**, *125*, 141–146. [CrossRef]
191. Center for Drug Evaluation, Research. Serious Breathing Difficulties with Gabapentin and Pregabalin. Available online: https://www.fda.gov/drugs/drug-safety-and-availability/fda-warns-about-serious-breathing-problems-seizure-and-nerve-pain-medicines-gabapentin-neurontin (accessed on 5 January 2021).
192. Ohnuma, T.; Raghunathan, K.; Moore, S.; Setoguchi, S.; Ellis, A.R.; Fuller, M.; Whittle, J.; Pyati, S.; Bryan, W.E.; Pepin, M.J.; et al. Dose-Dependent Association of Gabapentinoids with Pulmonary Complications After Total Hip and Knee Arthroplasties. *J. Bone Jt. Surg. Am. Vol.* **2019**, *102*, 221–229. [CrossRef] [PubMed]
193. Bykov, K.; Bateman, B.T.; Franklin, J.M.; Vine, S.M.; Patorno, E. Association of Gabapentinoids with the Risk of Opioid-Related Adverse Events in Surgical Patients in the United States. *JAMA Netw. Open* **2020**, *3*, e2031647. [CrossRef]
194. Liu, B.; Liu, R.; Wang, L. A meta-analysis of the preoperative use of gabapentinoids for the treatment of acute postoperative pain following spinal surgery. *Medicine* **2017**, *96*, e8031. [CrossRef] [PubMed]
195. Han, C.; Kuang, M.-J.; Ma, J.-X.; Ma, X.-L. The Efficacy of Preoperative Gabapentin in Spinal Surgery: A Meta-Analysis of Randomized Controlled Trials. *Pain Physician* **2017**, *20*, 649–661. [PubMed]
196. Mao, Y.; Wu, L.; Ding, W. The efficacy of preoperative administration of gabapentin/pregabalin in improving pain after total hip arthroplasty: A meta-analysis. *BMC Musculoskelet. Disord.* **2016**, *17*, 1–11. [CrossRef] [PubMed]
197. Hannon, C.P.; Fillingham, Y.A.; Browne, J.A.; Schemitsch, E.H.; Buvanendran, A.; Hamilton, W.G.; Della Valle, C.J.; Deen, J.T.; Erens, G.A.; Lonner, J.H.; et al. Gabapentinoids in Total Joint Arthroplasty: The Clinical Practice Guidelines of the American Association of Hip and Knee Surgeons, American Society of Regional Anesthesia and Pain Medicine, American Academy of Orthopaedic Surgeons, Hip Society, and Knee Society. *J. Arthroplast.* **2020**, *35*, 2700–2703. [CrossRef]
198. Eipe, N.; Penning, J.; Yazdi, F.; Mallick, R.; Turner, L.; Ahmadzai, N.; Ansari, M.T. Perioperative use of pregabalin for acute pain—A systematic review and meta-analysis. *Pain* **2015**, *156*, 1284–1300. [CrossRef]
199. Doleman, B.; Heinink, T.P.; Read, D.J.; Faleiro, R.J.; Lund, J.N.; Williams, J.P. A systematic review and meta-regression analysis of prophylactic gabapentin for postoperative pain. *Anaesthesia* **2015**, *70*, 1186–1204. [CrossRef]
200. Chaparro, L.E.; Smith, S.A.; Moore, R.A.; Wiffen, P.J.; Gilron, I. Pharmacotherapy for the prevention of chronic pain after surgery in adults. *Cochrane Database Syst. Rev.* **2013**, *2013*, CD008307. [CrossRef]
201. Engelman, D.T.; Ben Ali, W.; Williams, J.B.; Perrault, L.P.; Reddy, V.S.; Arora, R.C.; Roselli, E.E.; Khoynezhad, A.; Gerdisch, M.; Levy, J.H.; et al. Guidelines for Perioperative Care in Cardiac Surgery. *JAMA Surg.* **2019**, *154*, 755. [CrossRef]
202. Baos, S.; Rogers, C.A.; Abbadi, R.; Alzetani, A.; Casali, G.; Chauhan, N.; Collett, L.; Culliford, L.; De Jesus, S.E.; Edwards, M.; et al. Effectiveness, cost-effectiveness and safety of gabapentin versus placebo as an adjunct to multimodal pain regimens in surgical patients: Protocol of a placebo controlled randomised controlled trial with blinding (GAP study). *BMJ Open* **2020**, *10*, e041176. [CrossRef]
203. Chincholkar, M. Gabapentinoids: Pharmacokinetics, pharmacodynamics and considerations for clinical practice. *Br. J. Pain* **2020**, *14*, 104–114. [CrossRef] [PubMed]
204. Toth, C. Substitution of Gabapentin Therapy with Pregabalin Therapy in Neuropathic Pain due to Peripheral Neuropathy. *Pain Med.* **2010**, *11*, 456–465. [CrossRef] [PubMed]
205. Branton, M.W.; Hopkins, T.J.; Nemec, E.C. Duloxetine for the reduction of opioid use in elective orthopedic surgery: A systematic review and meta-analysis. *Int. J. Clin. Pharm.* **2021**, 1–10. [CrossRef]
206. Zorrilla-Vaca, A.; Stone, A.; Caballero-Lozada, A.F.; Paredes, S.; Grant, M.C. Perioperative duloxetine for acute postoperative analgesia: A meta-analysis of randomized trials. *Reg. Anesth. Pain Med.* **2019**, *44*, 959–965. [CrossRef]
207. Koh, I.J.; Kim, M.S.; Sohn, S.; Song, K.Y.; Choi, N.Y.; In, Y. Duloxetine Reduces Pain and Improves Quality of Recovery Following Total Knee Arthroplasty in Centrally Sensitized Patients. *J. Bone Jt. Surg. Am. Vol.* **2019**, *101*, 64–73. [CrossRef] [PubMed]
208. YaDeau, J.T.; Brummett, C.M.; Mayman, D.J.; Lin, Y.; Goytizolo, E.A.; Padgett, D.E.; Alexiades, M.M.; Kahn, R.L.; Jules-Elysee, K.M.; Fields, K.G.; et al. Duloxetine and Subacute Pain after Knee Arthroplasty when Added to a Multimodal Analgesic Regimen. *Anesthesiology* **2016**, *125*, 561–572. [CrossRef]
209. Castro-Alves, L.J.; De Medeiros, A.C.P.O.; Neves, S.P.; De Albuquerque, C.L.C.; Modolo, N.S.; De Azevedo, V.L.; De Oliveira, G.S. Perioperative Duloxetine to Improve Postoperative Recovery after Abdominal Hysterectomy. *Anesth. Analg.* **2016**, *122*, 98–104. [CrossRef]
210. Nasr, D. Efficacy of perioperative duloxetine on acute and chronic postmastectomy pain. *Ain-Shams J. Anaesthesiol.* **2014**, *7*, 129. [CrossRef]
211. Sheth, K.R.; Bernthal, N.M.; Ho, H.S.; Bergese, S.D.; Apfel, C.C.; Stoicea, N.; Jahr, J.S. Perioperative bleeding and non-steroidal anti-inflammatory drugs. *Medicine* **2020**, *99*, e20042. [CrossRef]

212. Fillingham, Y.A.; Hannon, C.P.; Roberts, K.C.; Hamilton, W.G.; Della Valle, C.J.; Deen, J.T.; Erens, G.A.; Lonner, J.H.; Pour, A.E.; Sterling, R.S. Nonsteroidal Anti-Inflammatory Drugs in Total Joint Arthroplasty: The Clinical Practice Guidelines of the American Association of Hip and Knee Surgeons, American Society of Regional Anesthesia and Pain Medicine, American Academy of Orthopaedic Surgeons, Hip Society, and Knee Society. *J. Arthroplast.* **2020**, *35*, 2704–2708. [CrossRef]
213. Martinez, L.; Ekman, E.; Nakhla, N. Perioperative Opioid-sparing Strategies: Utility of Conventional NSAIDs in Adults. *Clin. Ther.* **2019**, *41*, 2612–2628. [CrossRef] [PubMed]
214. Maslin, B.; Lipana, L.; Roth, B.; Kodumudi, G.; Vadivelu, N. Safety Considerations in the Use of Ketorolac for Postoperative Pain. *Curr. Drug Saf.* **2017**, *12*, 67–73. [CrossRef] [PubMed]
215. Gobble, R.M.; Hoang, H.L.T.; Kachniarz, B.; Orgill, D.P. Ketorolac Does Not Increase Perioperative Bleeding. *Plast. Reconstr. Surg.* **2014**, *133*, 741–755. [CrossRef]
216. Cassinelli, E.H.; Dean, C.L.; Garcia, R.M.; Furey, C.G.; Bohlman, H.H. Ketorolac Use for Postoperative Pain Management Following Lumbar Decompression Surgery. *Spine* **2008**, *33*, 1313–1317. [CrossRef]
217. Devin, C.J.; McGirt, M.J. Best evidence in multimodal pain management in spine surgery and means of assessing postoperative pain and functional outcomes. *J. Clin. Neurosci.* **2015**, *22*, 930–938. [CrossRef]
218. Jamjittrong, S.; Matsuda, A.; Matsumoto, S.; Kamonvarapitak, T.; Sakurazawa, N.; Kawano, Y.; Yamada, T.; Suzuki, H.; Miyashita, M.; Yoshida, H. Postoperative non-steroidal anti-inflammatory drugs and anastomotic leakage after gastrointestinal anastomoses: Systematic review and meta-analysis. *Ann. Gastroenterol. Surg.* **2020**, *4*, 64–75. [CrossRef]
219. Modasi, A.; Pace, D.; Godwin, M.; Smith, C.; Curtis, B. NSAID administration post colorectal surgery increases anastomotic leak rate: Systematic review/meta-analysis. *Surg. Endosc.* **2019**, *33*, 879–885. [CrossRef]
220. Huang, Y.; Tang, S.R.; Young, C.J. Nonsteroidal anti-inflammatory drugs and anastomotic dehiscence after colorectal surgery: A meta-analysis. *ANZ J. Surg.* **2017**, *88*, 959–965. [CrossRef] [PubMed]
221. Nussmeier, N.A.; Whelton, A.A.; Brown, M.T.; Langford, R.M.; Hoeft, A.; Parlow, J.L.; Boyce, S.W.; Verburg, K.M. Complications of the COX-2 Inhibitors Parecoxib and Valdecoxib after Cardiac Surgery. *N. Engl. J. Med.* **2005**, *352*, 1081–1091. [CrossRef] [PubMed]
222. Schug, S.A.; Joshi, G.P.; Camu, F.; Pan, S.; Cheung, R. Cardiovascular Safety of the Cyclooxygenase-2 Selective Inhibitors Parecoxib and Valdecoxib in the Postoperative Setting: An Analysis of Integrated Data. *Anesth. Analg.* **2009**, *108*, 299–307. [CrossRef] [PubMed]
223. Schug, A.S.; Parsons, B.; Li, C.; Xia, F. The safety profile of parecoxib for the treatment of postoperative pain: A pooled analysis of 28 randomized, double-blind, placebo-controlled clinical trials and a review of over 10 years of postauthorization data. *J. Pain Res.* **2017**, *10*, 2451–2459. [CrossRef]
224. Fanelli, A.; Ghisi, D.; Aprile, P.L.; Lapi, F. Cardiovascular and cerebrovascular risk with nonsteroidal anti-inflammatory drugs and cyclooxygenase 2 inhibitors: Latest evidence and clinical implications. *Ther. Adv. Drug Saf.* **2017**, *8*, 173–182. [CrossRef] [PubMed]
225. Scheiman, J.M.; Hindley, C.E. Strategies to optimize treatment with NSAIDs in patients at risk for gastrointestinal and cardiovascular adverse events. *Clin. Ther.* **2010**, *32*, 667–677. [CrossRef]
226. Massoth, C.; Zarbock, A.; Meersch, M. Risk Stratification for Targeted AKI Prevention After Surgery: Biomarkers and Bundled Interventions. *Semin. Nephrol.* **2019**, *39*, 454–461. [CrossRef]
227. Goren, O.; Matot, I. Perioperative acute kidney injury. *Br. J. Anaesth.* **2015**, *115*, ii3–ii14. [CrossRef]
228. Meersch, M.; Schmidt, C.; Zarbock, A. Perioperative Acute Kidney Injury. *Anesth. Analg.* **2017**, *125*, 1223–1232. [CrossRef]
229. Zarbock, A.; Koyner, J.L.; Hoste, E.A.J.; Kellum, J.A. Update on Perioperative Acute Kidney Injury. *Anesth. Analg.* **2018**, *127*, 1236–1245. [CrossRef]
230. Bihorac, A. Acute Kidney Injury in the Surgical Patient: Recognition and Attribution. *Nephron* **2015**, *131*, 118–122. [CrossRef]
231. Khan, D.A.; Knowles, S.R.; Shear, N.H. Sulfonamide Hypersensitivity: Fact and Fiction. *J. Allergy Clin. Immunol. Prract.* **2019**, *7*, 2116–2123. [CrossRef]
232. Wulf, N.R.; Matuszewski, K.A. Sulfonamide cross-reactivity: Is there evidence to support broad cross-allergenicity? *Am. J. Health Pharm.* **2013**, *70*, 1483–1494. [CrossRef] [PubMed]
233. Brackett, C.C. Sulfonamide allergy and cross-reactivity. *Curr. Allergy Asthma Rep.* **2007**, *7*, 41–48. [CrossRef] [PubMed]
234. Yska, J.P.; Gertsen, S.; Flapper, G.; Emous, M.; Wilffert, B.; Van Roon, E.N. NSAID Use after Bariatric Surgery: A Randomized Controlled Intervention Study. *Obes. Surg.* **2016**, *26*, 2880–2885. [CrossRef] [PubMed]
235. Zeid, H.A.; Kallab, R.; Najm, M.A.; Jabbour, H.; Noun, R.; Sleilati, F.; Chucri, S.; Dagher, C.; Sleilaty, G.; Naccache, N. Safety and Efficacy of Non-Steroidal Anti-Inflammatory Drugs (NSAIDs) Used for Analgesia After Bariatric Surgery: A Retrospective Case-Control Study. *Obes. Surg.* **2018**, *29*, 911–916. [CrossRef] [PubMed]
236. Thorell, A.; MacCormick, A.D.; Awad, S.; Reynolds, N.; Roulin, D.; Demartines, N.; Vignaud, M.; Alvarez, A.; Singh, P.M.; Lobo, D.N. Guidelines for Perioperative Care in Bariatric Surgery: Enhanced Recovery after Surgery (ERAS) Society Recommendations. *World J. Surg.* **2016**, *40*, 2065–2083. [CrossRef]
237. American Society of Anesthesiologists. Anesthesia 101: Types of Anesthesia. Available online: https://www.asahq.org/whensecondscount/anesthesia-101/types-of-anesthesia/ (accessed on 21 September 2020).
238. Lee, J.H. Anesthesia for ambulatory surgery. *Korean J. Anesthesiol.* **2017**, *70*, 398–406. [CrossRef]
239. New York Society of Regional Anesthesia (NYSORA). Neuraxial Techniques. Available online: https://www.nysora.com/techniques/neuraxial-and-perineuraxial-techniques/ (accessed on 21 September 2020).

240. American Society of Regional Anesthesia, Pain Medicine. Regional Anesthesia for Surgery. Available online: https://www.asra.com/page/41/regional-anesthesia-for-surgery (accessed on 21 September 2020).
241. Urban, B.W.; Bleckwenn, M. Concepts and correlations relevant to general anaesthesia. *Br. J. Anaesth.* **2002**, *89*, 3–16. [CrossRef] [PubMed]
242. Brown, E.N.; Pavone, K.J.; Naranjo, M. Multimodal general anesthesia: Theory and practice. *Anesth. Analg.* **2018**, *127*, 1246–1258. [CrossRef] [PubMed]
243. Sun, E.C.; Memtsoudis, S.G.; Mariano, E.R. Regional Anesthesia. *Anesthesiology* **2019**, *131*, 1205–1206. [CrossRef]
244. Smith, L.M.; Cozowicz, C.; Uda, Y.; Memtsoudis, S.G.; Barrington, M.J. Neuraxial and Combined Neuraxial/General Anesthesia Compared to General Anesthesia for Major Truncal and Lower Limb Surgery. *Anesth. Analg.* **2017**, *125*, 1931–1945. [CrossRef]
245. Guay, J.; Choi, P.; Suresh, S.; Albert, N.; Kopp, S.; Pace, N.L. Neuraxial blockade for the prevention of postoperative mortality and major morbidity: An overview of Cochrane systematic reviews. *Cochrane Database Syst. Rev.* **2014**, *2014*, CD010108. [CrossRef] [PubMed]
246. Pérez-González, O.; Cuéllar-Guzmán, L.F.; Soliz, J.; Cata, J.P. Impact of Regional Anesthesia on Recurrence, Metastasis, and Immune Response in Breast Cancer Surgery. *Reg. Anesth. Pain Med.* **2017**, *42*, 751–756. [CrossRef]
247. Le-Wendling, L.; Nin, O.; Capdevila, X. Cancer Recurrence and Regional Anesthesia: The Theories, the Data, and the Future in Outcomes. *Pain Med.* **2016**, *17*, pme12893-75. [CrossRef] [PubMed]
248. Joshi, G.; Kehlet, H.; Beloeil, H.; Bonnet, F.; Fischer, B.; Hill, A.; Lavandhomme, P.; Lirk, P.; Pogatzki-Zhan, E.; Raeder, J.; et al. Guidelines for perioperative pain management: Need for re-evaluation. *Br. J. Anaesth.* **2017**, *119*, 720–722. [CrossRef] [PubMed]
249. Albrecht, E.; Chin, K.J. Advances in regional anaesthesia and acute pain management: A narrative review. *Anaesthesia* **2020**, *75*, e101–e110. [CrossRef]
250. Emelife, P.I.; Eng, M.R.; Menard, B.L.; Meyers, A.S.; Cornett, E.M.; Urman, R.D.; Kaye, A.D. Adjunct medications for peripheral and neuraxial anesthesia. *Best Pract. Res. Clin. Anaesthesiol.* **2018**, *32*, 83–99. [CrossRef]
251. Desai, N.; Kirkham, K.R.; Albrecht, E. Local anaesthetic adjuncts for peripheral regional anaesthesia: A narrative review. *Anaesthesia* **2021**, *76*, 100–109. [CrossRef]
252. Ranganath, Y.S.; Seering, M.S.; Marian, A.A. American Society of Regional Anesthesia News. Curb Your Enthusiasm: Local Anesthetic Adjuvants for Peripheral Nerve Blocks. 2020. Available online: https://www.asra.com/asra-news/article/301/curb-your-enthusiasm-local-anesthetic-ad (accessed on 23 November 2020).
253. Gola, W.; Zając, M.; Cugowski, A. Adjuvants in peripheral nerve blocks—The current state of knowledge. *Anestezjol. Intensywna Ter.* **2020**, *52*, 323–329. [CrossRef]
254. Bailard, N.S.; Ortiz, J.; Flores, R.A. Additives to local anesthetics for peripheral nerve blocks: Evidence, limitations, and recommendations. *Am. J. Health Pharm.* **2014**, *71*, 373–385. [CrossRef]
255. Joshi, G.; Gandhi, K.; Shah, N.; Gadsden, J.; Corman, S.L. Peripheral nerve blocks in the management of postoperative pain: Challenges and opportunities. *J. Clin. Anesth.* **2016**, *35*, 524–529. [CrossRef]
256. Suksompong, S.; Von Bormann, S.; Von Bormann, B. Regional Catheters for Postoperative Pain Control: Review and Observational Data. *Anesthesiol. Pain Med.* **2020**, *10*, e99745. [CrossRef]
257. Prabhakar, A.; Ward, C.T.; Watson, M.; Sanford, J.; Fiza, B.; Moll, V.; Kaye, R.J.; Hall, O.M.; Cornett, E.M.; Urman, R.D.; et al. Liposomal bupivacaine and novel local anesthetic formulations. *Best Pract. Res. Clin. Anaesthesiol.* **2019**, *33*, 425–432. [CrossRef]
258. New York Society of Regional Anesthesia (NYSORA). Controlled-Release Local Anesthetics. 8 June 2018. Available online: https://www.nysora.com/foundations-of-regional-anesthesia/pharmacology/controlled-release-local-anesthetics/ (accessed on 21 September 2020).
259. Orebaugh, S.L.; Dewasurendra, A. Has the future arrived? Liposomal bupivacaine versus perineural catheters and additives for interscalene brachial plexus block. *Curr. Opin. Anaesthesiol.* **2020**, *33*, 704–709. [CrossRef]
260. Onwochei, D.N.; West, S.; Pawa, A. If Wishes Were Horses, Beggars Would Ride. *Reg. Anesth. Pain Med.* **2017**, *42*, 546. [CrossRef]
261. Gabriel, R.A.; Swisher, M.W.; Sztain, J.F.; Furnish, T.J.; Ilfeld, B.M.; Said, E.T. State of the art opioid-sparing strategies for post-operative pain in adult surgical patients. *Expert Opin. Pharmacother.* **2019**, *20*, 949–961. [CrossRef]
262. McCann, M.E. Liposomal Bupivacaine. *Anesthesiology* **2021**, *134*, 139–142. [CrossRef] [PubMed]
263. Hamilton, T.W.; Athanassoglou, V.; Mellon, S.; Strickland, L.H.H.; Trivella, M.; Murray, D.; Pandit, H.G. Liposomal bupivacaine infiltration at the surgical site for the management of postoperative pain. *Cochrane Database Syst. Rev.* **2017**, *2*, CD011419. [CrossRef] [PubMed]
264. Ilfeld, B.M.; Gabriel, R.A.; Eisenach, J.C. Liposomal Bupivacaine Infiltration for Knee Arthroplasty. *Anesthesiology* **2018**, *129*, 623–626. [CrossRef] [PubMed]
265. Zhou, S.-C.; Liu, B.-G.; Wang, Z.-H. Efficacy of liposomal bupivacaine vs. traditional anaesthetic infiltration for pain management in total hip arthroplasty: A systematic review and meta-analysis. *Eur. Rev. Med. Pharmacol. Sci.* **2020**, *24*, 11305–11314.
266. Schwarzkopf, R.; Drexler, M.; Ma, M.W.; Schultz, V.M.; Le, K.T.; Rutenberg, T.F.; Rinehart, J.B. Is There a Benefit for Liposomal Bupivacaine Compared to a Traditional Periarticular Injection in Total Knee Arthroplasty Patients with a History of Chronic Opioid Use? *J. Arthroplast.* **2016**, *31*, 1702–1705. [CrossRef]
267. Kuang, M.-J.; Du, Y.; Ma, J.-X.; He, W.; Fu, L.; Ma, X.-L. The Efficacy of Liposomal Bupivacaine Using Periarticular Injection in Total Knee Arthroplasty: A Systematic Review and Meta-Analysis. *J. Arthroplast.* **2017**, *32*, 1395–1402. [CrossRef]

268. Hyland, S.J.; Deliberato, D.G.; Fada, R.A.; Romanelli, M.J.; Collins, C.L.; Wasielewski, R.C. Liposomal Bupivacaine Versus Standard Periarticular Injection in Total Knee Arthroplasty with Regional Anesthesia: A Prospective Randomized Controlled Trial. *J. Arthroplast.* **2019**, *34*, 488–494. [CrossRef]
269. Abildgaard, J.T.; Chung, A.S.; Tokish, J.M.; Hattrup, S.J. Clinical Efficacy of Liposomal Bupivacaine. *JBJS Rev.* **2019**, *7*, e8. [CrossRef] [PubMed]
270. Bravin, L.N.; Ernest, E.P.; Dietz, M.J.; Frye, B.M. Liposomal Bupivacaine Offers No Benefit Over Ropivacaine for Multimodal Periarticular Injection in Total Knee Arthroplasty. *Orthopedics* **2019**, *43*, 91–96. [CrossRef] [PubMed]
271. Hussain, N.; Brull, R.; Sheehy, B.T.; Kushelev, M.; Essandoh, M.K.; Abdallah, F.W. The mornings after—Periarticular liposomal bupivacaine infiltration does not improve analgesic outcomes beyond 24 hours following total knee arthroplasty: A systematic review and meta-analysis. *Reg. Anesth. Pain Med.* **2021**, *46*, 61–72. [CrossRef]
272. Ilfeld, B.M.; Eisenach, J.C.; Gabriel, R.A. Clinical Effectiveness of Liposomal Bupivacaine Administered by Infiltration or Peripheral Nerve Block to Treat Postoperative Pain. *Anesthesiology* **2021**, *134*, 283–344. [CrossRef] [PubMed]
273. Vandepitte, C.; Kuroda, M.; Witvrouw, R.; Anne, L.; Bellemans, J.; Corten, K.; Vanelderen, P.; Mesotten, D.; Leunen, I.; Heylen, M.; et al. Addition of Liposome Bupivacaine to Bupivacaine HCl Versus Bupivacaine HCl Alone for Interscalene Brachial Plexus Block in Patients Having Major Shoulder Surgery. *Reg. Anesth. Pain Med.* **2017**, *42*, 334–341. [CrossRef]
274. Chen, J.; Zhou, C.; Ma, C.; Sun, G.; Yuan, L.; Hei, Z.; Guo, C.; Yao, W. Which is the best analgesia treatment for total knee arthroplasty: Adductor canal block, periarticular infiltration, or liposomal bupivacaine? A network meta-analysis. *J. Clin. Anesth.* **2021**, *68*, 110098. [CrossRef] [PubMed]
275. Hussain, N.; Brull, R.; Sheehy, B.; Essandoh, M.K.; Stahl, D.L.; Weaver, T.E.; Abdallah, F.W. Perineural Liposomal Bupivacaine Is Not Superior to Nonliposomal Bupivacaine for Peripheral Nerve Block Analgesia. *Anesthesiology* **2021**, *134*, 147–164. [CrossRef] [PubMed]
276. Neal, J.M.; Barrington, M.J.; Fettiplace, M.R.; Gitman, M.; Memtsoudis, S.G.; Mörwald, E.E.; Rubin, D.S.; Weinberg, G. The Third American Society of Regional Anesthesia and Pain Medicine Practice Advisory on Local Anesthetic Systemic Toxicity. *Reg. Anesth. Pain Med.* **2018**, *43*, 113–123. [CrossRef] [PubMed]
277. New York Society of Regional Anesthesia (NYSORA). Local Anesthetic Systemic Toxicity. 24 June 2018. Available online: https://www.nysora.com/foundations-of-regional-anesthesia/complications/local-anesthetic-systemic-toxicity/ (accessed on 21 September 2020).
278. BrugadaDrugs.org. Drugs Preferably Avoided by Brugada Syndrome Patients. Available online: https://www.brugadadrugs.org/pref_avoid/ (accessed on 28 February 2020).
279. New York Society of Regional Anesthesia (NYSORA). Home—NYSORA. Available online: http://www.nysora.com (accessed on 21 September 2020).
280. American Society of Regional Anesthesia, Pain Medicine. Resources. Available online: https://www.asra.com/education (accessed on 29 December 2020).
281. Gustafsson, U.O.; Scott, M.J.; Hubner, M.; Nygren, J.; Demartines, N.; Francis, N.; Rockall, T.A.; Young-Fadok, T.M.; Hill, A.G.; Soop, M.; et al. Guidelines for Perioperative Care in Elective Colorectal Surgery: Enhanced Recovery after Surgery (ERAS®) Society Recommendations: 2018. *World J. Surg.* **2019**, *43*, 659–695. [CrossRef] [PubMed]
282. Tran, D.Q.; Salinas, F.V.; Benzon, H.T.; Neal, J.M. Lower extremity regional anesthesia: Essentials of our current understanding. *Reg. Anesth. Pain Med.* **2019**, *44*, 143–180. [CrossRef] [PubMed]
283. Neilio, J.; Kunze, L.; Drew, J.M. Contemporary Perioperative Analgesia in Total Knee Arthroplasty: Multimodal Protocols, Regional Anesthesia, and Peripheral Nerve Blockade. *J. Knee Surg.* **2018**, *31*, 600–604. [CrossRef] [PubMed]
284. Ariza, F.; Rodriguez-Mayoral, H.; Villarreal, K. Epidural analgesia in abdominal major surgery. *Colomb. J. Anesthesiol.* **2018**, *46*, 175–176. [CrossRef]
285. Elsharkawy, H.; Pawa, A.; Mariano, E.R. Interfascial Plane Blocks. *Reg. Anesth. Pain Med.* **2018**, *43*, 341–346. [CrossRef]
286. Ilfeld, B.M. Continuous Peripheral Nerve Blocks. *Anesth. Analg.* **2017**, *124*, 308–335. [CrossRef] [PubMed]
287. Lee, H.-S. Recent advances in topical anesthesia. *J. Dent. Anesth. Pain Med.* **2016**, *16*, 237–244. [CrossRef]
288. Dunn, L.K.; Durieux, M.E. Perioperative Use of Intravenous Lidocaine. *Anesthesiology* **2017**, *126*, 729–737. [CrossRef]
289. Earls, B.; Bellil, L. Systemic Lidocaine: An Effective and Safe Modality for Postoperative Pain Management and Early Recovery—Anesthesia Patient Safety Foundation. Anesthesia Patient Safety Foundation Newsletter. 2018. Available online: https://www.apsf.org/article/systemic-lidocaine-an-effective-and-safe-modality-for-postoperative-pain-management-and-early-recovery/ (accessed on 14 September 2020).
290. American Society of Regional Anesthesia, Pain Medicine. Clinical Implications of IV Lidocaine Infusion in Preoperative/Acute Pain Settings. Available online: https://www.asra.com/asra-news/article/114/clinical-implications-of-iv-lidocaine-in (accessed on 21 September 2020).
291. Weibel, S.; Jelting, Y.; Pace, N.L.; Helf, A.; Eberhart, L.H.; Hahnenkamp, K.; Hollmann, M.W.; Poepping, D.M.; Schnabel, A.; Kranke, P. Continuous intravenous perioperative lidocaine infusion for postoperative pain and recovery in adults. *Cochrane Database Syst. Rev.* **2018**, *6*, CD009642. [CrossRef]
292. Khan, J.S.; Yousuf, M.; Victor, J.C.; Sharma, A.; Siddiqui, N. An estimation for an appropriate end time for an intraoperative intravenous lidocaine infusion in bowel surgery: A comparative meta-analysis. *J. Clin. Anesth.* **2016**, *28*, 95–104. [CrossRef] [PubMed]

293. Zhu, Y.; Wang, F.; Yang, L.; Zhu, T. Effects of perioperative intravenous lidocaine infusion for postoperative pain and recovery in elderly patients undergoing surgery: A systematic review and meta-analysis of randomized controlled trials. *BMC* in process. [CrossRef]
294. Dewinter, G.; Moens, P.; Fieuws, S.; Vanaudenaerde, B.; Van De Velde, M.; Rex, S. Systemic lidocaine fails to improve postoperative morphine consumption, postoperative recovery and quality of life in patients undergoing posterior spinal arthrodesis. A double-blind, randomized, placebo-controlled trial. *Br. J. Anaesth.* **2017**, *118*, 576–585. [CrossRef]
295. Lii, T.R.; Aggarwal, A.K. Comparison of intravenous lidocaine versus epidural anesthesia for traumatic rib fracture pain: A retrospective cohort study. *Reg. Anesth. Pain Med.* **2020**, *45*, 628–633. [CrossRef] [PubMed]
296. Greenwood, E.; Nimmo, S.; Paterson, H.; Homer, N.; Foo, I. Intravenous lidocaine infusion as a component of multimodal analgesia for colorectal surgery—Measurement of plasma levels. *Perioper. Med.* **2019**, *8*, 1–5. [CrossRef]
297. Oh, T.K.; Chung, S.H.; Park, J.; Shin, H.; Chang, C.B.; Kim, T.K.; Do, S.-H. Effects of Perioperative Magnesium Sulfate Administration on Postoperative Chronic Knee Pain in Patients Undergoing Total Knee Arthroplasty: A Retrospective Evaluation. *J. Clin. Med.* **2019**, *8*, 2231. [CrossRef]
298. Shin, H.-J.; Kim, E.-Y.; Na, H.-S.; Kim, T.; Kim, M.-H.; Do, S.-H. Magnesium sulphate attenuates acute postoperative pain and increased pain intensity after surgical injury in staged bilateral total knee arthroplasty: A randomized, double-blinded, placebo-controlled trial. *Br. J. Anaesth.* **2016**, *117*, 497–503. [CrossRef]
299. Pockett, S. Spinal Cord Synaptic Plasticity and Chronic Pain. *Anesth. Analg.* **1995**, *80*, 173–179. [CrossRef]
300. Zhu, A.; Benzon, H.A.; Anderson, T.A. Evidence for the Efficacy of Systemic Opioid-Sparing Analgesics in Pediatric Surgical Populations. *Anesth. Analg.* **2017**, *125*, 1569–1587. [CrossRef] [PubMed]
301. Beaussier, M.; Delbos, A.; Maurice-Szamburski, A.; Ecoffey, C.; Mercadal, L. Perioperative Use of Intravenous Lidocaine. *Drugs* **2018**, *78*, 1229–1246. [CrossRef]
302. Daykin, H. The efficacy and safety of intravenous lidocaine for analgesia in the older adult: A literature review. *Br. J. Pain* **2016**, *11*, 23–31. [CrossRef]
303. Eipe, M.N.; Gupta, F.S.; Penning, F.J. Intravenous lidocaine for acute pain: An evidence-based clinical update. *BJA Educ.* **2016**, *16*, 292–298. [CrossRef]
304. Cooke, C.; Kennedy, E.D.; Foo, I.; Nimmo, S.; Speake, D.; Paterson, H.M.; Ventham, N.T. Meta-analysis of the effect of perioperative intravenous lidocaine on return of gastrointestinal function after colorectal surgery. *Tech. Coloproctol.* **2019**, *23*, 15–24. [CrossRef]
305. Missair, A.; Cata, J.P.; Votta-Velis, G.; Johnson, M.; Borgeat, A.; Tiouririne, M.; Gottumukkala, V.; Buggy, D.; Vallejo, R.; De Marrero, E.B.; et al. Impact of perioperative pain management on cancer recurrence: An ASRA/ESRA special article. *Reg. Anesth. Pain Med.* **2019**, *44*, 13–28. [CrossRef] [PubMed]
306. Dai, Y.; Jiang, R.; Su, W.; Wang, M.; Liu, Y.; Zuo, Y. Impact of perioperative intravenous lidocaine infusion on postoperative pain and rapid recovery of patients undergoing gastrointestinal tumor surgery: A randomized, double-blind trial. *J. Gastrointest. Oncol.* **2020**, *11*, 1274–1282. [CrossRef] [PubMed]
307. Yazici, K.K.; Kaya, M.; Aksu, B.; Ünver, S. The Effect of Perioperative Lidocaine Infusion on Postoperative Pain and Postsurgical Recovery Parameters in Gynecologic Cancer Surgery. *Clin. J. Pain* **2021**, *37*, 126–132. [CrossRef] [PubMed]
308. Mehta, S.D.; Smyth, D.; Vasilopoulos, T.; Friedman, D.; Sappenfield, J.W.; Alex, G. Ketamine infusion reduces narcotic requirements following gastric bypass surgery: A randomized controlled trial. *Surg. Obes. Relat. Dis.* **2020**. [CrossRef]
309. Helander, E.M.; Menard, B.L.; Harmon, C.M.; Homra, B.K.; Allain, A.V.; Bordelon, G.J.; Wyche, M.Q.; Padnos, I.W.; Lavrova, A.; Kaye, A.D. Multimodal Analgesia, Current Concepts, and Acute Pain Considerations. *Curr. Pain Headache Rep.* **2017**, *21*, 3. [CrossRef] [PubMed]
310. Radvansky, B.M.; Shah, K.; Parikh, A.; Sifonios, A.N.; Le, V.; Eloy, J.D. Role of Ketamine in Acute Postoperative Pain Management: A Narrative Review. *BioMed Res. Int.* **2015**, *2015*, 1–10. [CrossRef]
311. Rodríguez-Rubio, L.; Nava, E.; Del Pozo, J.S.G.; Jordán, J. Influence of the perioperative administration of magnesium sulfate on the total dose of anesthetics during general anesthesia. A systematic review and meta-analysis. *J. Clin. Anesth.* **2017**, *39*, 129–138. [CrossRef]
312. Park, J.-Y.; Hong, J.H.; Kim, D.-H.; Yu, J.; Hwang, J.-H.; Kim, Y.-K. Magnesium and Bladder Discomfort after Transurethral Resection of Bladder Tumor. *Anesthesiology* **2020**, *133*, 64–77. [CrossRef]
313. Kim, R.K.; Hwang, J.H.; Tsui, B.C. Utilization of Magnesium in Opioid-Free Anesthesia for Peroral Endoscopic Myotomy: A Case Report. *A&A Pract.* **2021**, *15*, e01372. [CrossRef]
314. De Oliveira, G.S.; Castro-Alves, L.J.; Khan, J.H.; McCarthy, R.J. Perioperative Systemic Magnesium to Minimize Postoperative Pain. *Anesthesiology* **2013**, *119*, 178–190. [CrossRef]
315. Zhu, H.; Ren, A.; Zhou, K.; Chen, Q.; Zhang, M.; Liu, J. Impact of Dexmedetomidine Infusion on Postoperative Acute Kidney Injury in Elderly Patients Undergoing Major Joint Replacement: A Retrospective Cohort Study. *Drug Des. Dev. Ther.* **2020**, *14*, 4695–4701. [CrossRef]
316. Grant, M.C.; Isada, T.; Ruzankin, P.; Gottschalk, A.; Whitman, G.; Lawton, J.S.; Dodd, O.J.; Barodka, V. Opioid-Sparing Cardiac Anesthesia. *Anesth. Analg.* **2020**, *131*, 1852–1861. [CrossRef]
317. Wieruszewski, P.M.; Wittwer, E.D. It's All in the Details: Dexmedetomidine and Acute Kidney Injury After Cardiac Surgery. *J. Cardiothorac. Vasc. Anesth.* **2020**, *34*, 2549. [CrossRef] [PubMed]
318. Lee, S. Dexmedetomidine: Present and future directions. *Korean J. Anesthesiol.* **2019**, *72*, 323–330. [CrossRef]

319. Naik, B.I.; Nemergut, E.C.; Kazemi, A.; Fernández, L.; Cederholm, S.K.; McMurry, T.L.; Durieux, M.E. The Effect of Dexmedetomidine on Postoperative Opioid Consumption and Pain After Major Spine Surgery. *Anesth. Analg.* **2016**, *122*, 1646–1653. [CrossRef]
320. Lundorf, L.J.; Nedergaard, H.K.; Møller, A.M. Perioperative dexmedetomidine for acute pain after abdominal surgery in adults. *Cochrane Database Syst. Rev.* **2016**, *2*, CD010358. [CrossRef]
321. Ge, D.-J.; Qi, B.; Tang, G.; Li, J.-Y. Intraoperative Dexmedetomidine Promotes Postoperative Analgesia and Recovery in Patients after Abdominal Hysterectomy: A Double-Blind, Randomized Clinical Trial. *Sci. Rep.* **2016**, *6*, 21514. [CrossRef]
322. Cheung, C.W.; Qiu, Q.; Ying, A.C.L.; Choi, S.W.; Law, W.L.; Irwin, M. The effects of intra-operative dexmedetomidine on postoperative pain, side-effects and recovery in colorectal surgery. *Anaesthesia* **2014**, *69*, 1214–1221. [CrossRef]
323. Bajracharya, J.L.; Subedi, A.; Pokharel, K.; Bhattarai, B. The effect of intraoperative lidocaine versus esmolol infusion on postoperative analgesia in laparoscopic cholecystectomy: A randomized clinical trial. *BMC Anesthesiol.* **2019**, *19*, 198–199. [CrossRef]
324. Bahr, M.P.; Williams, B.A. Esmolol, Antinociception, and Its Potential Opioid-Sparing Role in Routine Anesthesia Care. *Reg. Anesth. Pain Med.* **2018**, *43*, 815–818. [CrossRef] [PubMed]
325. Gelineau, A.M.; King, M.R.; Ladha, K.S.; Burns, S.M.; Houle, T.; Anderson, T.A. Intraoperative Esmolol as an Adjunct for Perioperative Opioid and Postoperative Pain Reduction. *Anesth. Analg.* **2018**, *126*, 1035–1049. [CrossRef]
326. Klag, E.A.; Kuhlmann, N.A.; Tramer, J.S.; Franovic, S.; Muh, S.J. Dexamethasone decreases postoperative opioid and antiemetic use in shoulder arthroplasty patients: A prospective, randomized controlled trial. *J. Shoulder Elb. Surg.* **2021**. [CrossRef]
327. McHardy, P.G.; Singer, O.; Awad, I.T.; Safa, B.; Henry, P.D.; Kiss, A.; Au, S.K.; Kaustov, L.; Choi, S. Comparison of the effects of perineural or intravenous dexamethasone on low volume interscalene brachial plexus block: A randomised equivalence trial. *Br. J. Anaesth.* **2020**, *124*, 84–91. [CrossRef]
328. Cortés-Flores, A.; Jiménez-Tornero, J.; Morgan-Villela, G.; Delgado-Gómez, M.; Del Valle, C.J.Z.-F.; García-Rentería, J.; Rendón-Félix, J.; Fuentes-Orozco, C.; Macías-Amezcua, M.; Ambriz-González, G.; et al. Effects of preoperative dexamethasone on postoperative pain, nausea, vomiting and respiratory function in women undergoing conservative breast surgery for cancer: Results of a controlled clinical trial. *Eur. J. Cancer Care* **2017**, *27*, e12686. [CrossRef]
329. Kahn, R.L.; Cheng, J.; Gadulov, Y.; Fields, K.G.; YaDeau, J.T.; Gulotta, L.V. Perineural Low-Dose Dexamethasone Prolongs Interscalene Block Analgesia with Bupivacaine Compared With Systemic Dexamethasone. *Reg. Anesth. Pain Med.* **2018**, *43*, 572–579. [CrossRef]
330. Holland, D.; Amadeo, R.J.J.; Wolfe, S.; Girling, L.; Funk, F.; Collister, M.; Czaplinski, E.; Ferguson, C.; Leiter, J.; Old, J.; et al. Effect of dexamethasone dose and route on the duration of interscalene brachial plexus block for outpatient arthroscopic shoulder surgery: A randomized controlled trial. *Can. J. Anaesth.* **2017**, *65*, 34–45. [CrossRef]
331. Kirkham, K.R.; Jacot-Guillarmod, A.; Albrecht, E. Optimal Dose of Perineural Dexamethasone to Prolong Analgesia after Brachial Plexus Blockade. *Anesth. Analg.* **2018**, *126*, 270–279. [CrossRef]
332. Pehora, C.; Pearson, A.M.; Kaushal, A.; Crawford, M.W.; Johnston, B. Dexamethasone as an adjuvant to peripheral nerve block. *Cochrane Database Syst. Rev.* **2017**, *11*, CD011770. [CrossRef] [PubMed]
333. Abdallah, F.W.; Johnson, J.; Chan, V.; Murgatroyd, H.; Ghafari, M.; Ami, N.; Jin, R.; Brull, R. Intravenous Dexamethasone and Perineural Dexamethasone Similarly Prolong the Duration of Analgesia after Supraclavicular Brachial Plexus Block. *Reg. Anesth. Pain Med.* **2015**, *40*, 125–132. [CrossRef] [PubMed]
334. Machado, F.C.; Palmeira, C.C.D.A.; Torres, J.N.L.; Vieira, J.E.; Ashmawi, H.A. Intraoperative use of methadone improves control of postoperative pain in morbidly obese patients: A randomized controlled study. *J. Pain Res.* **2018**, *11*, 2123–2129. [CrossRef]
335. Murphy, G.S.; Wu, C.L.; Mascha, E.J. Methadone. *Anesth. Analg.* **2019**, *129*, 1456–1458. [CrossRef]
336. Komen, H.; Brunt, L.M.; Deych, E.; Blood, J.; Kharasch, E.D. Intraoperative Methadone in Same-Day Ambulatory Surgery. *Anesth. Analg.* **2019**, *128*, 802–810. [CrossRef]
337. Machado, F.C.; Vieira, J.E.; De Orange, F.A.; Ashmawi, H.A. Intraoperative Methadone Reduces Pain and Opioid Consumption in Acute Postoperative Pain. *Anesth. Analg.* **2019**, *129*, 1723–1732. [CrossRef] [PubMed]
338. Murphy, G.S.; Szokol, J.W.; Avram, M.J.; Greenberg, S.B.; Marymont, J.H.; Shear, T.; Parikh, K.N.; Patel, S.S.; Gupta, D.K. Intraoperative Methadone for the Prevention of Postoperative PainA Randomized, Double-blinded Clinical Trial in Cardiac Surgical Patients. *Anesthesiology* **2015**, *122*, 1112–1122. [CrossRef] [PubMed]
339. Murphy, G.S.; Szokol, J.W.; Avram, M.J.; Greenberg, S.B.; Shear, T.D.; Deshur, M.A.; Vender, J.S.; Benson, J.; Newmark, R.L. Clinical Effectiveness and Safety of Intraoperative Methadone in Patients Undergoing Posterior Spinal Fusion Surgery. *Anesthesiology* **2017**, *126*, 822–833. [CrossRef]
340. Gottschalk, A.; Durieux, M.E.; Nemergut, E.C. Intraoperative Methadone Improves Postoperative Pain Control in Patients Undergoing Complex Spine Surgery. *Anesth. Analg.* **2011**, *112*, 218–223. [CrossRef]
341. Hussain, N.; Grzywacz, V.P.; Ferreri, C.A.; Atrey, A.; Banfield, L.; Shaparin, N.; Vydyanathan, A. Investigating the Efficacy of Dexmedetomidine as an Adjuvant to Local Anesthesia in Brachial Plexus Block. *Reg. Anesth. Pain Med.* **2017**, *42*, 184–196. [CrossRef]
342. Hanna, V.; Senderovich, H. Methadone in Pain Management: A Systematic Review. *J. Pain* **2020**. [CrossRef]
343. McNicol, E.D.; Ferguson, M.C.; Schumann, R. Methadone for neuropathic pain in adults. *Cochrane Database Syst. Rev.* **2017**, *5*, 012499. [CrossRef]
344. Tripathi, S.; Hunter, J. Neuromuscular blocking drugs in the critically ill. *Contin. Educ. Anaesth. Crit. Care Pain* **2006**, *6*, 119–123. [CrossRef]

345. Treanor, N.; Vezina, V.; Lui, A. ESRA19-0218 'Fast-track' patients to phase II recovery and decrease pacu duration in ambulatory arthroscopic shoulder surgery with combined peripheral nerve block and monitored anesthesia care. *E-Poster Discuss.* **2019**, *44*, A136. [CrossRef]
346. Wood, C. Effect of sublingual versus intravenous opioid administration on total opioid administration in patients following total knee arthroplasty. In Proceedings of the Great Lakes Pharmacy Residency Conference, Pursue University, West Lafayette, IN, USA, 25 April 2019.
347. Fan, M.; Chen, Z. A systematic review of non-pharmacological interventions used for pain relief after orthopedic surgical procedures. *Exp. Ther. Med.* **2020**, *20*, 1. [CrossRef] [PubMed]
348. Olsen, S.W.; Rosenkilde, C.; Lauridsen, J.; Hasfeldt, D. Effects of Nonpharmacologic Distraction Methods on Children's Postoperative Pain—A Nonmatched Case-Control Study. *J. PeriAnesth. Nurs.* **2020**, *35*, 147–154. [CrossRef] [PubMed]
349. Song, M.; Li, N.; Zhang, X.; Shang, Y.; Yan, L.; Chu, J.; Sun, R.; Xu, Y. Music for reducing the anxiety and pain of patients undergoing a biopsy: A meta-analysis. *J. Adv. Nurs.* **2017**, *74*, 1016–1029. [CrossRef] [PubMed]
350. Rafer, L.; Austin, F.; Frey, J.; Mulvey, C.; Vaida, S.; Prozesky, J. Effects of jazz on postoperative pain and stress in patients undergoing elective hysterectomy. *Adv. Mind Body Med.* **2015**, *29*, 6–11.
351. Liu, Y.; Petrini, M.A. Effects of music therapy on pain, anxiety, and vital signs in patients after thoracic surgery. *Complement. Ther. Med.* **2015**, *23*, 714–718. [CrossRef]
352. Wang, Y.; Tang, H.; Guo, Q.; Liu, J.; Liu, X.; Luo, J.; Yang, W. Effects of Intravenous Patient-Controlled Sufentanil Analgesia and Music Therapy on Pain and Hemodynamics After Surgery for Lung Cancer: A Randomized Parallel Study. *J. Altern. Complement. Med.* **2015**, *21*, 667–672. [CrossRef]
353. Ardon, A.E.; Prasad, A.; McClain, R.L.; Melton, M.S.; Nielsen, K.C.; Greengrass, R. Regional Anesthesia for Ambulatory Anesthesiologists. *Anesthesiol. Clin.* **2019**, *37*, 265–287. [CrossRef]
354. Amundson, A.W.; Panchamia, J.K.; Jacob, A.K. Anesthesia for Same-Day Total Joint Replacement. *Anesthesiol. Clin.* **2019**, *37*, 251–264. [CrossRef]
355. Beaussier, M.; Sciard, D.; Sautet, A. New modalities of pain treatment after outpatient orthopaedic surgery. *Orthop. Traumatol. Surg. Res.* **2016**, *102*, S121–S124. [CrossRef] [PubMed]
356. Pasero, C.; Quinlan-Colwell, A.; Rae, D.; Broglio, K.; Drew, D. American Society for Pain Management Nursing Position Statement: Prescribing and Administering Opioid Doses Based Solely on Pain Intensity. *Pain Manag. Nurs.* **2016**, *17*, 170–180. [CrossRef] [PubMed]
357. Pasero, C. One Size Does Not Fit All: Opioid Dose Range Orders. *J. PeriAnesth. Nurs.* **2014**, *29*, 246–252. [CrossRef] [PubMed]
358. Drew, D.J.; Gordon, D.B.; Morgan, B.; Manworren, R.C. "As-Needed" Range Orders for Opioid Analgesics in the Management of Pain: A Consensus Statement of the American Society for Pain Management Nursing and the American Pain Society. *Pain Manag. Nurs.* **2018**, *19*, 207–210. [CrossRef]
359. Smetzer, J.L.; Cohen, M.R. Pain Scales Don't Weigh Every Risk. *J. Pain Palliat. Care Pharmacother.* **2003**, *17*, 67–70. [CrossRef]
360. Van Boekel, R.L.M.; Vissers, K.C.P.; Van Der Sande, R.; Bronkhorst, E.; Lerou, J.G.C.; Steegers, M.A.H. Moving beyond pain scores: Multidimensional pain assessment is essential for adequate pain management after surgery. *PLoS ONE* **2017**, *12*, e0177345. [CrossRef]
361. Scher, C.; Petti, E.; Meador, L.; Van Cleave, J.H.; Liang, E.; Reid, M.C. Multidimensional Pain Assessment Tools for Ambulatory and Inpatient Nursing Practice. *Pain Manag. Nurs.* **2020**, *21*, 416–422. [CrossRef]
362. Hirsh, A.T.; Anastas, T.M.; Miller, M.M.; Quinn, P.D.; Kroenke, K. Patient race and opioid misuse history influence provider risk perceptions for future opioid-related problems. *Am. Psychol.* **2020**, *75*, 784–795. [CrossRef]
363. Anderson, K.O.; Green, C.R.; Payne, R. Racial and Ethnic Disparities in Pain: Causes and Consequences of Unequal Care. *J. Pain* **2009**, *10*, 1187–1204. [CrossRef]
364. Green, C.R.; Anderson, K.O.; Baker, T.A.; Campbell, L.C.; Decker, S.; Fillingim, R.B.; Kaloukalani, D.A.; Lasch, K.E.; Myers, C.; Tait, R.C.; et al. The Unequal Burden of Pain: Confronting Racial and Ethnic Disparities in Pain. *Pain Med.* **2003**, *4*, 277–294. [CrossRef] [PubMed]
365. George, S.; Johns, M. Review of nonopioid multimodal analgesia for surgical and trauma patients. *Am. J. Health Pharm.* **2020**, *77*, 2052–2063. [CrossRef] [PubMed]
366. Ho, A.M.-H.; Ho, A.K.; Mizubuti, G.B.; Klar, G.; Karmakar, M.K. Regional analgesia for patients with traumatic rib fractures: A narrative review. *J. Trauma Acute Care Surg.* **2020**, *88*, e22–e30. [CrossRef]
367. Saranteas, T.; Koliantzaki, I.; Savvidou, O.; Tsoumpa, M.; Eustathiou, G.; Kontogeorgakos, V.; Souvatzoglou, R. Acute pain management in trauma: Anatomy, ultrasound-guided peripheral nerve blocks and special considerations. *Minerva Anestesiol.* **2019**, *85*, 763–773. [CrossRef]
368. Hamrick, K.L.; Beyer, C.A.; Lee, J.A.; Cocanour, C.S.; Duby, J.J. Multimodal Analgesia and Opioid Use in Critically Ill Trauma Patients. *J. Am. Coll. Surg.* **2019**, *228*, 769–775.e1. [CrossRef]
369. Czernicki, M.; Kunnumpurath, S.; Park, W.; Kunnumpurath, A.; Kodumudi, G.; Tao, J.; Kodumudi, V.; Vadivelu, N.; Urman, R.D. Perioperative Pain Management in the Critically Ill Patient. *Curr. Pain Headache Rep.* **2019**, *23*, 34. [CrossRef] [PubMed]
370. Rubio-Haro, R.; Morales-Sarabia, J.; Ferrer-Gomez, C.; De Andrés, J. Regional analgesia techniques for pain management in patients admitted to the intensive care unit. *Minerva Anestesiol.* **2019**, *85*, 1118–1128. [CrossRef] [PubMed]

371. Corcoran, E.; Kinirons, B. Regional anaesthesia in the elderly patient a current perspective. *Curr. Opin. Anaesthesiol.* **2021**, *34*, 48–53. [CrossRef]
372. Villatte, G.; Mathonnet, M.; Villeminot, J.; Savary, M.; Theissen, A.; Ostermann, S.; Erivan, R.; Raynaud-Simon, A.; Slim, K. Interest of enhanced recovery programs in the elderly during total hip arthroplasty A systematic review. *Geriatr. Psychol. Neuropsychiatr. Vieil.* **2019**, *17*, 234–242.
373. Belcaid, I.; Eipe, N. Perioperative Pain Management in Morbid Obesity. *Drugs* **2019**, *79*, 1163–1175. [CrossRef] [PubMed]
374. Brown, H.L. Opioid Management in Pregnancy and Postpartum. *Obstet. Gynecol. Clin. North Am.* **2020**, *47*, 421–427. [CrossRef] [PubMed]
375. Peahl, A.F.; Smith, R.; Johnson, T.R.; Morgan, D.M.; Pearlman, M.D. Better late than never: Why obstetricians must implement enhanced recovery after cesarean. *Am. J. Obstet. Gynecol.* **2019**, *221*, 117-e1–117-e7. [CrossRef] [PubMed]
376. ACOG Committee. Opinion No. 742 Summary: Postpartum Pain Management. *Obstet. Gynecol.* **2018**, *132*, 252–253. [CrossRef] [PubMed]
377. Sutton, C.D.; Carvalho, B. Optimal Pain Management After Cesarean Delivery. *Anesthesiol. Clin.* **2017**, *35*, 107–124. [CrossRef]
378. Wu, M.-S.; Chen, K.-H.; Chen, I.-F.; Huang, S.K.; Tzeng, P.-C.; Yeh, M.-L.; Lee, F.-P.; Lin, J.-G.; Chen, C. The Efficacy of Acupuncture in Post-Operative Pain Management: A Systematic Review and Meta-Analysis. *PLoS ONE* **2016**, *11*, e0150367. [CrossRef]
379. Sun, J.-N.; Chen, W.; Zhang, Y.; Zhang, Y.; Feng, S.; Chen, X.-Y. Does cognitive behavioral education reduce pain and improve joint function in patients after total knee arthroplasty? A randomized controlled trial. *Int. Orthop.* **2020**, *44*, 2027–2035. [CrossRef]
380. Nicholls, J.L.; Azam, M.A.; Burns, L.C.; Englesakis, M.; Sutherland, A.M.; Weinrib, A.Z.; Katz, J.; Clarke, H. Psychological treatments for the management of postsurgical pain: A systematic review of randomized controlled trials. *Patient Relat. Outcome Meas.* **2018**, *9*, 49–64. [CrossRef] [PubMed]
381. Yu, R.; Zhuo, Y.; Feng, E.; Wang, W.; Lin, W.; Lin, F.; Li, Z.; Lin, L.; Xiao, L.; Wang, H.; et al. The effect of musical interventions in improving short-term pain outcomes following total knee replacement: A meta-analysis and systematic review. *J. Orthop. Surg. Res.* **2020**, *15*, 1–16. [CrossRef] [PubMed]
382. Thybo, K.H.; Hägi-Pedersen, D.; Dahl, J.B.; Wetterslev, J.; Nersesjan, M.; Jakobsen, J.C.; Pedersen, N.A.; Overgaard, S.; Schrøder, H.M.; Schmidt, H.; et al. Effect of Combination of Paracetamol (Acetaminophen) and Ibuprofen vs Either Alone on Patient-Controlled Morphine Consumption in the First 24 Hours After Total Hip Arthroplasty. *JAMA* **2019**, *321*, 562–571. [CrossRef]
383. Derry, C.J.; Derry, S.; Moore, R.A. Single dose oral ibuprofen plus paracetamol (acetaminophen) for acute postoperative pain. *Cochrane Database Syst. Rev.* **2013**, *2013*, CD010210. [CrossRef]
384. Ong, C.K.S.; Seymour, R.A.; Lirk, P.; Merry, A.F. Combining Paracetamol (Acetaminophen) with Nonsteroidal Antiinflammatory Drugs: A Qualitative Systematic Review of Analgesic Efficacy for Acute Postoperative Pain. *Anesth. Analg.* **2010**, *110*, 1170–1179. [CrossRef]
385. Prescott, L.F. Paracetamol: Past, present, and future. *Am. J. Ther.* **2000**, *7*, 143–147. [CrossRef] [PubMed]
386. Langford, R.A.; Hogg, M.; Bjorksten, A.R.; Williams, D.L.; Leslie, K.; Jamsen, K.; Kirkpatrick, C. Comparative Plasma and Cerebrospinal Fluid Pharmacokinetics of Paracetamol After Intravenous and Oral Administration. *Anesth. Analg.* **2016**, *123*, 610–615. [CrossRef] [PubMed]
387. Stundner, O.; Poeran, J.; Ladenhauf, H.N.; Berger, M.M.; Levy, S.B.; Zubizarreta, N.; Mazumdar, M.; Bekeris, J.; Liu, J.; Galatz, L.M.; et al. Effectiveness of intravenous acetaminophen for postoperative pain management in hip and knee arthroplasties: A population-based study. *Reg. Anesth. Pain Med.* **2019**, *44*, 565–572. [CrossRef] [PubMed]
388. Nichols, D.C.; Nadpara, P.A.; Taylor, P.D.; Brophy, G.M. Intravenous Versus Oral Acetaminophen for Pain Control in Neurocritical Care Patients. *Neurocrit. Care* **2016**, *25*, 400–406. [CrossRef]
389. White, P.F. Cost-effective multimodal analgesia in the perioperative period: Use of intravenous vs. oral acetaminophen. *J. Clin. Anesth.* **2020**, *61*, 109625. [CrossRef] [PubMed]
390. Vincent, W.R.; Huiras, P.; Empfield, J.; Horbowicz, K.J.; Lewis, K.; McAneny, D.; Twitchell, D. Controlling postoperative use of i.v. acetaminophen at an academic medical center. *Am. J. Health Pharm.* **2018**, *75*, 548–555. [CrossRef] [PubMed]
391. Johnson, C.Y. The Growing Case Against IV Tylenol, Once Seen as a Solution to the OPIOID crisis. The Washington Post, 19 June 2018. Available online: https://www.washingtonpost.com/news/wonk/wp/2018/06/19/the-growing-case-against-iv-tylenol-once-seen-as-a-solution-to-the-opioid-crisis/ (accessed on 2 January 2021).
392. Foley, M.K.H.; Anderson, J.; Mallea, L.; Morrison, K.; Downey, M. Effects of Healing Touch on Postsurgical Adult Outpatients. *J. Holist. Nurs.* **2016**, *34*, 271–279. [CrossRef] [PubMed]
393. Arias, J.-I.; Aller, M.-A.; Arias, J. Surgical inflammation: A pathophysiological rainbow. *J. Transl. Med.* **2009**, *7*, 19. [CrossRef]
394. Matsuda, M.; Huh, Y.; Ji, R.-R. Roles of inflammation, neurogenic inflammation, and neuroinflammation in pain. *J. Anesth.* **2019**, *33*, 131–139. [CrossRef] [PubMed]
395. Mammoto, T.; Fujie, K.; Taguchi, N.; Ma, E.; Shimizu, T.; Hashimoto, K. Short-Term Effects of Early Postoperative Celecoxib Administration for Pain, Sleep Quality, and Range of Motion After Total Knee Arthroplasty: A Randomized Controlled Trial. *J. Arthroplast.* **2021**, *36*, 526–531. [CrossRef]
396. Oxford League Table of Analgesic Efficacy. Available online: http://www.bandolier.org.uk/booth/painpag/Acutrev/Analgesics/lftab.html (accessed on 28 February 2021).
397. Yurashevich, M.; Pedro, C.; Fuller, M.; Habib, A. Intra-operative ketorolac 15 mg versus 30 mg for analgesia following cesarean delivery: A retrospective study. *Int. J. Obstet. Anesth.* **2020**, *44*, 116–121. [CrossRef] [PubMed]

398. Motov, S.; Masoudi, A.; Drapkin, J.; Sotomayor, C.; Kim, S.; Butt, M.; Likourezos, A.; Fassassi, C.; Hossain, R.; Brady, J.; et al. Randomized Trial Comparing 3 Doses of Oral Ibuprofen for Management of Pain in Adult EM Patients. *J. Emerg. Med.* **2020**, *59*, 759–760. [CrossRef]
399. Motov, S.; Yasavolian, M.; Likourezos, A.; Pushkar, I.; Hossain, R.; Drapkin, J.; Cohen, V.; Filk, N.; Smith, A.; Huang, F.; et al. Comparison of Intravenous Ketorolac at Three Single-Dose Regimens for Treating Acute Pain in the Emergency Department: A Randomized Controlled Trial. *Ann. Emerg. Med.* **2017**, *70*, 177–184. [CrossRef]
400. Zhou, T.J.; Tang, J.; White, P.F. Propacetamol Versus Ketorolac for Treatment of Acute Postoperative Pain After Total Hip or Knee Replacement. *Anesth. Analg.* **2001**, *92*, 1569–1575. [CrossRef]
401. CPIC. Clinical Pharmacogenetics Implementation Consortium Guidelines. 11 August 2020. Available online: https://cpicpgx.org/guidelines/ (accessed on 28 February 2021).
402. Abdallah, F.W.; Hussain, N.; Weaver, T.; Brull, R. Analgesic efficacy of cannabinoids for acute pain management after surgery: A systematic review and meta-analysis. *Reg. Anesth. Pain Med.* **2020**, *45*, 509–519. [CrossRef]
403. McDonagh, M.S.; Selph, S.S.; Buckley, D.I.; Holmes, R.S.; Mauer, K.; Ramirez, S.; Hsu, F.C.; Dana, T.; Fu, R.; Chou, R. Nonopioid Pharmacologic Treatments for Chronic Pain. In *Nonopioid Pharmacologic Treatments for Chronic Pain*; Agency for Healthcare Research and Quality: Rockville, MD, USA, 2020.
404. Mun, C.J.; Letzen, J.E.; Peters, E.N.; Campbell, C.M.; Vandrey, R.; Gajewski-Nemes, J.; DiRenzo, D.; Caufield-Noll, C.; Finan, P.H. Cannabinoid effects on responses to quantitative sensory testing among individuals with and without clinical pain: A systematic review. *Pain* **2020**, *161*, 244–260. [CrossRef]
405. Moore, A.B.; Navarrett, S.; Herzig, S.J. Potentially Inappropriate Use of Intravenous Opioids in Hospitalized Patients. *J. Hosp. Med.* **2019**, *14*, 678–680. [CrossRef]
406. Choi, Y.Y.; Park, J.S.; Park, S.Y.; Kim, H.J.; Yeo, J.; Kim, J.-C.; Park, S.; Choi, G.-S. Can intravenous patient-controlled analgesia be omitted in patients undergoing laparoscopic surgery for colorectal cancer? *Ann. Surg. Treat. Res.* **2015**, *88*, 86–91. [CrossRef]
407. McEvoy, M.D.; Wanderer, J.P.; King, A.B.; Geiger, T.M.; Tiwari, V.; Terekhov, M.; Ehrenfeld, J.M.; Furman, W.R.; Lee, L.A.; Sandberg, W.S. A perioperative consult service results in reduction in cost and length of stay for colorectal surgical patients: Evidence from a healthcare redesign project. *Perioper. Med.* **2016**, *5*, 3. [CrossRef]
408. Institute for Safe Medication Practices (ISMP). Safety Issues with PCA Part I—How Errors Occur. 10 July 2003. Available online: https://www.ismp.org/resources/safety-issues-pca-part-i-how-errors-occur (accessed on 17 January 2021).
409. Institute for Safe Medication Practices (ISMP). Safety Issues with PCA Part II—How to Prevent Errors. 24 July 2003. Available online: https://www.ismp.org/resources/safety-issues-pca-part-ii-how-prevent-errors (accessed on 17 January 2021).
410. Smith, H.S. Opioid Metabolism. *Mayo Clin. Proc.* **2009**, *84*, 613–624. [CrossRef]
411. Coller, J.K.; Christrup, L.L.; Somogyi, A.A. Role of active metabolites in the use of opioids. *Eur. J. Clin. Pharmacol.* **2008**, *65*, 121–139. [CrossRef] [PubMed]
412. Smith, H.S. The Metabolism of Opioid Agents and the Clinical Impact of Their Active Metabolites. *Clin. J. Pain* **2011**, *27*, 824–838. [CrossRef]
413. Overholser, B.R.; Foster, D.R. Opioid pharmacokinetic drug-drug interactions. *Am. J. Manag. Care* **2011**, *17*, 276–287.
414. Crews, K.R.; Monte, A.A.; Huddart, R.; Caudle, K.E.; Kharasch, E.D.; Gaedigk, A.; Dunnenberger, H.M.; Leeder, J.S.; Callaghan, J.T.; Samer, C.F.; et al. Clinical Pharmacogenetics Implementation Consortium Guideline for CYP2D6, OPRM1, and COMT Genotypes and Select Opioid Therapy. *Clin. Pharmacol. Ther.* **2021**. [CrossRef]
415. Davison, S.N. Clinical Pharmacology Considerations in Pain Management in Patients with Advanced Kidney Failure. *Clin. J. Am. Soc. Nephrol.* **2019**, *14*, 917–931. [CrossRef]
416. Crews, K.R.; Gaedigk, A.; Dunnenberger, H.M.; Leeder, J.S.; Klein, T.E.; Caudle, K.E.; Haidar, C.E.; Shen, D.D.; Callaghan, J.T.; Sadhasivam, S.; et al. Clinical Pharmacogenetics Implementation Consortium Guidelines for Cytochrome P450 2D6 Genotype and Codeine Therapy: 2014 Update. *Clin. Pharmacol. Ther.* **2014**, *95*, 376–382. [CrossRef] [PubMed]
417. Miotto, K.; Cho, A.K.; Khalil, M.A.; Blanco, K.; Sasaki, J.D.; Rawson, R. Trends in Tramadol. *Anesth. Analg.* **2017**, *124*, 44–51. [CrossRef] [PubMed]
418. Zhou, Y.; Ingelman-Sundberg, M.; Lauschke, V.M. Worldwide Distribution of Cytochrome P450 Alleles: A Meta-analysis of Population-scale Sequencing Projects. *Clin. Pharmacol. Ther.* **2017**, *102*, 688–700. [CrossRef]
419. Ren, Z.-Y.; Xu, X.-Q.; Bao, Y.-P.; He, J.; Shi, L.; Deng, J.-H.; Gao, X.-J.; Tang, H.-L.; Wang, Y.-M.; Lu, L. The impact of genetic variation on sensitivity to opioid analgesics in patients with postoperative pain: A systematic review and meta-analysis. *Pain Physician* **2015**, *18*, 131–152. [PubMed]
420. Comelon, M.; Raeder, J.; Drægni, T.; Lieng, M.; Lenz, H. Tapentadol versus oxycodone analgesia and side effects after laparoscopic hysterectomy. *Eur. J. Anaesthesiol.* **2021**. [CrossRef]
421. Wang, X.; Narayan, S.W.; Penm, J.; Patanwala, A.E. Efficacy and Safety of Tapentadol Immediate Release for Acute Pain. *Clin. J. Pain* **2020**, *36*, 399–409. [CrossRef]
422. Wei, J.; Lane, N.E.; Bolster, M.B.; Dubreuil, M.; Zeng, C.; Misra, D.; Lu, N.; Choi, H.K.; Lei, G.; Zhang, Y. Association of Tramadol Use With Risk of Hip Fracture. *J. Bone Miner. Res.* **2020**, *35*, 631–640. [CrossRef] [PubMed]
423. Romualdi, P.; Grilli, M.; Canonico, P.L.; Collino, M.; Dickenson, A.H. Pharmacological rationale for tapentadol therapy: A review of new evidence. *J. Pain Res.* **2019**, *12*, 1513–1520. [CrossRef] [PubMed]

424. Zeng, C.; Dubreuil, M.; LaRochelle, M.R.; Lu, N.; Wei, J.; Choi, H.K.; Lei, G.; Zhang, Y. Association of Tramadol with All-Cause Mortality among Patients with Osteoarthritis. *JAMA* **2019**, *321*, 969–982. [CrossRef]
425. Faria, J.; Barbosa, J.; Moreira, R.; Queirós, O.; Carvalho, F.; Dinis-Oliveira, R. Comparative pharmacology and toxicology of tramadol and tapentadol. *Eur. J. Pain* **2018**, *22*, 827–844. [CrossRef] [PubMed]
426. Vadivelu, N.; Chang, D.; Helander, E.M.; Bordelon, G.J.; Kai, A.; Kaye, A.D.; Hsu, D.; Bang, D.; Julka, I. Ketorolac, Oxymorphone, Tapentadol, and Tramadol. *Anesthesiol. Clin.* **2017**, *35*, e1–e20. [CrossRef]
427. Barbosa, J.; Faria, J.; Queirós, O.; Moreira, R.; Carvalho, F.; Dinis-Oliveira, R.J. Comparative metabolism of tramadol and tapentadol: A toxicological perspective. *Drug Metab. Rev.* **2016**, *48*, 577–592. [CrossRef]
428. "Weak" Opioid Analgesics. Codeine, Dihydrocodeine and Tramadol: No Less Risky Than Morphine. *Prescrire Int.* **2016**, *25*, 45–50. Available online: https://www.ncbi.nlm.nih.gov/pubmed/27042732 (accessed on 14 September 2020).
429. Brennan, M.J. The Clinical Implications of Cytochrome P450 Interactions with Opioids and Strategies for Pain Management. *J. Pain Symptom Manag.* **2012**, *44*, S15–S22. [CrossRef]
430. Pergolizzi, J.V. Quantifying the impact of drug-drug interactions associated with opioids. *Am. J. Manag. Care* **2011**, *17*, 288–292.
431. Li, P.H.; Ue, K.L.; Wagner, A.; Rutkowski, R; Rutkowski, K. Opioid Hypersensitivity: Predictors of Allergy and Role of Drug Provocation Testing. *J. Allergy Clin. Immunol. Pract.* **2017**, *5*, 1601–1606. [CrossRef] [PubMed]
432. Kalangara, J.; Vanijcharoenkarn, K.; Lynde, G.C.; McIntosh, N.; Kuruvilla, M. Approach to Perioperative Anaphylaxis in 2020: Updates in Diagnosis and Management. *Curr. Allergy Asthma Rep.* **2021**, *21*, 1–10. [CrossRef]
433. Baldo, B.A.; Pham, N.H. Histamine-Releasing and Allergenic Properties of Opioid Analgesic Drugs: Resolving the Two. *Anaesth. Intensiv. Care* **2012**, *40*, 216–235. [CrossRef] [PubMed]
434. Powell, M.Z.; Mueller, S.W.; Reynolds, P.M. Assessment of Opioid Cross-reactivity and Provider Perceptions in Hospitalized Patients with Reported Opioid Allergies. *Ann. Pharmacother.* **2019**, *53*, 1117–1123. [CrossRef]
435. Swarm, R.A.; Paice, J.A.; Anghelescu, D.L.; Are, M.; Bruce, J.Y.; Buga, S.; Chwistek, M.; Cleeland, C.; Craig, D.; Gafford, E.; et al. Adult Cancer Pain, Version 3.2019, NCCN Clinical Practice Guidelines in Oncology. *J. Natl. Compr. Cancer Netw.* **2019**, *17*, 977–1007. [CrossRef]
436. Said, E.T.; Drueding, R.E.; Martin, E.I.; Furnish, T.J.; Meineke, M.N.; Sztain, J.F.; Abramson, W.B.; Swisher, M.W.; Jacobsen, G.R.; Gosman, A.A.; et al. The Implementation of an Acute Pain Service for Patients Undergoing Open Ventral Hernia Repair with Mesh and Abdominal Wall Reconstruction. *World J. Surg.* **2021**, *45*, 1102–1108. [CrossRef]
437. Bui, B.T.; Grygiel, M.R.; Konstantatos, M.B.A.; Christelis, N.; Liew, M.B.S.; Hopkins, B.R.; Dooley, B.M. The impact of an innovative pharmacist-led inpatient opioid de-escalation intervention in post-operative orthopedic patients. *J. Opioid Manag.* **2020**, *16*, 167–176. [CrossRef]
438. Lovasi, O.; Lám, J.; Kósik, N. Az akutfájdalom-kezelő szolgálat szerepe a műtét utáni fájdalomcsillapításban. *Orvosi Hetil.* **2020**, *161*, 575–581. [CrossRef]
439. Mitra, S.; Jain, K.; Singh, J.; Jindal, S.; Saxena, P.; Singh, M.; Saroa, R.; Ahuja, V.; Kang, J.; Garg, S. Does an acute pain service improve the perception of postoperative pain management in patients undergoing lower limb surgery? A prospective controlled non-randomized study. *J. Anaesthesiol. Clin. Pharmacol.* **2020**, *36*, 187–194. [CrossRef]
440. Said, E.T.; Sztain, J.F.; Abramson, W.B.; Meineke, M.N.; Furnish, T.J.; Schmidt, U.H.; Manecke, G.R.; Gabriel, R.A. A Dedicated Acute Pain Service Is Associated with Reduced Postoperative Opioid Requirements in Patients Undergoing Cytoreductive Surgery With Hyperthermic Intraperitoneal Chemotherapy. *Anesth. Analg.* **2018**, *127*, 1044–1050. [CrossRef]
441. Zaccagnino, M.P.; Bader, A.M.; Sang, C.N.; Correll, D.J. The Perioperative Surgical Home. *Anesth. Analg.* **2017**, *125*, 1394–1402. [CrossRef] [PubMed]
442. Hall, K.R.; Stanley, A.Y. Literature Review: Assessment of Opioid-related Sedation and the Pasero Opioid Sedation Scale. *J. PeriAnesth. Nurs.* **2019**, *34*, 132–142. [CrossRef] [PubMed]
443. Jungquist, C.R.; Quinlan-Colwell, A.; Vallerand, A.; Carlisle, H.L.; Cooney, M.; Dempsey, S.J.; Dunwoody, D.; Maly, A.; Meloche, K.; Meyers, A.; et al. American Society for Pain Management Nursing Guidelines on Monitoring for Opioid-Induced Advancing Sedation and Respiratory Depression: Revisions. *Pain Manag. Nurs.* **2020**, *21*, 7–25. [CrossRef] [PubMed]
444. Jungquist, C.R.; Smith, K.; Nicely, K.L.W.; Polomano, R.C. Monitoring Hospitalized Adult Patients for Opioid-Induced Sedation and Respiratory Depression. *AJN Am. J. Nurs.* **2017**, *117*, S27–S35. [CrossRef]
445. Lam, T.; Nagappa, M.; Wong, J.; Singh, M.; Wong, D.; Chung, F. Continuous Pulse Oximetry and Capnography Monitoring for Postoperative Respiratory Depression and Adverse Events. *Anesth. Analg.* **2017**, *125*, 2019–2029. [CrossRef]
446. Steele, T.; Eidem, L.; Bond, J. Impact of Adoption of Smart Pump System with Continuous Capnography Monitoring on Opioid-Related Adverse Event Rates: Experience From a Tertiary Care Hospital. *J. Patient Saf.* **2019**, *16*, e194–e198. [CrossRef]
447. Kim, B.; Nolan, S.; Beaulieu, T.; Shalansky, S.; Ti, L. Inappropriate opioid prescribing practices: A narrative review. *Am. J. Health Pharm.* **2019**, *76*, 1231–1237. [CrossRef] [PubMed]
448. Parhami, I.; Massey, J.; Trimzi, I.; Huckshorn, K.; Gallucci, G. Risks Associated with Co-Prescribing Opioids and Benzodiazepines and Delaware's Prescription Drug Monitoring Program. *Del. Med. J.* **2015**, *87*, 270–274.
449. Weinstein, S.; Poultsides, L.; Baaklini, L.; Mörwald, E.; Cozowicz, C.; Saleh, J.; Arrington, M.; Poeran, J.; Zubizarreta, N.; Memtsoudis, S. Postoperative delirium in total knee and hip arthroplasty patients: A study of perioperative modifiable risk factors. *Br. J. Anaesth.* **2018**, *120*, 999–1008. [CrossRef] [PubMed]

424. Zeng, C.; Dubreuil, M.; LaRochelle, M.R.; Lu, N.; Wei, J.; Choi, H.K.; Lei, G.; Zhang, Y. Association of Tramadol with All-Cause Mortality among Patients with Osteoarthritis. *JAMA* **2019**, *321*, 969–982. [CrossRef]
425. Faria, J.; Barbosa, J.; Moreira, R.; Queirós, O.; Carvalho, F.; Dinis-Oliveira, R. Comparative pharmacology and toxicology of tramadol and tapentadol. *Eur. J. Pain* **2018**, *22*, 827–844. [CrossRef] [PubMed]
426. Vadivelu, N.; Chang, D.; Helander, E.M.; Bordelon, G.J.; Kai, A.; Kaye, A.D.; Hsu, D.; Bang, D.; Julka, I. Ketorolac, Oxymorphone, Tapentadol, and Tramadol. *Anesthesiol. Clin.* **2017**, *35*, e1–e20. [CrossRef]
427. Barbosa, J.; Faria, J.; Queirós, O.; Moreira, R.; Carvalho, F.; Dinis-Oliveira, R.J. Comparative metabolism of tramadol and tapentadol: A toxicological perspective. *Drug Metab. Rev.* **2016**, *48*, 577–592. [CrossRef]
428. "Weak" Opioid Analgesics. Codeine, Dihydrocodeine and Tramadol: No Less Risky Than Morphine. *Prescrire Int.* **2016**, *25*, 45–50. Available online: https://www.ncbi.nlm.nih.gov/pubmed/27042732 (accessed on 14 September 2020).
429. Brennan, M.J. The Clinical Implications of Cytochrome P450 Interactions with Opioids and Strategies for Pain Management. *J. Pain Symptom Manag.* **2012**, *44*, S15–S22. [CrossRef]
430. Pergolizzi, J.V. Quantifying the impact of drug-drug interactions associated with opioids. *Am. J. Manag. Care* **2011**, *17*, 288–292.
431. Li, P.H.; Ue, K.L.; Wagner, A.; Rutkowski, R.; Rutkowski, K. Opioid Hypersensitivity: Predictors of Allergy and Role of Drug Provocation Testing. *J. Allergy Clin. Immunol. Pract.* **2017**, *5*, 1601–1606. [CrossRef] [PubMed]
432. Kalangara, J.; Vanijcharoenkarn, K.; Lynde, G.C.; McIntosh, N.; Kuruvilla, M. Approach to Perioperative Anaphylaxis in 2020: Updates in Diagnosis and Management. *Curr. Allergy Asthma Rep.* **2021**, *21*, 1–10. [CrossRef]
433. Baldo, B.A.; Pham, N.H. Histamine-Releasing and Allergenic Properties of Opioid Analgesic Drugs: Resolving the Two. *Anaesth. Intensiv. Care* **2012**, *40*, 216–235. [CrossRef] [PubMed]
434. Powell, M.Z.; Mueller, S.W.; Reynolds, P.M. Assessment of Opioid Cross-reactivity and Provider Perceptions in Hospitalized Patients with Reported Opioid Allergies. *Ann. Pharmacother.* **2019**, *53*, 1117–1123. [CrossRef]
435. Swarm, R.A.; Paice, J.A.; Anghelescu, D.L.; Are, M.; Bruce, J.Y.; Buga, S.; Chwistek, M.; Cleeland, C.; Craig, D.; Gafford, E.; et al. Adult Cancer Pain, Version 3.2019, NCCN Clinical Practice Guidelines in Oncology. *J. Natl. Compr. Cancer Netw.* **2019**, *17*, 977–1007. [CrossRef]
436. Said, E.T.; Drueding, R.E.; Martin, E.I.; Furnish, T.J.; Meineke, M.N.; Sztain, J.F.; Abramson, W.B.; Swisher, M.W.; Jacobsen, G.R.; Gosman, A.A.; et al. The Implementation of an Acute Pain Service for Patients Undergoing Open Ventral Hernia Repair with Mesh and Abdominal Wall Reconstruction. *World J. Surg.* **2021**, *45*, 1102–1108. [CrossRef]
437. Bui, B.T.; Grygiel, M.R.; Konstantatos, M.B.A.; Christelis, N.; Liew, M.B.S.; Hopkins, B.R.; Dooley, B.M. The impact of an innovative pharmacist-led inpatient opioid de-escalation intervention in post-operative orthopedic patients. *J. Opioid Manag.* **2020**, *16*, 167–176. [CrossRef]
438. Lovasi, O.; Lám, J.; Kósik, N. Az akutfájdalom-kezelő szolgálat szerepe a műtét utáni fájdalomcsillapításban. *Orvosi Hetil.* **2020**, *161*, 575–581. [CrossRef]
439. Mitra, S.; Jain, K.; Singh, J.; Jindal, S.; Saxena, P.; Singh, M.; Saroa, R.; Ahuja, V.; Kang, J.; Garg, S. Does an acute pain service improve the perception of postoperative pain management in patients undergoing lower limb surgery? A prospective controlled non-randomized study. *J. Anaesthesiol. Clin. Pharmacol.* **2020**, *36*, 187–194. [CrossRef]
440. Said, E.T.; Sztain, J.F.; Abramson, W.B.; Meineke, M.N.; Furnish, T.J.; Schmidt, U.H.; Manecke, G.R.; Gabriel, R.A. A Dedicated Acute Pain Service Is Associated with Reduced Postoperative Opioid Requirements in Patients Undergoing Cytoreductive Surgery With Hyperthermic Intraperitoneal Chemotherapy. *Anesth. Analg.* **2018**, *127*, 1044–1050. [CrossRef]
441. Zaccagnino, M.P.; Bader, A.M.; Sang, C.N.; Correll, D.J. The Perioperative Surgical Home. *Anesth. Analg.* **2017**, *125*, 1394–1402. [CrossRef] [PubMed]
442. Hall, K.R.; Stanley, A.Y. Literature Review: Assessment of Opioid-related Sedation and the Pasero Opioid Sedation Scale. *J. PeriAnesth. Nurs.* **2019**, *34*, 132–142. [CrossRef] [PubMed]
443. Jungquist, C.R.; Quinlan-Colwell, A.; Vallerand, A.; Carlisle, H.L.; Cooney, M.; Dempsey, S.J.; Dunwoody, D.; Maly, A.; Meloche, K.; Meyers, A.; et al. American Society for Pain Management Nursing Guidelines on Monitoring for Opioid-Induced Advancing Sedation and Respiratory Depression: Revisions. *Pain Manag. Nurs.* **2020**, *21*, 7–25. [CrossRef] [PubMed]
444. Jungquist, C.R.; Smith, K.; Nicely, K.L.W.; Polomano, R.C. Monitoring Hospitalized Adult Patients for Opioid-Induced Sedation and Respiratory Depression. *AJN Am. J. Nurs.* **2017**, *117*, S27–S35. [CrossRef]
445. Lam, T.; Nagappa, M.; Wong, J.; Singh, M.; Wong, D.; Chung, F. Continuous Pulse Oximetry and Capnography Monitoring for Postoperative Respiratory Depression and Adverse Events. *Anesth. Analg.* **2017**, *125*, 2019–2029. [CrossRef]
446. Steele, T.; Eidem, L.; Bond, J. Impact of Adoption of Smart Pump System with Continuous Capnography Monitoring on Opioid-Related Adverse Event Rates: Experience From a Tertiary Care Hospital. *J. Patient Saf.* **2019**, *16*, e194–e198. [CrossRef]
447. Kim, B.; Nolan, S.; Beaulieu, T.; Shalansky, S.; Ti, L. Inappropriate opioid prescribing practices: A narrative review. *Am. J. Health Pharm.* **2019**, *76*, 1231–1237. [CrossRef] [PubMed]
448. Parhami, I.; Massey, J.; Trimzi, I.; Huckshorn, K.; Gallucci, G. Risks Associated with Co-Prescribing Opioids and Benzodiazepines and Delaware's Prescription Drug Monitoring Program. *Del. Med. J.* **2015**, *87*, 270–274.
449. Weinstein, S.; Poultsides, L.; Baaklini, L.; Mörwald, E.; Cozowicz, C.; Saleh, J.; Arrington, M.; Poeran, J.; Zubizarreta, N.; Memtsoudis, S. Postoperative delirium in total knee and hip arthroplasty patients: A study of perioperative modifiable risk factors. *Br. J. Anaesth.* **2018**, *120*, 999–1008. [CrossRef] [PubMed]

398. Motov, S.; Masoudi, A.; Drapkin, J.; Sotomayor, C.; Kim, S.; Butt, M.; Likourezos, A.; Fassassi, C.; Hossain, R.; Brady, J.; et al. Randomized Trial Comparing 3 Doses of Oral Ibuprofen for Management of Pain in Adult EM Patients. *J. Emerg. Med.* **2020**, *59*, 759–760. [CrossRef]
399. Motov, S.; Yasavolian, M.; Likourezos, A.; Pushkar, I.; Hossain, R.; Drapkin, J.; Cohen, V.; Filk, N.; Smith, A.; Huang, F.; et al. Comparison of Intravenous Ketorolac at Three Single-Dose Regimens for Treating Acute Pain in the Emergency Department: A Randomized Controlled Trial. *Ann. Emerg. Med.* **2017**, *70*, 177–184. [CrossRef]
400. Zhou, T.J.; Tang, J.; White, P.F. Propacetamol Versus Ketorolac for Treatment of Acute Postoperative Pain After Total Hip or Knee Replacement. *Anesth. Analg.* **2001**, *92*, 1569–1575. [CrossRef]
401. CPIC. Clinical Pharmacogenetics Implementation Consortium Guidelines. 11 August 2020. Available online: https://cpicpgx.org/guidelines/ (accessed on 28 February 2021).
402. Abdallah, F.W.; Hussain, N.; Weaver, T.; Brull, R. Analgesic efficacy of cannabinoids for acute pain management after surgery: A systematic review and meta-analysis. *Reg. Anesth. Pain Med.* **2020**, *45*, 509–519. [CrossRef]
403. McDonagh, M.S.; Selph, S.S.; Buckley, D.I.; Holmes, R.S.; Mauer, K.; Ramirez, S.; Hsu, F.C.; Dana, T.; Fu, R.; Chou, R. Nonopioid Pharmacologic Treatments for Chronic Pain. In *Nonopioid Pharmacologic Treatments for Chronic Pain*; Agency for Healthcare Research and Quality: Rockville, MD, USA, 2020.
404. Mun, C.J.; Letzen, J.E.; Peters, E.N.; Campbell, C.M.; Vandrey, R.; Gajewski-Nemes, J.; DiRenzo, D.; Caufield-Noll, C.; Finan, P.H. Cannabinoid effects on responses to quantitative sensory testing among individuals with and without clinical pain: A systematic review. *Pain* **2020**, *161*, 244–260. [CrossRef]
405. Moore, A.B.; Navarrett, S.; Herzig, S.J. Potentially Inappropriate Use of Intravenous Opioids in Hospitalized Patients. *J. Hosp. Med.* **2019**, *14*, 678–680. [CrossRef]
406. Choi, Y.Y.; Park, J.S.; Park, S.Y.; Kim, H.J.; Yeo, J.; Kim, J.-C.; Park, S.; Choi, G.-S. Can intravenous patient-controlled analgesia be omitted in patients undergoing laparoscopic surgery for colorectal cancer? *Ann. Surg. Treat. Res.* **2015**, *88*, 86–91. [CrossRef]
407. McEvoy, M.D.; Wanderer, J.P.; King, A.B.; Geiger, T.M.; Tiwari, V.; Terekhov, M.; Ehrenfeld, J.M.; Furman, W.R.; Lee, L.A.; Sandberg, W.S. A perioperative consult service results in reduction in cost and length of stay for colorectal surgical patients: Evidence from a healthcare redesign project. *Perioper. Med.* **2016**, *5*, 3. [CrossRef]
408. Institute for Safe Medication Practices (ISMP). Safety Issues with PCA Part I—How Errors Occur. 10 July 2003. Available online: https://www.ismp.org/resources/safety-issues-pca-part-i-how-errors-occur (accessed on 17 January 2021).
409. Institute for Safe Medication Practices (ISMP). Safety Issues with PCA Part II—How to Prevent Errors. 24 July 2003. Available online: https://www.ismp.org/resources/safety-issues-pca-part-ii-how-prevent-errors (accessed on 17 January 2021).
410. Smith, H.S. Opioid Metabolism. *Mayo Clin. Proc.* **2009**, *84*, 613–624. [CrossRef]
411. Coller, J.K.; Christrup, L.L.; Somogyi, A.A. Role of active metabolites in the use of opioids. *Eur. J. Clin. Pharmacol.* **2008**, *65*, 121–139. [CrossRef] [PubMed]
412. Smith, H.S. The Metabolism of Opioid Agents and the Clinical Impact of Their Active Metabolites. *Clin. J. Pain* **2011**, *27*, 824–838. [CrossRef]
413. Overholser, B.R.; Foster, D.R. Opioid pharmacokinetic drug-drug interactions. *Am. J. Manag. Care* **2011**, *17*, 276–287.
414. Crews, K.R.; Monte, A.A.; Huddart, R.; Caudle, K.E.; Kharasch, E.D.; Gaedigk, A.; Dunnenberger, H.M.; Leeder, J.S.; Callaghan, J.T.; Samer, C.F.; et al. Clinical Pharmacogenetics Implementation Consortium Guideline for CYP2D6, OPRM1, and COMT Genotypes and Select Opioid Therapy. *Clin. Pharmacol. Ther.* **2021**. [CrossRef]
415. Davison, S.N. Clinical Pharmacology Considerations in Pain Management in Patients with Advanced Kidney Failure. *Clin. J. Am. Soc. Nephrol.* **2019**, *14*, 917–931. [CrossRef]
416. Crews, K.R.; Gaedigk, A.; Dunnenberger, H.M.; Leeder, J.S.; Klein, T.E.; Caudle, K.E.; Haidar, C.E.; Shen, D.D.; Callaghan, J.T.; Sadhasivam, S.; et al. Clinical Pharmacogenetics Implementation Consortium Guidelines for Cytochrome P450 2D6 Genotype and Codeine Therapy: 2014 Update. *Clin. Pharmacol. Ther.* **2014**, *95*, 376–382. [CrossRef] [PubMed]
417. Miotto, K.; Cho, A.K.; Khalil, M.A.; Blanco, K.; Sasaki, J.D.; Rawson, R. Trends in Tramadol. *Anesth. Analg.* **2017**, *124*, 44–51. [CrossRef] [PubMed]
418. Zhou, Y.; Ingelman-Sundberg, M.; Lauschke, V.M. Worldwide Distribution of Cytochrome P450 Alleles: A Meta-analysis of Population-scale Sequencing Projects. *Clin. Pharmacol. Ther.* **2017**, *102*, 688–700. [CrossRef]
419. Ren, Z.-Y.; Xu, X.-Q.; Bao, Y.-P.; He, J.; Shi, L.; Deng, J.-H.; Gao, X.-J.; Tang, H.-L.; Wang, Y.-M.; Lu, L. The impact of genetic variation on sensitivity to opioid analgesics in patients with postoperative pain: A systematic review and meta-analysis. *Pain Physician* **2015**, *18*, 131–152. [PubMed]
420. Comelon, M.; Raeder, J.; Drægni, T.; Lieng, M.; Lenz, H. Tapentadol versus oxycodone analgesia and side effects after laparoscopic hysterectomy. *Eur. J. Anaesthesiol.* **2021**. [CrossRef]
421. Wang, X.; Narayan, S.W.; Penm, J.; Patanwala, A.E. Efficacy and Safety of Tapentadol Immediate Release for Acute Pain. *Clin. J. Pain* **2020**, *36*, 399–409. [CrossRef]
422. Wei, J.; Lane, N.E.; Bolster, M.B.; Dubreuil, M.; Zeng, C.; Misra, D.; Lu, N.; Choi, H.K.; Lei, G.; Zhang, Y. Association of Tramadol Use With Risk of Hip Fracture. *J. Bone Miner. Res.* **2020**, *35*, 631–640. [CrossRef] [PubMed]
423. Romualdi, P.; Grilli, M.; Canonico, P.L.; Collino, M.; Dickenson, A.H. Pharmacological rationale for tapentadol therapy: A review of new evidence. *J. Pain Res.* **2019**, *12*, 1513–1520. [CrossRef] [PubMed]

450. Rade, M.C.; YaDeau, J.T.; Ford, C.; Reid, M.C. Postoperative Delirium in Elderly Patients After Elective Hip or Knee Arthroplasty Performed Under Regional Anesthesia. *HSS J.* **2011**, *7*, 151–156. [CrossRef] [PubMed]
451. Rizk, P.; Morris, W.; Oladeji, P.; Huo, M. Review of Postoperative Delirium in Geriatric Patients Undergoing Hip Surgery. *Geriatr. Orthop. Surg. Rehabil.* **2016**, *7*, 100–105. [CrossRef]
452. Rogers, E.; Mehta, S.; Shengelia, R.; Reid, M.C. Four Strategies for Managing Opioid-Induced Side Effects in Older Adults. *Clin. Geriatr.* **2013**, *21*.
453. American Society of Anesthesiologists Task Force on Neuraxial Opioids. Practice Guidelines for the Prevention, Detection, and Management of Respiratory Depression Associated with Neuraxial Opioid Administration. *Anesthesiology* **2016**, *124*, 535–552. [CrossRef] [PubMed]
454. Müller-Lissner, S.; Bassotti, G.; Coffin, B.; Drewes, A.M.; Breivik, H.; Eisenberg, E.; Emmanuel, A.; Laroche, F.; Meissner, W.; Morlion, B. Opioid-Induced Constipation and Bowel Dysfunction: A Clinical Guideline. *Pain Med.* **2016**, *18*, 1837–1863. [CrossRef]
455. Drewes, A.M.; Munkholm, P.; Simrén, M.; Breivik, H.; Kongsgaard, U.E.; Hatlebakk, J.G.; Agreus, L.; Friedrichsen, M.; Christrup, L.L. Definition, diagnosis and treatment strategies for opioid-induced bowel dysfunction–Recommendations of the Nordic Working Group. *Scand. J. Pain* **2016**, *11*, 111–122. [CrossRef]
456. Alvaro, D.; Caraceni, A.T.; Coluzzi, F.; Gianni, W.; Lugoboni, F.; Marinangeli, F.; Massazza, G.; Pinto, C.; Varrassi, G. What to Do and What Not to Do in the Management of Opioid-Induced Constipation: A Choosing Wisely Report. *Pain Ther.* **2020**, *9*, 657–667. [CrossRef]
457. Yue, C.; Liu, Y.; Zhang, X.; Xu, B.; Sheng, H. Randomised controlled trial of a comprehensive protocol for preventing constipation following total hip arthroplasty. *J. Clin. Nurs.* **2020**, *29*, 2863–2871. [CrossRef]
458. Woelk, C.J. The hand that writes the opioid. *Can. Fam. Physician Med. Fam. Can.* **2007**, *53*, 1015–1017.
459. Schwenk, E.S.; Grant, A.E.; Torjman, M.C.; McNulty, S.E.; Baratta, J.L.; Viscusi, E.R. The Efficacy of Peripheral Opioid Antagonists in Opioid-Induced Constipation and Postoperative Ileus. *Reg. Anesth. Pain Med.* **2017**, *42*, 767–777. [CrossRef] [PubMed]
460. Nishie, K.; Yamamoto, S.; Yamaga, T.; Horigome, N.; Hanaoka, M. Peripherally acting μ-opioid antagonist for the treatment of opioid-induced constipation: Systematic review and meta-analysis. *J. Gastroenterol. Hepatol.* **2018**, *34*, 818–829. [CrossRef] [PubMed]
461. Nemeth, Z.H.; Bogdanovski, D.A.; Paglinco, S.R.; Barratt-Stopper, P.; Rolandelli, R.H. Cost and efficacy examination of alvimopan for the prevention of postoperative ileus. *J. Investig. Med.* **2017**, *65*, 949–952. [CrossRef]
462. Kelley, S.R.; Wolff, B.G.; Lovely, J.K.; Larson, D.W. Fast-track pathway for minimally invasive colorectal surgery with and without alvimopan (Entereg)TM: Which is more cost-effective? *Am. Surg.* **2013**, *79*, 630–633. Available online: https://www.ncbi.nlm.nih.gov/pubmed/23711275 (accessed on 14 September 2020). [CrossRef] [PubMed]
463. Goodstein, T.; Launer, B.; White, S.; Lyon, M.; George, N.; Deronde, K.; Burke, M.; O'Donnell, C.; Lyda, C.; Kiser, T.H.; et al. A Retrospective Study of Patients Undergoing Radical Cystectomy and Receiving Peri-Operative Naloxegol or Alvimopan: Comparison of Length of Stay. *J. Surg.* **2018**, *6*, 129–134. [CrossRef]
464. Marciniak, C.M.; Toledo, S.; Lee, J.; Jesselson, M.; Bateman, J.; Grover, B.; Tierny, J. Lubiprostonevs Sennain postoperative orthopedic surgery patients with opioid-induced constipation: A double-blind, active-comparator trial. *World J. Gastroenterol.* **2014**, *20*, 16323–16333. [CrossRef] [PubMed]
465. De Boer, H.D.; Detriche, O.; Forget, P. Opioid-related side effects: Postoperative ileus, urinary retention, nausea and vomiting, and shivering. A review of the literature. *Best Pract. Res. Clin. Anaesthesiol.* **2017**, *31*, 499–504. [CrossRef] [PubMed]
466. Tubog, T.D.; Harenberg, J.L.; Buszta, K.; Hestand, J.D. Prophylactic Nalbuphine to Prevent Neuraxial Opioid-Induced Pruritus: A Systematic Review and Meta-Analysis of Randomized Controlled Trials. *J. PeriAnesth. Nurs.* **2019**, *34*, 491–501.e8. [CrossRef] [PubMed]
467. Jannuzzi, R.G. Nalbuphine for Treatment of Opioid-induced Pruritus. *Clin. J. Pain* **2016**, *32*, 87–93. [CrossRef] [PubMed]
468. McNicol, E.D.; Ferguson, M.C.; Hudcova, J. Patient controlled opioid analgesia versus non-patient controlled opioid analgesia for postoperative pain. *Cochrane Database Syst. Rev.* **2015**, *2015*, CD003348. [CrossRef]
469. Mancini, R.; Filicetti, M. Pain management of opioid-tolerant patients undergoing surgery. *Am. J. Health Pharm.* **2010**, *67*, 872–875. [CrossRef]
470. Oliver, J.; Coggins, C.; Compton, P.; Hagan, S.; Matteliano, D.; Stanton, M.; Marie, B.S.; Strobbe, S.; Turner, H.N. American Society for Pain Management Nursing Position Statement: Pain Management in Patients with Substance Use Disorders. *Pain Manag. Nurs.* **2012**, *13*, 169–183. [CrossRef]
471. Li, W.T.; Bell, K.L.; Yayac, M.; Barmann, J.A.; Star, A.M.; Austin, M.S. A Postdischarge Multimodal Pain Management Cocktail Following Total Knee Arthroplasty Reduces Opioid Consumption in the 30-Day Postoperative Period: A Group-Randomized Trial. *J. Arthroplast.* **2021**, *36*, 164–172.e2. [CrossRef]
472. MacPherson, R.; Pattullo, G. Management of postsurgical pain in the community. *Aust. Prescr.* **2020**, *43*, 191–194. [CrossRef]
473. Hill, M.V.; McMahon, M.L.; Stucke, R.S.; Barth, R.J. Wide Variation and Excessive Dosage of Opioid Prescriptions for Common General Surgical Procedures. *Ann. Surg.* **2017**, *265*, 709–714. [CrossRef] [PubMed]
474. Vu, J.V.; Howard, R.A.; Gunaseelan, V.; Brummett, C.M.; Waljee, J.F.; Englesbe, M.J. Statewide Implementation of Postoperative Opioid Prescribing Guidelines. *N. Engl. J. Med.* **2019**, *381*, 680–682. [CrossRef] [PubMed]
475. Hill, M.V.; Stucke, R.S.; Billmeier, S.E.; Kelly, J.L.; Barth, R.J. Guideline for Discharge Opioid Prescriptions after Inpatient General Surgical Procedures. *J. Am. Coll. Surg.* **2018**, *226*, 996–1003. [CrossRef] [PubMed]

476. Thiels, C.A.; Ubl, D.S.; Yost, K.J.; Dowdy, S.C.; Mabry, T.M.; Gazelka, H.M.; Cima, R.R.; Habermann, E.B. Results of a Prospective, Multicenter Initiative Aimed at Developing Opioid-prescribing Guidelines after Surgery. *Ann. Surg.* **2018**, *268*, 457–468. [CrossRef]
477. Kelley-Quon, L.I.; Kirkpatrick, M.G.; Ricca, R.L.; Baird, R.; Harbaugh, C.M.; Brady, A.; Garrett, P.; Wills, H.; Argo, J.; Diefenbach, K.A.; et al. Guidelines for Opioid Prescribing in Children and Adolescents After Surgery. *JAMA Surg.* **2021**, *156*, 76. [CrossRef]
478. Genord, C.; Frost, T.; Eid, D. Opioid exit plan: A pharmacist's role in managing acute postoperative pain. *J. Am. Pharm. Assoc.* **2017**, *57*, S92–S98. [CrossRef]
479. Brandal, D.; Keller, M.S.; Lee, C.; Grogan, T.; Fujimoto, Y.; Gricourt, Y.; Yamada, T.; Rahman, S.; Hofer, I.; Kazanjian, K.; et al. Impact of Enhanced Recovery After Surgery and Opioid-Free Anesthesia on Opioid Prescriptions at Discharge From the Hospital. *Anesth. Analg.* **2017**, *125*, 1784–1792. [CrossRef] [PubMed]
480. Loomis, E.; McNaughton, D.B.; Genord, C.K. A Quality Improvement Initiative Addressing Safe Opioid Prescribing and Disposal Post-Cesarean Delivery. *Pain Manag. Nurs.* in press.
481. Kumar, K.; Gulotta, L.V.; Dines, J.S.; Allen, A.A.; Cheng, J.; Fields, K.G.; YaDeau, J.T.; Wu, C.L. Unused Opioid Pills after Outpatient Shoulder Surgeries Given Current Perioperative Prescribing Habits. *Am. J. Sports Med.* **2017**, *45*, 636–641. [CrossRef] [PubMed]
482. Chalmers, B.P.; Mayman, D.J.; Jerabek, S.A.; Sculco, P.K.; Haas, S.B.; Ast, M.P. Reduction of Opioids Prescribed Upon Discharge After Total Knee Arthroplasty Significantly Reduces Consumption: A Prospective Study Comparing Two States. *J. Arthroplast.* **2021**, *36*, 160–163. [CrossRef] [PubMed]
483. Wyles, C.C.; Hevesi, M.; Ubl, D.S.; Habermann, E.B.; Gazelka, H.M.; Trousdale, R.T.; Turner, N.S.; Pagnano, M.W.; Mabry, T.M. Implementation of Procedure-Specific Opioid Guidelines. *JBJS Open Access* **2020**, *5*, e0050. [CrossRef] [PubMed]
484. Pena, J.J.; Chen, C.J.; Clifford, H.; Xue, Z.; Wang, S.; Argenziano, M.; Landau, R.; Meng, M.-L. Introduction of an Analgesia Prescription Guideline Can Reduce Unused Opioids After Cardiac Surgery: A Before and After Cohort Study. *J. Cardiothorac. Vasc. Anesth.* **2020**. [CrossRef] [PubMed]
485. Solouki, S.; Vega, M.; Agalliu, I.; Abraham, N.E. Patient Satisfaction and Refill Rates after Decreasing Opioids Prescribed for Urogynecologic Surgery. *Female Pelvic Med. Reconstr. Surg.* **2020**, *26*, e78–e82. [CrossRef]
486. Fleischman, A.N.; Tarabichi, M.; Foltz, C.; Makar, G.; Hozack, W.J.; Austin, M.S.; Chen, A.F.; Star, A.M.; Greenky, M.; Henstenburg, B.; et al. Cluster-Randomized Trial of Opiate-Sparing Analgesia after Discharge from Elective Hip Surgery. *J. Am. Coll. Surg.* **2019**, *229*, 335–345.e5. [CrossRef]
487. Hartford, L.B.; Van Koughnett, J.A.M.; Murphy, P.B.; Knowles, S.A.; Wigen, R.B.; Allen, L.J.; Clarke, C.F.M.; Brackstone, M.; Gray, D.K.; Maciver, A.H. The Standardization of Outpatient Procedure (STOP) Narcotics: A Prospective Health Systems Intervention to Reduce Opioid Use in Ambulatory Breast Surgery. *Ann. Surg. Oncol.* **2019**, *26*, 3295–3304. [CrossRef]
488. Holte, A.J.; Carender, C.N.; Noiseux, N.O.; Otero, J.E.; Brown, T.S. Restrictive Opioid Prescribing Protocols Following Total Hip Arthroplasty and Total Knee Arthroplasty Are Safe and Effective. *J. Arthroplast.* **2019**, *34*, S135–S139. [CrossRef] [PubMed]
489. Choo, K.J.; Grace, T.R.; Khanna, K.; Barry, J.; Hansen, E.N. A Goal-directed Quality Improvement Initiative to Reduce Opioid Prescriptions After Orthopaedic Procedures. *JAAOS Glob. Res. Rev.* **2019**, *3*, e109. [CrossRef] [PubMed]
490. Wyles, C.C.; Hevesi, M.; Trousdale, E.R.; Ubl, D.S.; Gazelka, H.M.; Habermann, E.B.; Trousdale, R.T.; Pagnano, M.W.; Mabry, T.M. The 2018 Chitranjan S. Ranawat, MD Award: Developing and Implementing a Novel Institutional Guideline Strategy Reduced Postoperative Opioid Prescribing After TKA and THA. *Clin. Orthop. Relat. Res.* **2019**, *477*, 104–113. [CrossRef] [PubMed]
491. Mortensen, N.J.; Ashraf, S. Intestinal Anastomosis (Chapter 29). 2008. Available online: http://www.acssurgery.com/acs/Chapters/CH0529.htm (accessed on 13 December 2020).
492. Lawrence, A.E.; Carsel, A.J.; Leonhart, K.L.; Richards, H.W.; Harbaugh, C.M.; Waljee, J.F.; McLeod, D.J.; Walz, P.C.; Minneci, P.C.; Deans, K.J.; et al. Effect of Drug Disposal Bag Provision on Proper Disposal of Unused Opioids by Families of Pediatric Surgical Patients. *JAMA Pediatr.* **2019**, *173*, e191695. [CrossRef]
493. Hite, M.; Dippre, A.; Heldreth, A.; Cole, D.; Lockett, M.; Klauber-Demore, N.; Abbott, A.M. A Multifaceted Approach to Opioid Education, Prescribing, and Disposal for Patients with Breast Cancer Undergoing Surgery. *J. Surg. Res.* **2021**, *257*, 597–604. [CrossRef] [PubMed]
494. Ramel, C.L.; Habermann, E.B.; Thiels, C.A.; Dierkhising, R.A.; Cunningham, J.L. Provision of a Drug Deactivation System for Unused Opioid Disposal at Surgical Dismissal. *Mayo Clin. Proc. Innov. Qual. Outcomes* **2020**, *4*, 357–361. [CrossRef]
495. US Food and Drug Administration. Where and How to Dispose of Unused Medicines. 10 September 2020. Available online: https://www.fda.gov/consumers/consumer-updates/where-and-how-dispose-unused-medicines (accessed on 8 January 2021).
496. US Environmental Protection Agency. How to Dispose of Medicines Properly. In *April 2011.*. Available online: https://archive.epa.gov/region02/capp/web/pdf/ppcpflyer.pdf (accessed on 8 January 2021).
497. Wilson, N.; Kariisa, M.; Seth, P.; Smith, H.; Davis, N.L. Drug and Opioid-Involved Overdose Deaths—United States, 2017–2018. *MMWR. Morb. Mortal. Wkly. Rep.* **2020**, *69*, 290–297. [CrossRef]
498. Mudumbai, S.C.; Lewis, E.T.; Oliva, E.M.; Chung, P.D.; Harris, B.; Trafton, J.; Mariano, E.R.; Wagner, T.; Clark, J.D.; Stafford, R.S. Overdose Risk Associated with Opioid Use upon Hospital Discharge in Veterans Health Administration Surgical Patients. *Pain Med.* **2018**, *20*, 1020–1031. [CrossRef]
499. Han, J.K.; Hill, L.G.; Koenig, M.E.; Das, N. Naloxone Counseling for Harm Reduction and Patient Engagement. *Fam. Med.* **2017**, *49*, 730–733.

500. Punzal, M.; Santos, P.; Li, X.; Oyler, D.R.; Hall, A.M. Current practices in naloxone prescribing upon hospital discharge. *J. Opioid Manag.* **2019**, *15*, 357–361. [CrossRef]
501. Shah, A.; Hayes, C.J.; Martin, B.C. Characteristics of Initial Prescription Episodes and Likelihood of Long-Term Opioid Use—United States, 2006–2015. *MMWR. Morb. Mortal. Wkly. Rep.* **2017**, *66*, 265–269. [CrossRef]
502. Stapler, S.J.; Brockhaus, K.K.; Battaglia, M.A.; Mahoney, S.T.; McClure, A.M.; Cleary, R.K. A single institution analysis of targeted colorectal surgery enhanced recovery pathway strategies that decrease readmissions. *Dis. Colon Rectum.* in press.
503. L'Hermite, J.; Pagé, M.G.; Chevallier, T.; Occean, B.; Viel, E.; Bredeau, O.; Lefrant, J.-Y.; Cuvillon, P. Characterisation of pragmatic postoperative PAin trajectories over seven days and their association with CHronicity after 3 months: A prospective, pilot cohort study (PATCH study). *Anaesth. Crit. Care Pain Med.* **2020**, *40*, 100793. [CrossRef]
504. Ellis, J.L.; Ghiraldi, E.M.; Cohn, J.A.; Nitti, M.; Friedlander, J.I.; Ginzburg, S.; Sterious, S.N.; Abbosh, P.; Ohmann, E.; Uzzo, R.G.; et al. Prescribing Trends in Post-operative Pain Management After Urologic Surgery: A Quality Care Investigation for Healthcare Providers. *Urology* **2021**. [CrossRef] [PubMed]
505. Phillips, D.M. JCAHO Pain Management Standards Are Unveiled. *JAMA* **2000**, *284*, 428–429. [CrossRef]
506. Porter, J.; Jick, H. Addiction Rare in Patients Treated with Narcotics. *N. Engl. J. Med.* **1980**, *302*, 123. [CrossRef] [PubMed]
507. Society, A.P. Principles of analgesic use in the treatment of acute pain and cancer pain. *Am. Pain Soc.* **1999**, *9*, 601–612.
508. Scher, C.; Meador, L.; Van Cleave, J.H.; Reid, M.C. Moving Beyond Pain as the Fifth Vital Sign and Patient Satisfaction Scores to Improve Pain Care in the 21st Century. *Pain Manag. Nurs.* **2018**, *19*, 125–129. [CrossRef] [PubMed]
509. Lucas, C.E.; Vlahos, A.L.; Ledgerwood, A.M. Kindness Kills: The Negative Impact of Pain as the Fifth Vital Sign. *J. Am. Coll. Surg.* **2007**, *205*, 101–107. [CrossRef]
510. Chee, T.T.; Ryan, A.M.; Wasfy, J.H.; Borden, W.B. Current State of Value-Based Purchasing Programs. *Circulation* **2016**, *133*, 2197–2205. [CrossRef] [PubMed]
511. Adams, J.; Bledsoe, G.H.; Armstrong, J.H. Are Pain Management Questions in Patient Satisfaction Surveys Driving the Opioid Epidemic? *Am. J. Public Health* **2016**, *106*, 985–986. [CrossRef]
512. Anson, P. AMA Drops Pain as Vital Sign—Pain News Network. Pain News Network; 16 June 2016. Available online: https://www.painnewsnetwork.org/stories/2016/6/16/ama-drops-pain-as-vital-sign (accessed on 1 January 2021).
513. Thompson, C.A. HCAHPS survey to measure pain communication, not management. *Am. J. Health Pharm.* **2017**, *74*, 1924–1926. [CrossRef]
514. Wen, H.; Hockenberry, J.M.; Jeng, P.J.; Bao, Y. Prescription Drug Monitoring Program Mandates: Impact on Opioid Prescribing and Related Hospital Use. *Health Aff.* **2019**, *38*, 1550–1556. [CrossRef]
515. Hospital Compare. In the Center for Medicare and Medicaid Services. Available online: https://www.cms.gov/Medicare/Quality-Initiatives-Patient-Assessment-Instruments/HospitalQualityInits/HospitalCompare (accessed on 2 January 2021).
516. Leapfrog Hospital Safety Grade. In Leapfrod Group. 25 March 2016. Available online: https://www.leapfroggroup.org/data-users/leapfrog-hospital-safety-grade (accessed on 2 January 2021).
517. Huesch, M.D.; Currid-Halkett, E.; Doctor, J.N. Public hospital quality report awareness: Evidence from National and Californian Internet searches and social media mentions, 2012. *BMJ Open* **2014**, *4*, e004417. [CrossRef] [PubMed]
518. O'Hara, L.M.; Caturegli, I.; O'Hara, N.N.; O'Toole, R.V.; Dalury, D.F.; Harris, A.D.; Manson, T.T. What publicly available quality metrics do hip and knee arthroplasty patients care about most when selecting a hospital in Maryland: A discrete choice experiment. *BMJ Open* **2019**, *9*, e028202. [CrossRef] [PubMed]
519. National Quality Partners Playbook™: Opioid Stewardship. Available online: https://store.qualityforum.org/products/national-quality-partners-playbook%E2%84%A2-opioid-stewardship (accessed on 1 January 2021).
520. Ghafoor, V.L.; Phelps, P.K.; Pastor, I.J.; Meisel, S. Transformation of Hospital Pharmacist Opioid Stewardship. *Hosp. Pharm.* **2019**, *54*, 266–273. [CrossRef]
521. Quinlan, J.; Rann, S.; Bastable, R.; Levy, N. Perioperative opioid use and misuse. *Clin. Med.* **2019**, *19*, 441–445. [CrossRef]
522. Phelps, P.; Achey, T.S.; Mieure, K.D.; Cuellar, L.; MacMaster, H.; Pecho, R.; Ghafoor, V. A Survey of Opioid Medication Stewardship Practices at Academic Medical Centers. *Hosp. Pharm.* **2018**, *54*, 57–62. [CrossRef]
523. Rizk, E.; Swan, J.T.; Fink, E. Prioritization of quality indicators for opioid stewardship. *Am. J. Health Pharm.* **2019**, *76*, 1458–1459. [CrossRef]
524. Tichy, E.M.; Schumock, G.T.; Hoffman, J.M.; Suda, K.J.; Rim, M.H.; Tadrous, M.; Stubbings, J.; Cuellar, S.; Clark, J.S.; Wiest, M.D.; et al. National trends in prescription drug expenditures and projections for 2020. *Am. J. Health Pharm.* **2020**, *77*, 1213–1230. [CrossRef]
525. Hyland, S.J.; Kramer, B.J. Curbing the enthusiasm: Stewardship of high risk, high-cost drugs in perioperative settings. In Proceedings of the American College of Clinical Pharmacy Annual Meeting, Seattle, WA, USA, 22 October 2018.
526. Patel, G.P.; Hyland, S.J.; Birrer, K.L.; Wolfe, R.C.; Lovely, J.K.; Smith, A.N.; Dixon, R.L.; Johnson, E.G.; Gaviola, M.L.; Giancarelli, A.; et al. Perioperative clinical pharmacy practice: Responsibilities and scope within the surgical care continuum. *J. Am. Coll. Clin. Pharm.* **2019**, *3*, 501–519. [CrossRef]
527. Oddis, J.A. Report of the ASHP Opioid Task Force. *Am. J. Health Pharm.* **2020**, *77*, 1158–1165. [CrossRef]
528. Coulson, E.E.; Kral, L.A. The Clinical Pharmacist's Role in Perioperative Surgical Pain Management. *J. Pain Palliat. Care Pharmacother.* **2020**, *34*, 120–126. [CrossRef]

529. Hyland, S.J.; Kramer, B.J.; Fada, R.A.; Lucki, M.M. Clinical Pharmacist Service Associated With Improved Outcomes and Cost Savings in Total Joint Arthroplasty. *J. Arthroplast.* **2020**, *35*, 2307.e1–2317.e1. [CrossRef]
530. Poirier, R.H.; Brown, C.S.; Baggenstos, Y.T.; Walden, S.G.; Gann, N.Y.; Patty, C.M.; Sandoval, R.A.; McNulty, J.R. Impact of a pharmacist-directed pain management service on inpatient opioid use, pain control, and patient safety. *Am. J. Health Pharm.* **2018**, *76*, 17–25. [CrossRef]
531. Brown, R.F.; Brockhaus, K.; Rajkumar, D.; Battaglia, M.; Cleary, R.K. Postoperative Pain After Enhanced Recovery Pathway Robotic Colon and Rectal Surgery, Diseases of the Colon & Rectum: 26 January 2021–Volume Publish Ahead of Print–Issue. Available online: https://journals.lww.com/dcrjournal/Abstract/9000/Postoperative_Pain_After_Enhanced_Recovery_Pathway.99586.aspx (accessed on 13 January 2021). [CrossRef]
532. Hefti, E.; Remington, M.; Lavallee, C. Hospital consumer assessment of healthcare providers and systems scores relating to pain following the incorporation of clinical pharmacists into patient education prior to joint replacement surgery. *Pharm. Pract.* **2017**, *15*, 1071. [CrossRef]
533. Liu, Y.; Hu, Q.; Yang, J. Oliceridine for the Management of Acute Postoperative Pain. *Ann. Pharmacother.* **2021**. [CrossRef]
534. Bergese, S.D.; Brzezinski, M.; Hammer, G.B.; Beard, T.L.; Pan, P.H.; Mace, S.E.; Berkowitz, R.D.; Cochrane, K.; Wase, L.; Minkowitz, H.S.; et al. ATHENA: A Phase 3, Open-Label Study Of The Safety And Effectiveness Of Oliceridine (TRV130), A G-Protein Selective Agonist At The µ-Opioid Receptor, In Patients With Moderate To Severe Acute Pain Requiring Parenteral Opioid Therapy. *J. Pain Res.* **2019**, *12*, 3113–3126. [CrossRef] [PubMed]
535. Hakim, L.; Nahar, N.; Saha, M.; Islam, M.S.; Reza, H.M.; Sharker, S.M. Local drug delivery from surgical thread for area-specific anesthesia. *Biomed. Phys. Eng. Express* **2020**, *6*, 015028. [CrossRef] [PubMed]
536. Gabriel, R.A.; Ilfeld, B.M. Acute postoperative pain management with percutaneous peripheral nerve stimulation: The SPRINT neuromodulation system. *Expert Rev. Med. Devices* **2021**, 1–6. [CrossRef] [PubMed]
537. Inoue, R.; Nishizawa, D.; Hasegawa, J.; Nakayama, K.; Fukuda, K.; Ichinohe, T.; Mieda, T.; Tsujita, M.; Nakagawa, H.; Kitamura, A.; et al. Effects of rs958804 and rs7858836 single-nucleotide polymorphisms of the ASTN2 gene on pain-related phenotypes in patients who underwent laparoscopic colectomy and mandibular sagittal split ramus osteotomy. *Neuropsychopharmacol. Rep.* **2021**. [CrossRef]
538. Kost, J.A.; Ruaño, G. Pharmacogenetics and the Personalization of Pain Management: A Potential Role in Precision Opioid Treatment. *Conn. Med.* **2020**, *84*, 13–18. Available online: http://search.ebscohost.com/login.aspx?direct=true&profile=ehost&scope=site&authtype=crawler&jrnl=00106178&AN=141394148&h=WC%2F%2Fj3BfxC2wXRUHETAEgOc8WWLzGjPsSIu5o%2B5CYrADbW1dD9RcXpItvR%2FougtY3a4MTecX%2FdaoMpY7Chi4Zg%3D%3D&crl=c (accessed on 1 January 2021).
539. Chen, Y.K.; Boden, K.A.; Schreiber, K.L. The role of regional anaesthesia and multimodal analgesia in the prevention of chronic postoperative pain: A narrative review. *Anaesthesia* **2021**, *76*, 8–17. [CrossRef] [PubMed]
540. Ardeljan, L.D.; Waldfogel, J.M.; Bicket, M.C.; Hunsberger, J.B.; Vecchione, T.M.; Arwood, N.; Eid, A.; Hatfield, L.A.; McNamara, L.; Duncan, R.; et al. Current state of opioid stewardship. *Am. J. Health Pharm.* **2020**, *77*, 636–643. [CrossRef] [PubMed]

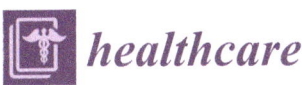

Article

Enhanced Recovery: A Decade of Experience and Future Prospects at the Mayo Clinic

Jenna K. Lovely * and David W. Larson

Mayo Clinic, Rochester, MN 55902, USA; larson.david2@mayo.edu
* Correspondence: lovely.jenna@mayo.edu; Tel.: +1-507-255-6825

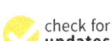

Citation: Lovely, J.K.; Larson, D.W. Enhanced Recovery: A Decade of Experience and Future Prospects at the Mayo Clinic. *Healthcare* **2021**, *9*, 549. https://doi.org/10.3390/healthcare9050549

Academic Editors: Richard H. Parrish II and John Kortbeek

Received: 1 March 2021
Accepted: 12 April 2021
Published: 8 May 2021

Publisher's Note: MDPI stays neutral with regard to jurisdictional claims in published maps and institutional affiliations.

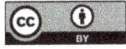

Copyright: © 2021 by the authors. Licensee MDPI, Basel, Switzerland. This article is an open access article distributed under the terms and conditions of the Creative Commons Attribution (CC BY) license (https://creativecommons.org/licenses/by/4.0/).

Abstract: This work aims to describe the implementation and subsequent learnings from the first decade after the full implementation of enhanced recovery pathway for colorectal surgery at a single institution. This paper will describe the diffusion efforts and plans through the Define, Measure, Analyze, Improve, Control (DMAIC) process of ongoing quality improvement and through research efforts. The information applies to all readers that provide surgical care within their organization as the fundamental principles of enhanced recovery for surgery are applicable regardless of the setting.

Keywords: enhanced recovery; surgical care; colorectal surgery; quality improvement

1. Problem Description

Starting in 2008, it was recognized that while well-established literature supported principles of enhanced recovery, full implementation of those principles had yet to be delivered to our patients. Enhanced recovery is referred to under different names, known as Enhanced Recovery After Surgery (ERAS^R), rapid recovery, or earlier referred to Fast-track programs [1–3]. Implementation has developed over 20 years after described by Kehlet in 1997 [4]. Several groups across the world have contributed to over 1000 PubMed search articles demonstrating benefits with Enhanced Recovery principles, while the ERAS® Society has developed numerous published guidelines covering specialty and sub-specialty surgeries [5–17]. The principles of enhanced recovery, when fully implemented, have been demonstrated to reduce the length of hospital stay (LOS), morbidity, and convalescence, without an increase in readmission rates or complications [4,18–20]. Enhanced recovery pathways (ERP) can be considered a Quality Improvement (QI) intervention and are an inter-professional and multimodal approach to care [21–26]. ERP seeks to optimize patient care before, during, and after surgery to minimize the surgical stress response. The pathways are multimodal and combine preoperative education, minimally invasive surgery, regional anesthetic techniques, multimodal opioid-sparing pain management, early feeding, and ambulation [27–34]. To address this problem of the gap from knowledge in literature and conceptual agreement to actualization in the practice [35], we first set out to develop and implement an institutional pathway for enhanced recovery. As the results of that implementation were known, we worked to address new problems and answer new research questions while also spreading to other surgical specialties.

After over a decade of a fully implemented enhanced recovery pathway [36,37], our institution has embarked on several innovations and quality improvement initiatives to continue to evolve toward the next new standard of innovative care [38–40]. The age-old project management challenges continue to impede delivering optimal care. Critical elements of the implementation [35,41,42] dissemination, and sustainability [43,44] are areas for all interested parties to engage.

The specific aim of this paper strives to provide those working to implement and adopt enhanced recovery pathways, the principles intended to stretch collaborative thinking and execute high value patient care.

2. Methods

2.1. Standards of Care

The first stage was to fully implement the institution developed enhanced recovery pathway. This pathway was based on evidence-based principles and where no specific literature, existed, then by consensus developed agreement with interdisciplinary team members. The lead surgeon, anesthesiologist, clinical pharmacist, and clinical nurse specialist designed with input for logistics from variety stakeholders. Using combined methodology of 5 Whys, Value Stream Mapping and Failure Mode Effect analysis, the entire process was set for clinical excellence and operationally LEAN. These standards were then implemented in stages. First with one surgeon in minimally invasive practice for two weeks, then with a second surgeon for timeframe of two months. Daily tracking of the process occurred by the clinical pharmacist with follow up within the day for other team members as needed. All pathway elements were tracked manually. Preliminary results for inpatient metrics and for 30 day outcomes to date were analyzed. The overwhelming improvements led to full adoption for two surgeons for all patients and procedures in 2010. The process and outcome measures continued to be tracked in a prospectively maintained database, with ongoing automation added where able within the electronic environment. After 3 months of overall data, all surgeons in the Division were invited to fully adopt and be supported with the tracking and monitoring plan for implementation in place. With adoption, it was recognized that a more formal implementation expectation was needed. We worked to publish our results and started new research studies to answer questions to the specific themes about risks and complications that those hesitant were claiming. The data for renal insufficiency, elderly patients and those with inflammatory bowel disease were internally reviewed and then further studied. No harm, only benefit was shown for the surgeons. This Design, Measure, Analyze, Improve, Control (DMAIC) process continued for each area of low compliance [45]. In 2011, the Division approved and committed to full implementation of enhanced recovery as a practice standard. The outcomes of that implementation are described and highlighted that diet and fluids were key to outcomes [36,38]. This is consistent with findings from others [46–48] The lessons learned demonstrated that standardized care is about discovering best practice, implementing it, publishing the results, and teaching it to others. These principles of care translate, for patients and providers, into less waste and unnecessary delays in the system, patient flow and improves patient experience [49].

Standardization of care leads to improved pattern recognition of complications versus non-standardized care. Enhanced recovery pathways bring the patient through highly choreographed preoperative care, intraoperative care, PACU, post-operative care, discharge, and post-discharge follow-up. This fact allows one to recognize deviations from this standard which typically represent complications resulting in earlier intervention and, ultimately better outcomes [38,40,50–52]. In the rectal cancer patient population specifically, we learned that the patterns recognized on days 2–3 may result in early recognition [40,53,54].

Another example may be when the Pharmacist may recognize that a certain amount of opioid medication was a signal for reassessment—patients requiring more than the usual needed attention. This attention can afford a new diagnosis of a complication or a reassessment in partnership with the pharmacist for another multimodal option and work to taper the opioid effectively [37,38,55,56].

Our Enhanced Recovery Pathway (ERP) provides for all the standard orders required for high value patient care during the first 48 h of post-op care until standardized discharge criteria have been met. After 48 h, the focus shifts to reassessment and recognizing alterations in patient status which may represent complications, or logistical barriers to discharge.

In the Colorectal surgery practice, providers can shortlist complications to focus on as in many other surgical specialties. Prevention, early recognition, and optimal management of complications are critical. This focused list of complications includes postoperative ileus, surgical site infection, bleeding, anastomotic leak, venous thrombosis, acute kidney injury, atrial fibrillation, or acute myocardial infarction. Focusing on these issues ensure prevention and recognition, and an early management treatment resulting in a smoother implementation of treatment.

2.2. Organizational Dynamics

Teams have a unique opportunity to learn from the past attempts and adaptions of existing ERPs and consider complication pathways and triage pathways for post-discharge care. Emphasizing the learning that can come from recognizing the patterns that are more easily seen with standard practices, i.e., the ability to catch the signal from the noise.

2.2.1. Leadership

Leadership is critical for supporting probabilistic thinking and logical pattern recognition. Critical aspects of organizational culture [42] make a difference in how much a surgical practice can achieve. Collectively an active 'just culture' and a dynamic 'continuous improvement' culture are needed as individual team members may struggle with parts [57]. The just culture model allows for coaching and improvements while not honoring or coddling performance issues. The inter-professional, multidisciplinary team approach has become commonplace. The advantages are evident on a variety of fronts. The challenge remains that when everyone's responsible, everyone is (duplicate work/waste at times) or no one is (breach of standards/potential safety risk). With teams, just as in team sports, everyone needs to know the game plan, yet not everyone does the same work. Clear roles and responsibilities need to be well articulated and then accountable as part of team-based care's overall success [58,59].

2.2.2. Diffusion

After initial implementation with colorectal surgeons in 2009 with minimally invasive teams, then expanded to the entire Division as a standard of practice for all patients undergoing colorectal surgery in 2011. Next, team members worked to diffuse to Gynecologic surgery [60], Breast [61], Urology [62–64], Endocrine, Hepatobiliary [65,66], Thoracic [67,68] and Vascular [69,70] within one campus of the institution, then continued to expand enterprise-wide knowledge within the same organization while also collaborating with teams at external organizations. The framework of spread was used, and results from network collaboratives shared [38]. Internal audits continue to drive quality improvement efforts for the targeted areas by specialty. Knowing critical factors [71] for predicting prolonged LOS and complications most relate to diet and fluid compliance. Additional opportunity exists across all teams for improved adoption of diet and fluid management principles.

2.3. Quality Improvement Methods

It cannot be discounted that optimal Quality Improvement Methodologies are required to contextualize improvement efforts and assure full implementation, diffusion, and adoption has occurred and will continue to be sustained. Core QI methodologies strengthen the clinical programs and allow early recognition of issues. Like clinical care, the 'pulse of the practice' is the health and wellness of any patient care unit, Division, Department, or entire Health System ecosystem. Knowing the status (as a project management term) as the 'health' of the organization or program is how ongoing improvements, new research questions, and innovations can emerge readily.

The Design, Measure, Analyze, Improve, Control (DMAIC) model was used to strategize then implement the following tactics. The overall goal was to improve patients' recovery plans that lead to improved patient hospital length of stay. The first was to review the current state of enhanced recovery compliance. It is well established that high compliance with enhanced recovery principles leads to better outcomes [43,64,72]. A report within the Electronic Health Record (EHR) was developed to implement a new health system to replace previous custom software dashboards and point of care tools related to

ERP. The current compliance across the Colorectal Surgical Division remains >90% across the timeframe of the past two years, despite the transition to a new electronic health record. There is a slight variation between the Surgeons, yet no individual provider is below 80%. The various themes are consistent with previous emergency cases' challenges and patients admitted through ED and medical service before going to surgery. When reviewing critical elements of the entire pathway, opportunities exist with intraoperative fluid [73–75]. When examining options postoperatively, reemphasize diet compliance for all staff involved may help with additional compliance needs. Had there been a large discrepancy or actionable gap, our Practice Optimization team would have embarked on specific quality improvement tactics to improve. However, we recognized a more significant impact on two bookends of the current Practice. (1) opportunity to shift from Inpatient to Outpatient for specific procedures/patient population and (2) minimize issues related to an extended length of stay. The development of an outpatient enhanced recovery has been implemented, and the clinical outcomes of this are being collected in ongoing work and will be described in another paper.

The refreshing of standardized plans for each day post-op has been outlined for the team and implemented daily multidisciplinary rounds. In parallel to the re-emphasis of standardized discharge criteria, daily accountability for discharge planning, and an active Practice Optimization and Acceleration project with the team, a baseline LOS from 2019 has been decreased by 1.4 days LOS to again move to early implementation LOS median of 4 days that we had reported before [37].

3. Complications

3.1. Post Operative Ileus (POI)

For POI, enhanced recovery principles are designed to prevent POI [4]. The literature on this is robust—minimize NPO preoperatively, no nasogastric tube (NGT) postoperatively, and regular diet provided within 4 h of surgery [4,76]. Earlier work had identified estimated blood loss and total opioid dose as independently associated with duration of POI in a pre-ERP era [77], which we assessed as technique related for EBL and actionable by opioid sparing methods covered with multi-modal pain control techniques. When ERP is implemented effectively with early feeding as critical for patient, it minimizes POI to low rates and in our practice reduces rates by a factor of 3 compared to not following this standard [78]. While medications, such as alvimopan, have been studied with promising results compared to traditional practice [79], no additional advantages have been proven in units with highly compliant enhanced recovery pathways. We do not include alvimopan in the active enhanced recovery pathway for colorectal surgery as it increases the cost of care, without providing added benefit in our patient population of highly compliant enhanced recovery.

The other factor is to avoid fluid overload [36,46,73,75,80–82]. We continue to work with our surgical and anesthesiologist colleagues on achieving euvolemia and avoiding fluid overload to minimize POI and other complications.

3.2. Surgical Site Infection (SSI)

The increasing adoption of standardized ERP and growing rates of Minimally Invasive Surgery have reduced of the complication of SSI. Locally this has been supplemented by following high adherence to both ERP and a standardized SSI bundle [83]. Ongoing efforts to sustain high compliance with the bundle have continued. One controversy remains, which is the use of mechanical bowel prep with oral antibiotics before surgery. In the 2009 version of our enhanced recovery pathway, we instituted no bowel prep as the clinical standard [36]. During this high ERP compliance and standardized SSI bundle initiation, the SSI rates dropped and remained low [83]. With the Michigan Quality Improvement teams' work, mechanical bowel prep with oral antibiotics showed great benefit [84]. While it's unclear whether merely implementing a standard of practice with strict monitoring and key metrics being transparently shared had a Hawthorne effect or whether the evidence is translatable. No RCT in the era of enhanced recovery and MIS has occurred, and the SSI rates are low, making a feasible RCT challenging to perform. Our institution's power analysis with the following qualities and assumptions would require >17,000 patients for 90% power. Nationally, as MIS rates increase, the impact of bowel prep may not be as critical as once thought.

3.3. Acute Kidney Injury

There are various facets which if implemented may prevention acute kidney injury. Appropriately implemented criteria for the use of non-steroidal anti-inflammatory agents, such that patients with known renal dysfunction before surgery are not exposed can result in better outcomes. The topic continued to be a barrier to full implementation for specific team members and for others researching [85–89]. The key difference is pharmacists in our institution serve as the safety net for appropriate medication ordering as standardized order sets, and electronic decisions have been designed to help the initial ordering provider dose appropriately for these patients. By tracking the data as well as implementing the safe guard systems, we have not seen AKI as a barrier to implementation and rather a risk able to be mitigated [89].

Fluid overload preoperatively, in the OR, and postoperatively are to be avoided. One tactic, implemented through multiple plan, study, do, act cycles to improve fluid compliance, was that operationally, we changed to not starting IV fluids upon arrival to the facility day of surgery but instead waiting until the patient was in the OR. This operational change through orderset updates and preoperative nursing education focusing on allowing patients to drink fluids as per ASRA standards rather than IV decreased the amount of fluid by approximately 1.5 L preoperatively based on internal audits. Within the OR, the fluids volumes have remained higher than our enhanced recovery pathway recommendations, and we see differences in outcomes when the goals are unable to be achieved [73]. Recent data suggest that total volume of fluid given rather than the rate in mL/Kg/hour is more important in our high-volume practice in terms of LOS and complication risk (paper in submission).

Postoperatively, the discontinuation of IV fluids at 0800 days after surgery has effectively reduced the amount of IV fluid exposure. However, the institution is still challenged by historical dogma to react to requests for more fluid from other team members. Low urine output, for example, is expected and not harmful in the colorectal patient population we serve, while fluid overload has been proven harmful. While there is still dogma for giving more fluid, our research shows that not only is a lower urinary output expected and acceptable in the early postoperative period [90], reactionary IV fluid and fluid overload were not beneficial [78]. In a study attempting to reverse the fluid overload situation with furosemide, there was no benefit, and the practice was ceased [91]. High ileostomy output has a known pathway for assuring the patient is eating adequately and the timing of increased production as a pattern in the postoperative setting to be expected and not overreacted to in the first 24–48 h postoperatively.

For each of the other surgical complications, we have developed and implemented programs for each topic. For example—VTE prophylaxis standards are embedded into the order sets and monitoring plans [92] and specific to CRS discharge plans [93,94]. A postoperative bleeding pathway was developed and implemented; a postoperative atrial fibrillation pathway was developed and implemented [95]. Considering the nation's attention to the opioid crisis, we studied discharge prescriptions and the newly deemed complication of prolonged opioid use [59,60]. From the work, new discharge guidelines were established, and improved outpatient triage options were implemented. Each of these initiatives followed similar methods and quality improvement tactics for execution that were able to be disseminated with others [38].

3.4. Readmissions

To smooth implementation concerns, we measured readmission as a counterbalance in all cases. Others findings were informative [42,47,96,97]. In our reviews of readmission patterns, we recognized that the readmission risk continued to rise with each added hospital day, i.e., the longer length of stays correlated with high readmissions We studied the disease state patterns and complications for each as a guide for learners to see those patterns sooner. The probability of predicting a patient's trajectory became important as we attempt to keep patients informed about reasonable expectations [98].

The key themes are these: (a) A longer length of stay was correlated with a higher rate of readmission; (b) Once the patients meet our standard discharge criteria, there is no further advantage of inpatient/hospital care and (c) logistical barriers are known where at times, a patient needing a Skilled Nursing Facility may not get placement for several days after meeting discharge criteria clinically with the surgical team. This remains a challenge in our health care system.

4. Sustainability

As described in ERP implementation work [1,64] an organizational framework is needed to sustain the gains [44,48]. Ongoing work to display the required actionable information in the clinical workflows within the electronic health record. Overall compliance is known with reports, and the length of stay targets have been presented to the team leads with dashboard functionality. The themes for electronic tools are consistent with design principles for putting the information needed for decision-making in the decision-maker's hands when the decision needs to be made [99]. Tactically, this means standardized order sets for pre- and post-operative care, real-time patient information collated to simple list views for rounding and monitoring teams, and leadership reports and opinions for high-level summaries.

5. Future

Our next phase of research and implementation will expand on outpatient care opportunities to all segmental colectomy patients. Moreover, advancing minimally invasive techniques, improving fluid management, and continuing to work on complication pathways for the chance to provide high-value care to our patients and decrease morbidity.

6. Conclusions

Enhanced recovery improves care for patients and allows optimal standardization for institutions and care teams for optimal systematic approaches to excellence in patient care. We share the framework and experiences so that others may partner with their teams or ours to achieve more. After over a decade, compliance remains high. Ongoing innovations, essential quality improvement methods, and continued opportunities remain challenging work to pursue.

Author Contributions: Conceptualization, J.K.L. and D.W.L.; writing—original draft preparation, J.K.L.; writing—review and editing, J.K.L. and D.W.L. All authors have read and agreed to the published version of the manuscript.

Funding: This work received no external funding.

Institutional Review Board Statement: Institutional Review Board Statement: Approved as Exempt.

Informed Consent Statement: Not applicable.

Data Availability Statement: No new data were created or analyzed in this study. Data sharing is not applicable to this article.

Conflicts of Interest: The authors declare no conflict of interest.

References

1. Bonnet, F.; Rousset, J. Regional anaesthesia in fast track surgery and rehabilitation. *Reg. Anesth. Pain Med.* **2012**, *37*.
2. Tsikitis, V.L.; Holubar, S.D.; Dozois, E.J.; Cima, R.R.; Pemberton, J.H.; Larson, D.W. Advantages of fast-track recovery after laparoscopic right hemicolectomy for colon cancer. *Surg. Endosc.* **2010**, *24*, 1911–1916. [CrossRef]
3. Varadhan, K.K.; Lobo, D.N.; Ljungqvist, O. Enhanced recovery after surgery: The future of improving surgical care. *Crit. Care Clin.* **2010**, *26*, 527–547. [CrossRef]
4. Kehlet, H. Multimodal approach to control postoperative pathophysiology and rehabilitation. *Br. J. Anaesth.* **1997**, *78*, 606–617. [CrossRef]
5. Ljungqvist, O.; Scott, M.; Fearon, K.C. Enhanced Recovery After Surgery: A Review. *JAMA Surg.* **2017**, *152*, 292–298. [CrossRef]
6. Brindle, M.; Nelson, G.; Lobo, D.N.; Ljungqvist, O.; Gustafsson, U.O. Recommendations from the ERAS® Society for standards for the development of enhanced recovery after surgery guidelines. *BJS Open* **2020**, *4*, 157–163. [CrossRef]
7. Ljungqvist, O.; Young-Fadok, T.; Demartines, N. The History of Enhanced Recovery After Surgery and the ERAS Society. *J. Laparoendosc. Adv. Surg. Tech. A* **2017**, *27*, 860–862. [CrossRef]
8. Elias, K.M.; Stone, A.B.; McGinigle, K.; Tankou, J.; Scott, M.J.; Fawcett, W.J.; Demartines, N.; Lobo, D.N.; Ljungqvist, O.; Urman, R.D.; et al. The Reporting on ERAS Compliance, Outcomes, and Elements Research (RECOvER) Checklist: A Joint Statement by the ERAS® and ERAS® USA Societies. *World J. Surg.* **2019**, *43*, 1–8. [CrossRef]
9. Ljungqvist, O.; Thanh, N.X.; Nelson, G. ERAS-Value based surgery. *J. Surg. Oncol.* **2017**, *116*, 608–612. [CrossRef]
10. Tanious, M.K.; Ljungqvist, O.; Urman, R.D. Enhanced Recovery After Surgery: History, Evolution, Guidelines, and Future Directions. *Int. Anesthesiol. Clin.* **2017**, *55*, 1–11. [CrossRef]
11. Currie, A.; Soop, M.; Demartines, N.; Fearon, K.; Kennedy, R.; Ljungqvist, O. Enhanced Recovery After Surgery Interactive Audit System: 10 Years' Experience with an International Web-Based Clinical and Research Perioperative Care Database. *Clin. Colon Rectal Surg.* **2019**, *32*, 75–81, Erratum in **2019**, *32*, e1. [CrossRef] [PubMed]
12. Loughlin, S.M.; Alvarez, A.; Falcão, L.F.D.R.; Ljungqvist, O. The History of ERAS (Enhanced Recovery After Surgery) Society and its development in Latin America. *Rev. Col. Bras. Cir.* **2020**, *47*, e20202525. [CrossRef]
13. Pisarska, M.; Torbicz, G.; Gajewska, N.; Rubinkiewicz, M.; Wierdak, M.; Major, P.; Budzyński, A.; Ljungqvist, O.; Pędziwiatr, M. Compliance with the ERAS Protocol and 3-Year Survival After Laparoscopic Surgery for Non-metastatic Colorectal Cancer. *World J. Surg.* **2019**, *43*, 2552–2560. [CrossRef] [PubMed]
14. Nelson, G.; Bakkum-Gamez, J.; Kalogera, E.; Glaser, G.; Altman, A.; Meyer, L.A.; Taylor, J.S.; Iniesta, M.; Lasala, J.; Mena, G.; et al. Guidelines for perioperative care in gynecologic/oncology: Enhanced Recovery after Surgery (ERAS) Society recommendations—2019 update. *Int. J. Gynecol. Cancer* **2019**, *29*. [CrossRef] [PubMed]
15. Caughey, A.B.; Wood, S.L.; Macones, G.A.; Wrench, I.J.; Huang, J.; Norman, M.; Pettersson, K.; Fawcett, W.J.; Shalabi, M.M.; Metcalfe, A.; et al. Guidelines for intraoperative care in cesarean delivery: Enhanced Recovery After Surgery Society Recommendations (Part 2). *Am. J. Obstet. Gynecol.* **2018**, *219*, 533–544. [CrossRef]
16. Engelman, D.T.; Ben Ali, W.; Williams, J.B.; Perrault, L.P.; Reddy, V.S.; Arora, R.C.; Roselli, E.E.; Khoynezhad, A.; Gerdisch, M.; Levy, J.H.; et al. Guidelines for Perioperative Care in Cardiac Surgery: Enhanced Recovery after Surgery Society Recommendations. *JAMA Surg.* **2019**, *154*, 755–766. [CrossRef]
17. Gibb, A.C.N.; Crosby, M.A.; McDiarmid, C.; Urban, D.; Lam, J.Y.K.; Wales, P.W.; Brockel, M.; Raval, M.; Offringa, M.; Skarsgard, E.D.; et al. Creation of an Enhanced Recovery after Surgery (ERAS) Guideline for neonatal intestinal surgery patients: A knowledge synthesis and consensus generation approach and protocol study. *BMJ Open* **2018**, *8*, e023651. [CrossRef]
18. Nygren, J.; Thacker, J.; Carli, F.; Fearon, K.C.H.; Norderval, S.; Lobo, D.N.; Ljungqvist, O.; Soop, M.; Ramirez, J. Guidelines for perioperative care in elective rectal/pelvic surgery: Enhanced Recovery After Surgery (ERAS®) Society recommendations. *Clin. Nutr.* **2012**, *31*, 801–816. [CrossRef]
19. Gustafsson, U.O.; Scott, M.J.; Schwenk, W.; Demartines, N.; Roulin, D.; Francis, N.; McNaught, C.E.; MacFie, J.; Liberman, A.S.; Soop, M.; et al. Guidelines for perioperative care in elective colonic surgery: Enhanced Recovery After Surgery (ERAS®) Society recommendations. *Clin. Nutr.* **2012**, *31*, 783–800. [CrossRef]
20. Miller, T.E.; Thacker, J.K.; White, W.D.; Mantyh, C.; Migaly, J.; Jin, J.; Roche, A.M.; Eisenstein, E.L.; Edwards, R.; Anstrom, K.J.; et al. Reduced length of hospital stay in colorectal surgery after implementation of an enhanced recovery protocol. *Anesth. Analg.* **2014**, *118*, 1052–1061. [CrossRef]
21. Fischer, C.; Wick, E. An AHRQ national quality improvement project for implementation of enhanced recovery after surgery. *Semin. Colon Rectal Surg.* **2020**, *31*, 100778. [CrossRef]
22. Brethauer, S.A.; Grieco, A.; Fraker, T.; Evans-Labok, K.; Smith, A.; McEvoy, M.D.; Saber, A.A.; Morton, J.M.; Petrick, A. Employing Enhanced Recovery Goals in Bariatric Surgery (ENERGY): A national quality improvement project using the Metabolic and Bariatric Surgery Accreditation and Quality Improvement Program. *Surg. Obes. Relat. Dis.* **2019**, *15*, 1977–1989. [CrossRef]
23. Heathcote, S.S.; Duggan, K.; Rosbrugh, J.; Hill, B.; Shaker, R.; Hope, W.W.; Fillion, M.M. Enhanced Recovery after Surgery (ERAS) Protocols Expanded over Multiple Service Lines Improves Patient Care and Hospital Cost. *Am Surg.* **2019**, *85*, 1044–1050. [CrossRef] [PubMed]
24. Pachella, L.A.; Mehran, R.J.; Curtin, K.; Schneider, S.M. Preoperative Carbohydrate Loading in Patients Undergoing Thoracic Surgery: A Quality-Improvement Project. *J. PeriAnesthesia Nurs.* **2019**, *34*, 1250–1256. [CrossRef]

25. Liu, J.Y.; Wick, E.C. Enhanced Recovery After Surgery and Effects on Quality Metrics. *Surg. Clin. N. Am.* **2018**, *98*, 1119–1127. [CrossRef]
26. Jakobsen, D.H.; Kehle, H. A simple method to secure data-driven improvement of perioperative care. *Br. J. Nurs.* **2020**, *29*, 516–519. [CrossRef] [PubMed]
27. Beverly, A.; Kaye, A.D.; Ljungqvist, O.; Urman, R.D. Essential Elements of Multimodal Analgesia in Enhanced Recovery after Surgery (ERAS) Guidelines. *Anesthesiol. Clin.* **2017**, *35*, e115–e143. [CrossRef]
28. Wick, E.C.; Grant, M.C.; Wu, C.L. Postoperative Multimodal Analgesia Pain Management With Nonopioid Analgesics and Techniques: A Review. *JAMA Surg.* **2017**, *152*, 691–697. [CrossRef]
29. Simpson, J.C.; Bao, X.; Agarwala, A. Pain Management in Enhanced Recovery after Surgery (ERAS) Protocols. *Clin. Colon Rectal Surg.* **2019**, *32*, 121–128. [CrossRef] [PubMed]
30. Mitra, S.; Carlyle, D.; Kodumudi, G.; Kodumudi, V.; Vadivelu, N. New Advances in Acute Postoperative Pain Management. *Curr. Pain Headache Rep.* **2018**, *22*, 35. [CrossRef]
31. Weimann, A.; Braga, M.; Carli, F.; Higashiguchi, T.; Hübner, M.; Klek, S.; Laviano, A.; Ljungqvist, O.; Lobo, D.N.; Martindale, R.; et al. ESPEN guideline: Clinical nutrition in surgery. *Clin. Nutr.* **2017**, *36*, 623–650. [CrossRef]
32. Gianotti, L.; Sandini, M.; Romagnoli, S.; Carli, F.; Ljungqvist, O. Enhanced recovery programs in gastrointestinal surgery: Actions to promote optimal perioperative nutritional and metabolic care. *Clin. Nutr.* **2020**, *39*, 2014–2024. [CrossRef] [PubMed]
33. Mc Loughlin, S.; Terrasa, S.A.; Ljungqvist, O.; Sanchez, G.; Garcia Fornari, G.; Alvarez, A.O. Nausea and vomiting in a colorectal ERAS program: Impact on nutritional recovery and the length of hospital stay. *Clin. Nutr. ESPEN* **2019**, *34*, 73–80. [CrossRef]
34. Aahlin, E.K.; von Meyenfeldt, M.; Dejong, C.H.; Ljungqvist, O.; Fearon, K.C.; Lobo, D.N.; Demartines, N.; Revhaug, A.; Wigmore, S.J.; Lassen, K. Functional recovery is considered the most important target: A survey of dedicated professionals. *Perioper. Med.* **2014**, *3*, 5. [CrossRef] [PubMed]
35. Maessen, J.; Dejong, C.H.C.; Hausel, J.; Nygren, J.; Lassen, K.; Andersen, J.; Kessels, A.G.H.; Revhaug, A.; Kehlet, H.; Ljungqvist, O.; et al. A protocol is not enough to implement an enhanced recovery programme for colorectal resection. *Br. J. Surg.* **2007**, *94*, 224–231. [CrossRef]
36. Lovely, J.K.; Maxson, P.M.; Jacob, A.K.; Cima, R.R.; Horlocker, T.T.; Hebl, J.R.; Harmsen, W.S.; Huebner, M.; Larson, D.W. Case-matched series of enhanced versus standard recovery pathway in minimally invasive colorectal surgery. *Br. J. Surg.* **2012**, *99*, 120–126. [CrossRef] [PubMed]
37. Larson, D.W.; Lovely, J.K.; Cima, R.R.; Dozois, E.J.; Chua, H.; Wolff, B.G.; Pemberton, J.H.; Devine, R.R.; Huebner, M. Outcomes after implementation of a multimodal standard care pathway for laparoscopic colorectal surgery. *Br. J. Surg.* **2014**, *101*, 1023–1030. [CrossRef]
38. Larson, D.W.; Lovely, J.K.; Welsh, J.; Annaberdyev, S.; Corning Coffey, C.; Murray, B.; Rose, D.; Prabhakar, L.; Torgenson, M.; Dankbar, E.; et al. A Collaborative for Implementation of an Evidence-Based Clinical Pathway for Enhanced Recovery in Colon and Rectal Surgery in an Affiliated Network of Healthcare Organizations. *Jt. Comm. J. Qual. Patient Saf.* **2018**, *44*, 204–211. [CrossRef]
39. Quiram, B.J.; Crippa, J.; Grass, F.; Lovely, J.K.; Behm, K.T.; Colibaseanu, D.T.; Merchea, A.; Kelley, S.R.; Harmsen, W.S.; Larson, D.W. Impact of enhanced recovery on oncological outcomes following minimally invasive surgery for rectal cancer. *Br. J. Surg.* **2019**, *106*, 922–929. [CrossRef]
40. Khreiss, W.; Huebner, M.; Cima, R.R.; Dozois, E.R.; Chua, H.K.; Pemberton, J.H.; Harmsen, W.S.; Larson, D.W. Improving conventional recovery with enhanced recovery in minimally invasive surgery for rectal cancer. *Dis. Colon Rectum* **2014**, *57*, 557–563. [CrossRef] [PubMed]
41. Elhassan, A.; Ahmed, A.; Awad, H.; Humeidan, M.; Nguyen, V.; Cornett, E.M.; Urman, R.D.; Kaye, A.D. The Evolution of Surgical Enhanced Recovery Pathways: A Review. *Curr. Pain Headache Rep.* **2018**, *22*, 74. [CrossRef]
42. Slakey, D.P.; Silver, D.S.; Chazin, S.M.; Katoozian, P.Y.; Sikora, K.S.; Ruther, M.M. Making enhanced recovery the norm not the exception. *Am. J. Surg.* **2020**, *219*, 472–476. [CrossRef]
43. Williamsson, C.; Karlsson, T.; Westrin, M.; Ansari, D.; Andersson, R.; Tingstedt, B. Sustainability of an Enhanced Recovery Program for Pancreaticoduodenectomy with Pancreaticogastrostomy. *Scand. J. Surg.* **2019**, *108*, 17–22. [CrossRef] [PubMed]
44. Wolfe, D.; Knighton, A.J.; Brunisholz, K.D.; Belnap, T.; Allen, T.L.; Srivastava, R. Sustaining Implementation Gains. *Qual. Manag. Health Care* **2019**, *28*, 250–251. [CrossRef]
45. Li, N.; Laux, C.M.; Antony, J. How to use lean Six Sigma methodology to improve service process in higher education: A case study. *Int. J. Lean Six Sigma* **2019**, *10*, 883–908. [CrossRef]
46. Joliat, G.R.; Ljungqvist, O.; Wasylak, T.; Peters, O.; Demartines, N. Beyond surgery: Clinical and economic impact of Enhanced Recovery after Surgery programs. *BMC Health Serv. Res.* **2018**, *18*, 1008. [CrossRef]
47. Fabrizio, A.C.; Grant, M.C.; Siddiqui, Z.; Alimi, Y.; Gearhart, S.L.; Wu, C.; Efron, J.E.; Wick, E.C. Is enhanced recovery enough for reducing 30-d readmissions after surgery? *J. Surg. Res.* **2017**, *217*, 45–53. [CrossRef]
48. Stone, A.B.; Yuan, C.T.; Rosen, M.A.; Grant, M.C.; Benishek, L.E.; Hanahan, E.; Lubomski, L.H.; Ko, C.; Wick, E.C. Barriers to and facilitators of implementing enhanced recovery pathways using an implementation framework: A systematic review. *JAMA Surg.* **2018**, *153*, 270–279. [CrossRef] [PubMed]
49. Li, D.; Jensen, C.C. Patient Satisfaction and Quality of Life with Enhanced Recovery Protocols. *Clin. Colon Rectal Surg.* **2019**, *32*, 138–144. [CrossRef]

50. Currie, A.; Burch, J.; Jenkins, J.T.; Faiz, O.; Kennedy, R.H.; Ljungqvist, O.; Demartines, N.; Hjern, F.; Norderval, S.; Lassen, K.; et al. The impact of enhanced recovery protocol compliance on elective colorectal cancer resection: Results from an international registry. *Ann. Surg.* **2015**, *261*, 1153–1159. [CrossRef]
51. Gramlich, L.M.; Sheppard, C.E.; Wasylak, T.; Gilmour, L.E.; Ljungqvist, O.; Basualdo-Hammond, C.; Nelson, G. Implementation of Enhanced Recovery After Surgery: A strategy to transform surgical care across a health system. *Implement. Sci.* **2017**, *12*, 1–17. [CrossRef]
52. Grass, F.; Crippa, J.; Mathis, K.L.; Kelley, S.R.; Larson, D.W. Feasibility and safety of robotic resection of complicated diverticular disease. *Surg. Endosc.* **2019**, *33*, 4171–4176. [CrossRef]
53. Lemini, R.; Spaulding, A.C.; Naessens, J.M.; Li, Z.; Merchea, A.; Crook, J.E.; Larson, D.W.; Colibaseanu, D.T. ERAS protocol validation in a propensity-matched cohort of patients undergoing colorectal surgery. *Int. J. Colorectal Dis.* **2018**, *33*, 1543–1550. [CrossRef]
54. Huebner, M.; Hübner, M.; Cima, R.R.; Larson, D.W. Timing of complications and length of stay after rectal cancer surgery. *J. Am. Coll. Surg.* **2014**, *218*, 914–919. [CrossRef] [PubMed]
55. Lovely, J.K.; Hyland, S.J.; Smith, A.N.; Nelson, G.; Ljungqvist, O.; Parrish, R.H. Clinical pharmacist perspectives for optimizing pharmacotherapy within Enhanced Recovery After Surgery (ERAS®) programs. *Int. J. Surg.* **2019**, *63*, 58–62. [CrossRef]
56. Patel, G.P.; Hyland, S.J.; Birrer, K.L.; Wolfe, R.C.; Lovely, J.K.; Smith, A.N.; Dixon, R.L.; Johnson, E.G.; Gaviola, M.L.; Giancarelli, A.; et al. Perioperative clinical pharmacy practice: Responsibilities and scope within the surgical care continuum. *J. Am. Coll. Clin. Pharm.* **2020**, *3*, 501–519. [CrossRef]
57. Swensen, S.J.; Dilling, J.A.; Milliner, D.S.; Zimmerman, R.S.; Maples, W.J.; Lindsay, M.E.; Bartley, G.B. Quality: The Mayo Clinic approach. *Am. J. Med. Qual.* **2009**, *24*, 428–440. [CrossRef]
58. Burton, R.M.; Obel, B. The science of organizational design: Fit between structure and coordination. *J. Organ. Des.* **2018**, *7*, 5. [CrossRef]
59. Timmel, J.; Kent, P.S.; Holzmueller, C.G.; Paine, L.; Schulick, R.D.; Pronovost, P.J. Impact of the Comprehensive Unit-based Safety Program (CUSP) on safety culture in a surgical inpatient unit. *Jt. Comm. J. Qual. Patient Saf.* **2010**, *36*, 252–260. [CrossRef]
60. Kalogera, E.; Bakkum-Gamez, J.N.; Jankowski, C.J.; Trabuco, E.; Lovely, J.K.; Dhanorker, S.; Grubbs, P.L.; Weaver, A.L.; Haas, L.R.; Borah, B.J.; et al. Enhanced recovery in gynecologic surgery. *Obstet. Gynecol.* **2013**, *122*, 319–328. [CrossRef] [PubMed]
61. Batdorf, N.J.; Lemaine, V.; Lovely, J.K.; Ballman, K.V.; Goede, W.J.; Martinez-Jorge, J.; Booth-Kowalczyk, A.L.; Grubbs, P.L.; Bungum, L.D.; Saint-Cyr, M. Enhanced recovery after surgery in microvascular breast reconstruction. *J. Plast. Reconstr. Aesthetic Surg.* **2015**, *68*, 395–402. [CrossRef]
62. Williams, S.B.; Cumberbatch, M.G.K.; Kamat, A.M.; Jubber, I.; Kerr, P.S.; McGrath, J.S.; Djaladat, H.; Collins, J.W.; Packiam, V.T.; Steinberg, G.D.; et al. Reporting Radical Cystectomy Outcomes Following Implementation of Enhanced Recovery After Surgery Protocols: A Systematic Review and Individual Patient Data Meta-analysis. *Eur. Urol.* **2020**, *78*. [CrossRef]
63. Cerantola, Y.; Valerio, M.; Persson, B.; Jichlinski, P.; Ljungqvist, O.; Hubner, M.; Kassouf, W.; Muller, S.; Baldini, G.; Carli, F.; et al. Guidelines for perioperative care after radical cystectomy for bladder cancer: Enhanced recovery after surgery (ERAS®) society recommendations. *Clin. Nutr.* **2013**, *32*, 879–887. [CrossRef]
64. Carter-Brooks, C.M.; Du, A.L.; Ruppert, K.M.; Romanova, A.L.; Zyczynski, H.M. Implementation of a urogynecology-specific enhanced recovery after surgery (ERAS) pathway. *Am. J. Obstet. Gynecol.* **2018**, *219*, 495.e1–495.e10. [CrossRef]
65. Agarwal, V.; Divatia, J.V. Enhanced recovery after surgery in liver resection: Current concepts and controversies. *Korean J. Anesthesiol.* **2019**, *72*, 119–129. [CrossRef] [PubMed]
66. Melloul, E.; Hübner, M.; Scott, M.; Snowden, C.; Prentis, J.; Dejong, C.H.C.; Garden, O.J.; Farges, O.; Kokudo, N.; Vauthey, J.N.; et al. Guidelines for Perioperative Care for Liver Surgery: Enhanced Recovery After Surgery (ERAS) Society Recommendations. *World J. Surg.* **2016**, *40*, 2425–2440. [CrossRef] [PubMed]
67. Low, D.E.; Allum, W.; De Manzoni, G.; Ferri, L.; Immanuel, A.; Kuppusamy, M.K.; Law, S.; Lindblad, M.; Maynard, N.; Neal, J.; et al. Guidelines for Perioperative Care in Esophagectomy: Enhanced Recovery After Surgery (ERAS®) Society Recommendations. *World J. Surg.* **2019**, *43*, 299–330. [CrossRef]
68. Batchelor, T.J.P.; Rasburn, N.J.; Abdelnour-Berchtold, E.; Brunelli, A.; Cerfolio, R.J.; Gonzalez, M.; Ljungqvist, O.; Petersen, R.H.; Popescu, W.M.; Slinger, P.D.; et al. Guidelines for enhanced recovery after lung surgery: Recommendations of the Enhanced Recovery after Surgery (ERAS®) Society and the European Society of Thoracic Surgeons (ESTS). *Eur. J. Cardio-Thorac. Surg.* **2019**, *55*, 91–115. [CrossRef] [PubMed]
69. Brustia, P.; Renghi, A.; Aronici, M.; Gramaglia, L.; Porta, C.; Musiani, A.; Martelli, M.; Casella, F.; De Simeis, M.L.; Coppi, G.; et al. Fast-track in abdominal aortic surgery: Experience in over 1000 patients. *Ann. Vasc. Surg.* **2015**, *29*, 1151–1159. [CrossRef]
70. Witcher, A.; Axley, J.; Novak, Z.; Laygo-Prickett, M.; Guthrie, M.; Xhaja, A.; Chu, D.I.; Brokus, S.D.; Spangler, E.L.; Passman, M.A.; et al. Implementation of an enhanced recovery program for lower extremity bypass. *J. Vasc. Surg.* **2021**, *73*. [CrossRef]
71. Huebner, M.; Larson, D.W.; Cima, R.R.; Habermann, E. 785 Impact of Key Factors of Enhanced Recovery Pathway and Preexisting Comorbidities on Complications and Length of Stay Following Colorectal Surgery. *Gastroenterology* **2013**, *144*, S-1061. [CrossRef]
72. Paton, F.; Chambers, D.; Wilson, P.; Eastwood, A.; Craig, D.; Fox, D.; Jayne, D.; McGinnes, E. Effectiveness and implementation of enhanced recovery after surgery programmes: A rapid evidence synthesis. *BMJ Open* **2014**, *4*, e005015. [CrossRef]

73. Grass, F.; Lovely, J.K.; Crippa, J.; Hübner, M.; Mathis, K.L.; Larson, D.W. Potential association between perioperative fluid management and occurrence of postoperative ileus. *Dis. Colon Rectum* **2020**, *63*, 68–74. [CrossRef]
74. Zhu, A.C.C.; Agarwala, A.; Bao, X. Perioperative Fluid Management in the Enhanced Recovery after Surgery (ERAS) Pathway. *Clin. Colon Rectal Surg.* **2019**, *32*, 114–120. [CrossRef]
75. Grass, F.; Hübner, M.; Mathis, K.L.; Hahnloser, D.; Dozois, E.J.; Kelley, S.R.; Demartines, N.; Larson, D.W. Challenges to accomplish stringent fluid management standards 7 years after enhanced recovery after surgery implementation—The surgeon's perspective. *Surgery (United States)* **2020**, *168*, 313–319. [CrossRef] [PubMed]
76. Bisch, S.; Nelson, G.; Altman, A. Impact of nutrition on enhanced recovery after surgery (ERAS) in gynecologic oncology. *Nutrients* **2019**, *11*, 1088. [CrossRef]
77. Artinyan, A.; Nunoo-Mensah, J.W.; Balasubramaniam, S.; Gauderman, J.; Essani, R.; Gonzalez-Ruiz, C.; Kaiser, A.M.; Beart, R.W. Prolonged postoperative ileus - Definition, risk factors, and predictors after surgery. *World J. Surg.* **2008**, *32*, 1495–1500. [CrossRef]
78. Grass, F.; Hübner, M.; Lovely, J.K.; Crippa, J.; Mathis, K.L.; Larson, D.W. Ordering a normal diet at the end of surgery—Justified or overhasty? *Nutrients* **2018**, *10*, 1758. [CrossRef] [PubMed]
79. Kelley, S.R.; Wolff, B.G.; Lovely, J.K.; Larson, D.W. Fast-track pathway for minimally invasive colorectal surgery with and without alvimopan (entereg)^{TM}: Which is more cost-effective? *Am. Surg.* **2013**, *79*, 630–633. [CrossRef]
80. Chen, F.; Rasouli, M.R.; Ellis, A.R.; Ohnuma, T.; Bartz, R.R.; Krishnamoorthy, V.; Haines, K.L.; Raghunathan, K. Associations Between Perioperative Crystalloid Volume and Adverse Outcomes in Five Surgical Populations. *J. Surg. Res.* **2020**, *251*, 26–32. [CrossRef]
81. Evans, T.; Koek, S.; Ballal, M. Perioperative restrictive intravenous fluid therapy in eras in pancreaticoduodenectomy. *HPB* **2018**, *20*, S240–S241. [CrossRef]
82. Guan, Z.; Gao, Y.; Qiao, Q.; Wang, Q.; Liu, J. Effects of intraoperative goal-directed fluid therapy and restrictive fluid therapy combined with enhanced recovery after surgery protocol on complications after thoracoscopic lobectomy in high-risk patients: Study protocol for a prospective randomized controlled trial. *Trials* **2021**, *22*, 1–8. [CrossRef]
83. Cima, R.; Dankbar, E.; Lovely, J.; Pendlimari, R.; Aronhalt, K.; Nehring, S.; Hyke, R.; Tyndale, D.; Rogers, J.; Quast, L. Colorectal surgery surgical site infection reduction program: A national surgical quality improvement program-driven multidisciplinary single-institution experience. *J. Am. Coll. Surg.* **2013**, *216*, 23–33. [CrossRef]
84. Waits, S.A.; Fritze, D.; Banerjee, M.; Zhang, W.; Kubus, J.; Englesbe, M.J.; Campbell, D.A.; Hendren, S. Developing an argument for bundled interventions to reduce surgical site infection in colorectal surgery. *Surgery (United States)* **2014**, *155*, 602–606. [CrossRef]
85. Hollis, R.H.; Kennedy, G.D. Postoperative Complications After Colorectal Surgery: Where Are We in the Era of Enhanced Recovery? *Curr. Gastroenterol. Rep.* **2020**, *22*, 1–7. [CrossRef]
86. Wiener, J.G.D.; Goss, L.; Wahl, T.S.; Terry, M.A.; Burge, K.G.; Chu, D.I.; Richman, J.S.; Cannon, J.; Kennedy, G.D.; Morris, M.S. The association of enhanced recovery pathway and acute kidney injury in patients undergoing colorectal surgery. *Dis. Colon Rectum* **2020**, *63*, 233–241. [CrossRef]
87. Hassinger, T.E.; Turrentine, F.E.; Thiele, R.H.; Sarosiek, B.M.; McMurry, T.L.; Friel, C.M.; Hedrick, T.L. Acute kidney injury in the age of enhanced recovery protocols. *Dis. Colon Rectum* **2018**, *61*, 946–954. [CrossRef]
88. Hanna, P.T.; Peterson, M.; Albersheim, J.; Drawz, P.; Zabell, J.; Konety, B.; Weight, C. Acute Kidney Injury following Enhanced Recovery after Surgery in Patients Undergoing Radical Cystectomy. *J. Urol.* **2020**, *204*. [CrossRef] [PubMed]
89. Grass, F.; Lovely, J.K.; Crippa, J.; Mathis, K.L.; Hübner, M.; Larson, D.W. Early Acute Kidney Injury Within an Established Enhanced Recovery Pathway: Uncommon and Transitory. *World J. Surg.* **2019**, *43*, 1207–1215. [CrossRef] [PubMed]
90. Hübner, M.; Lovely, J.K.; Huebner, M.; Slettedahl, S.W.; Jacob, A.K.; Larson, D.W. Intrathecal analgesia and restrictive perioperative fluid management within enhanced recovery pathway: Hemodynamic implications. *J. Am. Coll. Surg.* **2013**, *216*, 1124–1134. [CrossRef] [PubMed]
91. Danelich, I.M.; Bergquist, J.R.; Bergquist, W.J.; Osborn, J.L.; Wright, S.S.; Tefft, B.J.; Sturm, A.W.; Langworthy, D.R.; Mandrekar, J.; Devine, R.M.; et al. Early diuresis after colon and rectal surgery does not reduce length of hospital stay: Results of a randomized trial. *Dis. Colon Rectum* **2018**, *61*, 1187–1195. [CrossRef]
92. Morgenthaler, T.I.; Lovely, J.K.; Cima, R.R.; Berardinelli, C.F.; Fedraw, L.A.; Wallerich, T.J.; Hinrichs, D.J.; Varkey, P. Using a framework for spread of best practices to implement successful venous thromboembolism prophylaxis throughout a large hospital system. *Am. J. Med. Qual.* **2012**, *27*, 30–38. [CrossRef]
93. McKenna, N.P.; Shariq, O.A.; Bews, K.A.; Mathis, K.L.; Lightner, A.L. Venous thromboembolism in inflammatory bowel disease: Is it the disease, the operation, or both? *Dis. Colon Rectum* **2018**, *61*, e138.
94. McKenna, N.P.; Bews, K.A.; Behm, K.T.; Mathis, K.L.; Lightner, A.L.; Habermann, E.B. Do patients with inflammatory bowel disease have a higher postoperative risk of venous thromboembolism or do they undergo more high-risk operations? *Ann. Surg.* **2020**, *271*, 325–331. [CrossRef]
95. Danelich, I.M.; Lose, J.M.; Wright, S.S.; Asirvatham, S.J.; Ballinger, B.A.; Larson, D.W.; Lovely, J.K. Practical management of postoperative atrial fibrillation after noncardiac surgery. *J. Am. Coll. Surg.* **2014**, *219*, 831–841. [CrossRef]
96. Ostermann, S.; Morel, P.; Chalé, J.J.; Bucher, P.; Konrad, B.; Meier, R.P.H.; Ris, F.; Schiffer, E.R.C. Randomized Controlled Trial of Enhanced Recovery Program Dedicated to Elderly Patients after Colorectal Surgery. *Dis. Colon Rectum* **2019**, *62*, 1105–1116. [CrossRef]

97. Chin, A.B.; Galante, D.J.; Hobson, D.B.; Efron, J.E.; Gearhart, S.L.; Safar, B.; Fang, S.H.; Wu, C.; Wick, E.C. Readmission after Enhanced Recovery in Colorectal Patients. *J. Am. Coll. Surg.* **2015**, *221*, S36. [CrossRef]
98. Grass, F.; Crippa, J.; Lovely, J.K.; Ansell, J.; Behm, K.T.; Achilli, P.; Hübner, M.; Kelley, S.R.; Mathis, K.L.; Dozois, E.J.; et al. Readmissions within 48 Hours of Discharge: Reasons, Risk Factors, and Potential Improvements. *Dis. Colon Rectum* **2020**, *63*, 1142–1150. [CrossRef]
99. Michard, F.; Gan, T.J.; Kehlet, H. Digital innovations and emerging technologies for enhanced recovery programmes. *Br. J. Anaesth.* **2017**, *119*, 31–39. [CrossRef]

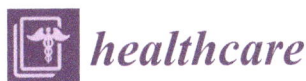 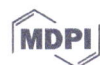

Project Report

Expanding Pharmacotherapy Data Collection, Analysis, and Implementation in ERAS® Programs—the Methodology of an Exploratory Feasibility Study

Eric Johnson [1], Richard Parrish II [2,*], Gregg Nelson [3], Kevin Elias [4], Brian Kramer [5] and Marian Gaviola [6]

1. Department of Pharmacy Services, University of Kentucky, Lexington, KY 40506, USA; eric.johnson@uky.edu
2. Department of Biomedical Sciences, Mercer University School of Medicine, Macon, GA 31207, USA
3. Department of Obstetrics and Gynecology, University of Calgary, Calgary, AB T2N 1N4, Canada; Gregg.Nelson@albertahealthservices.ca
4. Department of Obstetrics, Gynecology and Reproductive Biology, Harvard Medical School, Boston, MA 02115, USA; kelias@bwh.harvard.edu
5. Department of Pharmacy Services, Grant Medical Center, Columbus, OH 43215, USA; bkramer321@gmail.com
6. College of Pharmacy, University of North Texas, Denton, TX 76203, USA; marian.gaviola@gmail.com
* Correspondence: parrish_rh@mercer.edu

Received: 12 June 2020; Accepted: 29 July 2020; Published: 3 August 2020

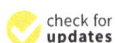

Abstract: Surgical organizations dedicated to the improvement of patient outcomes have led to a worldwide paradigm shift in perioperative patient care. Since 2012, the Enhanced Recovery After Surgery (ERAS®) Society has published guidelines pertaining to perioperative care in numerous disciplines including elective colorectal and gynecologic/oncology surgery patients. The ERAS® and ERAS-USA® Societies use standardized methodology for collecting and assessing various surgical parameters in real-time during the operative process. These multi-disciplinary groups have constructed a bundled framework of perioperative care that entails 22 specific components of clinical interventions, which are logged in a central database, allowing a system of audit and feedback. Of these 22 recommendations, nine of them specifically involve the use of medications or pharmacotherapy. This retrospective comparative pharmacotherapy project will address the potential need to (1) collect more specific pharmacotherapy data within the existing ERAS Interactive Audit System® (EIAS) program, (2) understand the relationship between medication regimen and patient outcomes, and (3) minimize variability in pharmacotherapy use in the elective colorectal and gynecologic/oncology surgical cohort. Primary outcomes measures include data related to surgical site infections, venous thromboembolism, and post-operative nausea and vomiting as well as patient satisfaction, the frequency and severity of post-operative complications, length of stay, and hospital re-admission at 7 and 30 days, respectively. The methodology of this collaborative research project is described.

Keywords: collaboration; enhanced recovery; infection, surgical wound; perioperative care; pharmacy, clinical; post-operative nausea and vomiting; prophylaxis; surgeon; surgery; colorectal; surgery; gynecological; thromboembolism; venous

1. Introduction

Since 2012, the Enhanced Recovery After Surgery (ERAS®) Society has published guidelines pertaining to perioperative care in numerous disciplines including elective colorectal [1] and gynecologic/oncology [2–4] surgery patients. These bundled guidelines contain recommendations on the use of pharmacologic therapy, including prophylaxis for (1) surgical site infection (SSI), (2) thromboembolism (VTE), and (3) postoperative nausea and vomiting (PONV), among others. While the guidelines contain high-quality evidence of the use of pharmacotherapy in each of these ERAS program elements, the specifics of agent selection and dosing regimens are absent. These dosing variables include medication administration time in relation to the procedure, dose of medication used, and duration of therapy. The literature suggests that the lack of effective prophylaxis to address these three endpoints is associated with significant clinical morbidity, and they may be independent drivers of hospital length of stay. Suboptimal preventive pharmacotherapy may lead to increased complication rates and delayed patient discharge from the facility.

The ERAS® and ERAS-USA® Societies use a standardized methodology for collecting and assessing various surgical parameters in real-time during the operative process [5]. By utilizing a retrospective multi-center research design, this project will address the potential need to (1) collect more specific pharmacotherapy data within the existing ERAS Interactive Audit System® (EIAS) program, (2) understand the relationship between medication regimen and patient outcomes, and (3) minimize variability in pharmacotherapy use in the elective colorectal and gynecologic/oncology surgical cohort. The specific aims of this project include:

1. Creation of a pharmacotherapy database and execution of a retrospective analysis to compile perioperative medication-specific data related to significant improvements in patient outcomes.
2. Estimation of the impact of prophylaxis medications on length of stay, postoperative complications, and hospital readmission rates at 7 and 30 days for the following indications:

    a. Surgical site infections;
    b. Thromboembolism;
    c. Post-operative nausea and vomiting.

3. Provide guidance on optimal medication use regarding regimen selection, dosing, timing, and duration of therapy.

2. Research Strategy

The development and evolution of Enhanced Recovery Programs have led to significant improvements in the care of surgical patients, as well as a decrease in important benchmarks such as hospital length of stay (LOS) and postoperative complications [6]. As a result, surgical organizations dedicated to the improvement of patient outcomes have led a paradigm shift in perioperative patient care. Specific groups, like the Enhanced Recovery After Surgery (ERAS®) Society and ERAS® USA, have constructed a bundled framework of care entailing 22 specific components of perioperative clinical interventions, which are logged in a central database, allowing a system of audit and feedback. Of these 22 recommendations, nine of them specifically involve the use of medications or pharmacotherapy. They include the following: (1) pre-anesthetic medication; (2) prophylaxis against venous thromboembolism (VTE); (3) antimicrobial prophylaxis and skin preparation; (4) standard anesthetic protocol; (5) post-operative nausea and vomiting (PONV) prophylaxis; (6) perioperative fluid management; (7) prevention of postoperative ileus (including use of postoperative laxatives); (8) postoperative analgesia, and (9) postoperative glucose control [7]. While these recommendations address global concepts of perioperative patient care, the ERAS protocols do not specify particular pharmacotherapeutic medication classes, agents, or doses. As a result of the inherent variability in medication use, the optimal pharmacotherapeutic agents within ERAS® pathways are unknown. Furthermore, variance in the timing of medication administration leaves practitioners searching for the exact method of replicating the significant outcomes found in ERAS publications.

In its current form, EIAS® collects limited information related to medication administration for ERAS® patients. Despite this dearth, patient outcomes have consistently improved in institutions that have adopted ERAS® pathways. Whether these improvements are due to individual therapeutic agents or the application of a bundled approach is unknown. Practitioners and pharmacists are challenged to make evidence-based pharmacotherapeutic recommendations of agents within the protocol. Inevitably, debates on implementation often center on more costly versions of medications such as intravenous acetaminophen or liposomal bupivacaine as means to limit opioid use.

We plan to integrate de-identified patient data from two separate ERAS® centers in North America with pharmacotherapy data collected retrospectively from each site. From this registry, we will seek answers to comparative pharmacotherapy questions embedded in the ERAS® pathway. Specifically, we plan to evaluate the following: (1) timing of preoperative and post-operative thromboprophylaxis and the impact on post-operative VTE; (2) specific agents and doses of antimicrobials used in surgical antimicrobial prophylaxis, and (3) optimal and efficacious regimens in the successful prevention of PONV.

3. Approach

Our Enhanced Recovery Comparative Pharmacotherapy Collaborative (ERCPC) group plans to evaluate the role that specific pharmacotherapeutic regimens within the ERAS® protocol play in regard to the improved outcomes, readmission, and hospital LOS. In addition, data regarding patient experience or satisfaction scores will be collected. This information will be obtained through patient registry of the EIAS®. The two institutions that have provided written support for access to their patients' data are the Foothills Medical Centre (FMC) of Calgary, Alberta, Canada and the Brigham & Women's Hospital of Boston, MA, USA. Both institutions have robust ERAS® practices and are leading researchers in the practice of enhanced surgical recovery.

Data from patient healthcare records at each site will be collected and entered into a centralized REDCap database. The project's data dictionary is included in a Supplementary Material File attachment. Patient demographics, intraoperative anesthetic techniques, and procedure details will also be collected. Drug-related variables will be compared to determine the effect of agent use on outcome measures. Potential hurdles that we anticipate are low event rates with some primary outcomes measures, specifically VTE. Recent literature suggests that the incidence of VTE in colorectal surgery patients is approximately 2.2% [8,9]. While a population of 500 colorectal patients would have an estimated incidence of 11 cases, we may be challenged to obtain a difference between groups if numerous different regimens are used. Gynecologic and colorectal malignancy patients show a similarly low incidence; however, it is slightly higher at approximately 3% [10] and is purported to be on the rise [11]. By combining the two patient populations, we estimate a sufficient number of thromboembolic events from which we will be able to ascertain a statistical difference. Additionally, because we will be evaluating the pharmacotherapeutic interventions from ERAS®, it is possible that ERAS® components not captured in our analysis may play more significant roles in reducing negative outcomes compared to the agents that we evaluate. However, if no difference is found, this may too provide justification for the use of different regimens within the ERAS pathway. Finally, we have strong physician support from experienced researchers who are eager to participate in this project.

4. Specific Research Questions

1. Determine the *optimal antimicrobial agents used in surgical prophylaxis*, including pre-operative dose, timing of preoperative dose, intraoperative repeat doses, postoperative duration of therapy, classification of surgical site infection (if present), and infection organism (if applicable) [12].
2. Provide evidence to define *optimal prophylaxis regimens to prevent PONV* in this surgical population. Specific parameters of analysis include PONV risk factors, preoperative Apfel risk score [13], prophylaxis regimen (dose, timing), postoperative nausea, and duration of Post Anesthesia Care Unit (PACU) LOS [14].
3. Evaluate the effect that *venous thromboembolism (VTE) prophylaxis* provides in preventing post-operative VTE in high-risk oncology populations. Specific points of evaluation include

prophylaxis agent used (unfractionated heparin versus low-molecular weight heparin verses direct thrombin inhibitors), perioperative timing of dose, post-operative duration of therapy, thromboembolic risk factors, and patient weight [15,16].

5. Conclusions

Our ERCPC group plans to evaluate the impact that specific pharmacotherapeutic regimens within the ERAS® protocol have on primary clinical outcomes (surgical site infections, venous thromboembolism, and post-operative nausea and vomiting) as well as their relationship to and impact on readmission, complications, and hospital LOS. We plan to integrate de-identified patient data from two separate ERAS® centers in North America with pharmacotherapy data collected retrospectively from each site. From this registry, we will seek answers to comparative pharmacotherapy questions embedded in the ERAS® pathway. Specifically, we plan to evaluate the following: (1) specific agents and doses of antimicrobials used in surgical antimicrobial prophylaxis; (2) timing of preoperative and post-operative thromboprophylaxis and the impact on post-operative VTE, and (3) optimal and efficacious regimens in the successful prevention of PONV.

Supplementary Materials: The following are available online at http://www.mdpi.com/2227-9032/8/3/252/s1, File: Enhanced Recovery Comparative Pharmacotherapy Collaborative (ERCPC) Data Dictionary of Pharmacotherapy Elements.

Author Contributions: Conceptualization, E.J., R.P.II and M.G.; methodology, E.J., R.P.II, G.N., K.E., B.K. and M.G.; writing—original draft preparation, E.J. and R.P.II; writing—review and editing, E.J., R.P.II, G.N., K.E., B.K. and M.G.; project administration, R.P. and M.G. All authors have read and agreed to the published version of the manuscript.

Funding: This research received no external funding.

Acknowledgments: The Enhanced Recovery Comparative Pharmacotherapy Collaborative (ERCPC) appreciates the work of site-basedd contributors and participants.

Conflicts of Interest: The authors declare no conflict of interest.

References

1. Gustafsson, U.O.; Scott, M.J.; Hubner, M.; Nygren, J.; Demartines, N.; Francis, N.; Rockall, T.A.; Young-Fadok, T.M.; Hill, A.G.; Soop, M.; et al. Guidelines for perioperative care in elective colorectal surgery: Enhanced Recovery After Surgery (ERAS®) Society recommendations: 2018. *World J. Surg.* **2019**, *43*, 659–695. [CrossRef] [PubMed]
2. Nelson, G.; Bakkum-Gamez, J.; Kalogera, E.; Glaser, G.; Altman, A.; Meyer, L.A.; Taylor, J.S.; Iniesta, M.; Lasala, J.; Mena, G.; et al. Guidelines for perioperative care in gynecologic/oncology: Enhanced Recovery After Surgery (ERAS) Society recommendations—2019 update. *Int. J. Gynecol. Cancer* **2019**, *29*, 651–668. [CrossRef] [PubMed]
3. Nelson, G.; Altman, A.D.; Nick, A.; Meyer, L.A.; Ramirez, P.T.; Achtari, C.; Antrobus, J.; Huang, J.; Scott, M.; Wijk, L.; et al. Guidelines for pre- and intra-operative care in gynecologic/oncology surgery: Enhanced Recovery After Surgery (ERAS®) Society recommendations—Part I. *Gynecol. Oncol.* **2016**, *140*, 313–322. [CrossRef] [PubMed]
4. Nelson, G.; Altman, A.D.; Nick, A.; Meyer, L.A.; Ramirez, P.T.; Achtari, C.; Antrobus, J.; Huang, J.; Scott, M.; Wijk, L.; et al. Guidelines for postoperative care in gynecologic/oncology surgery: Enhanced Recovery After Surgery (ERAS®) Society recommendations—Part II. *Gynecol. Oncol.* **2016**, *140*, 323–332. [CrossRef] [PubMed]
5. Elias, K.M.; Stone, A.B.; McGinigle, K.; Tankou, J.I.; Scott, M.J.; Fawcett, W.J.; Demartines, N.; Lobo, D.N.; Ljungqvist, O.; Urman, R.D. The reporting on ERAS compliance, outcomes, and elements research (RECOvER) checklist: A joint statement by the ERAS® and ERAS® USA Societies. *World J. Surg.* **2019**, *43*, 1–8. [CrossRef] [PubMed]
6. Lassen, K.; Soop, M.; Nygren, J.; Cox, P.; Hendry, P.; Spies, C.; von Meyenfeldt, M.F.; Fearon, K.C.H.; Revhaug, A.; Nordeval, S.; et al. Consensus review of optimal perioperative care in colorectal surgery:

Enhanced Recovery After Surgery (ERAS) Group recommendations. *Arch. Surg.* **2009**, *144*, 961–969. [CrossRef] [PubMed]
7. Lovely, J.; Hyland, S.; Smith, A.; Nelson, G.; Ljungqvist, O.; Parrish, R.H., II. Clinical pharmacist perspectives for optimizing pharmacotherapy within Enhanced Recovery After Surgery (ERAS®) programs. *Int. J. Surg.* **2019**, *63*, 58–62. [CrossRef] [PubMed]
8. Caprini, J.; Arcelus, J.; Hasty, J.; Tamhane, A.; Fabrega, F. Clinical assessment of venous thromboembolic risk in surgical patients. *Semin. Thromb. Hemost.* **1991**, *17*, 304–312. [PubMed]
9. Nelson, D.W.; Simianu, V.V.; Bastawrous, A.L.; Billingham, R.P.; Fichera, A.; Florence, M.G.; Johnson, E.K.; Johnson, M.G.; Thirlby, R.C.; Flum, D.R.; et al. Thromboembolic complications and prophylaxis patterns in colorectal surgery. *JAMA Surg.* **2015**, *150*, 712–720. [CrossRef] [PubMed]
10. Schmeler, K.; Wilson, G.; Cain, K.; Munsell, M.; Ramirez, P.; Soliman, P.; Nick, A.M.; Frumovitz, M.; Coleman, R.L.; Kroll, M.H.; et al. Venous thromboembolism (VTE) rates following the implementation of extended duration prophylaxis for patients undergoing surgery for gynecologic malignancies. *Gynecol. Oncol.* **2013**, *128*, 204–208. [CrossRef] [PubMed]
11. Rees, P.; Clouston, H.; Duff, S.; Kirwan, C. Colorectal cancer and thrombosis. *Int. J. Colorectal Dis.* **2018**, *33*, 105–108. [CrossRef] [PubMed]
12. Bratzler, D.W.; Dellinger, E.P.; Olsen, K.M.; Perl, T.M.; Auwaerter, P.G.; Bolon, M.K.; Fish, D.N.; Napolitano, L.M.; Sawyer, R.G.; Slain, D.; et al. Clinical practice guidelines for antimicrobial prophylaxis in surgery. *Am. J. Health-Syst. Pharm.* **2013**, *70*, 195–283. [CrossRef] [PubMed]
13. Apfel, C.; Heidrich, F.; Jukar-Rao, S.; Jalota, L.; Hornuss, C.; Whelan, R.; Zhang, K.; Cakmakkaya, O. Evidence-based analysis of risk factors for postoperative nausea and vomiting. *Br. J. Anaesth.* **2012**, *109*, 742–753. [CrossRef] [PubMed]
14. Gan, T.J.; Belani, K.G.; Bergese, S.; Chung, F.; Diemunsch, P.; Habib, A.S.; Jin, Z.; Kovac, A.L.; Meyer, T.A.; Urman, R.D.; et al. Fourth consensus guidelines for the management of postoperative nausea and vomiting. *Anesth. Analg.* **2020**. [CrossRef]
15. Farge, D.; Bounameaux, H.; Brenner, B.; Cajfinger, F.; Debourdeau, P.; Khorana, A.A.; Pabinger, I.; Solymoss, S.; Douketis, J.; Kakkar, A. International clinical practice guidelines including guidance for direct oral anticoagulants in the treatment and prophylaxis of venous thromboembolism in patients with cancer. *Lancet Oncol.* **2016**, *17*, e452–e466. [CrossRef]
16. Hornor, M.A.; Duane, T.M.; Ehlers, A.P.; Jensen, E.H.; Brown, P.S.; Pohl, D.; da Costa, P.M.; Ko, C.Y.; Laronga, C. American College of Surgeons' guidelines for the perioperative management of antithrombotic medication. *J. Am. Coll. Surg.* **2018**, *227*, 521–536. [CrossRef]

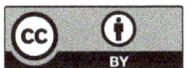

© 2020 by the authors. Licensee MDPI, Basel, Switzerland. This article is an open access article distributed under the terms and conditions of the Creative Commons Attribution (CC BY) license (http://creativecommons.org/licenses/by/4.0/).

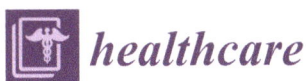 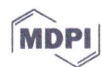

Commentary

The Perioperative Surgical Home in Pediatrics: Improve Patient Outcomes, Decrease Cancellations, Improve HealthCare Spending and Allocation of Resources during the COVID-19 Pandemic

Aysha Hasan [1,2,3,*], Remy Zimmerman [2], Kelly Gillock [2] and Richard H Parrish II [3,4,5]

1. Section of Anesthesiology, St. Christopher's Hospital for Children, Philadelphia, PA 19134, USA
2. College of Medicine, Drexel University, Philadelphia, PA 19129, USA; rjz34@drexel.edu (R.Z.); kelly.jean.gillock@drexel.edu (K.G.)
3. Tower Health, Reading, PA 19612, USA; parrish_rh@mercer.edu
4. Department of Pharmacy Services, St. Christopher's Hospital for Children, Philadelphia, PA 19134, USA
5. School of Medicine, Mercer University, Macon, GA 31207, USA
* Correspondence: Aysha.Hasan@TowerHealth.org

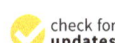

Received: 30 June 2020; Accepted: 6 August 2020; Published: 7 August 2020

Abstract: Cancellations or delays in surgical care for pediatric patients that present to the operating room create a great obstacle for both the physician and the patient. Perioperative outpatient management begins prior to the patient entering the hospital for the day of surgery, and many organizations practice using the perioperative surgical home (PSH), incorporating enhanced recovery concepts. This paper describes changes in standard operating procedures caused by the COVID-19 pandemic, and proposes the expansion of PSH, as a means of improving perioperative quality of care in pediatric populations.

Keywords: anesthesiology; COVID-19; nursing; pediatrics; pharmacy; surgeon; surgical home; perioperative; team-based care

---

Cancellations or delays in surgical care for pediatric patients that present to the operating room create a great obstacle for both the physician and the patient. Currently, in the United States (US), an estimated 343,670 elective operations have been cancelled weekly due to COVID-19 related concerns [1]. While this number focuses on adult cases, the fact remains that a majority of elective surgeries were affected by COVID-19, alluding to an unprecedented increase in cancellations and/or delays of both adult and pediatric surgeries. The medical dollars, hours and personnel wasted in delaying or canceling a case can be avoided by instituting the perioperative surgical home (PSH), especially during the new emergence of COVID-19, and with other chronic illnesses on the rise (i.e., obesity, diabetes) [2].

The PSH model (Figure 1) is a continuous patient-centered approach that involves a multidisciplinary team of physicians and healthcare providers, aimed at individualized attention that begins when the decision for operative care is made and ends approximately 30 days after hospital discharge [3]. Not only does this increase coordination between physicians, but it provides a standardized, evidence-based approach to patient care [4]. This streamlined model decreases unnecessary testing and cancellations, providing greater operative room access for in-patients, and contributing to decreased healthcare costs. PSH in a pediatric setting allows the child to be holistically evaluated by the perioperative team, including the pediatrician. Furthermore, anesthesiologists are well equipped to lead this team, as they play a critical role in preoperative, intraoperative and postoperative care, and are essential to postoperative pain management [5].

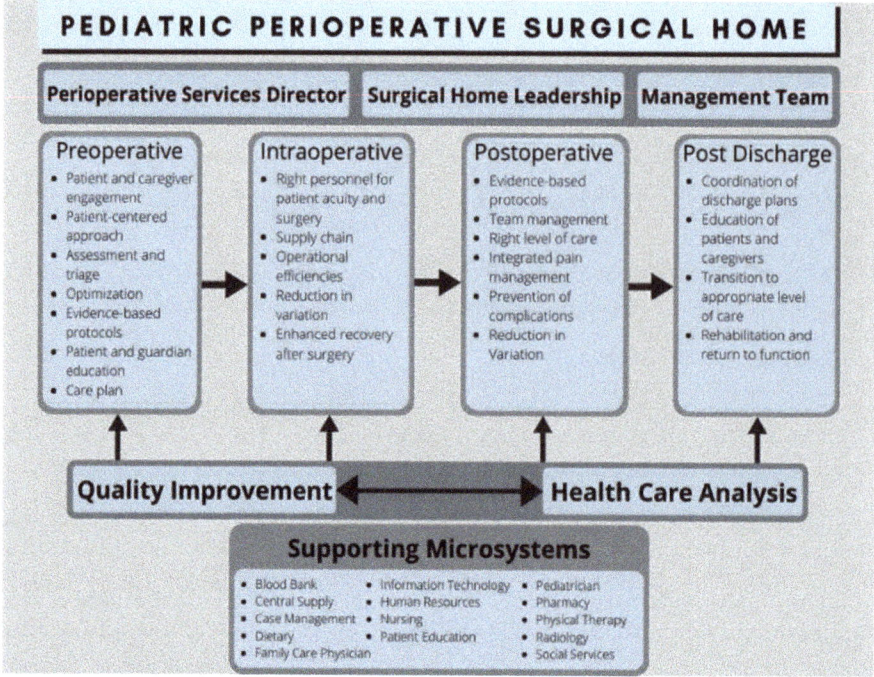

Figure 1. Diagram illustrating an overview of Pediatric Perioperative Surgical Home. This has been adapted for pediatric implementation from the American Society of Anesthesiologists' Perioperative Surgical Home Collaborative [6].

Despite being introduced recently with its first proposal in 2011, PSH has gained traction for its impact in the United States healthcare system, but the concept of perioperative medicine exists globally [7]. France, among other European countries, adopted Enhanced Recovery After Surgery (ERAS ®) guidelines, to implement structured protocols with the goal of improved patient outcomes; although, standardizations vary in regard to the applied specialty. In contrast, PSH focuses on patient-centered care, lowering healthcare costs, and improving patient experience via quality of care and patient satisfaction [8]. However, due to a plethora of factors, such as increasing healthcare costs, decreasing quality of patient care, and government incentives, both France and the United States are opting toward PSH, an individualized approach to perioperative medicine [3].

Incorporating pediatric-appropriate enhanced recovery concepts, perioperative outpatient management begins prior to the patient entering the hospital for the day of surgery [8]. Many health systems and surgical organizations practice using the PSH, in which the patient is seen in a team-based approach to address any issues that may delay or prohibit surgery. Pediatric PSH has not only been known to help reduce healthcare costs and increase patient and family satisfaction, but it also lowers school absences, reduces the impact on parents and patients, and decreases hospitalizations, emergency room visits and patient length of stay [9,10]. Kash et al. further validated this claim in a study analyzing US perioperative initiatives, including PSH models and PSH-like models, where 82% of those studied were reported to have significant positive results for cost and efficiency of hospital resources, as well as clinical outcomes [11]. While this study examines adult clinical care facilities, subsequent positive responses have been observed in pediatric settings; however, a scarcity of multicentered studies exist, due to fewer instances of implementation in pediatric hospitals.

The patient's perioperative period continues, as the patient optimizes their healthcare status with procedural education, medications, laboratory work, overcoming anxiety and inquire further with regards to their procedure. The patient enters the hospital fasting from the night before, and continues the process through admissions and entering the same day holding area. Similarly, inpatients begin this process typically the day they are admitted until they are down in the operating room. Statistically, only 4% of elective procedures were cancelled after seeing an anesthesiologist for preoperative evaluation, as compared to 11% of the patients being unseen [12].

In the current climate, we are facing, as healthcare practitioners, perioperative practice has changed drastically. Currently, many patients are required to be tested for pathogens such as coronavirus prior to entry into the operating room [13]. Patient access to primary care physicians is limited by volume, panic, fear and anxiety, exacerbated by mandated self-isolation and quarantine protocol [14]. Thus, by implementing PSH in pediatric hospitals, primary care physicians are incorporated within the perioperative team, allowing remote access to care. Patient fear and panic can be limited or avoided, while still providing adequate care.

In addition, patients and guardians are fearful and anxiety ridden, of not only the procedure they are undergoing, but also of the risk of acquiring an infection or other acute illness. Patients and their families are hesitant to admit to potential exposure of COVID-19 (large gatherings, unsafe hygiene, not wearing a mask in public, etc.) on the day of surgery for the fear of cancellation, thereby potentially increasing risk factors to providers and to themselves. The outcomes of a patient with COVID-19 receiving a surgical procedure with or without anesthesia are unknown, while in other upper respiratory infections, post-operative complications can be dire [15]. Patients may even avoid coming to the hospital altogether and avoid necessary procedures because of exposure concerns. Elective procedures are no longer performed at 100% capacity in facilities across the country, because fear dominates the healthcare sector [16]. A system conceived as onerous is designed to alleviate some of the fears, prepare the patients for surgery, test the asymptomatic patient for antibodies and high risk patients with swabs and antibody tests (in the COVID-19 era), to provide useful information to both the patient and healthcare team is already in place but underutilized. Beyond the COVID era we face today, the perioperative surgical home can capture potential infections, chronic underlying diseases that need further management, and risk assessment that can provide information to the practitioners, especially when the patient is on the operating room table. PSH is a centralized concept capable of overcoming many of these obstacles faced by the healthcare industry, especially those aimed toward the pediatric population.

PSH consists of the patient visiting the anesthesiologist in a clinic-based setting. It is comprised of helping the patient and parents understand the decision of proceeding with the proposed procedure, the risks and benefits of the procedure, and recovery afterwards. It has also helped advance the enhanced recovery after surgery initiative by beginning protocols, to enhance success in advance (i.e., adequate hydration) [17]. This model helps to identify and resolve risk stratification strategies prior to the day of surgery, allowing all teams involved from admissions, nursing, pharmacy, physicians and technical staff to be prepared for the patient, rather than hurrying to gather tools, medication and personnel the day of the procedure. It is also a vital component in pediatric hospitals. In the pediatric realm, patients are accompanied by a legal guardian that must also be involved in the patient's care, decisions and preparation of surgery. The PSH can facilitate coordination between families and healthcare providers especially, since many individuals are often required in the care of the pediatric patient [18]. It is worth mentioning that pediatric populations may suffer from rare or congenital disorders that often require specialists or individualized care for psychosocial concerns [18,19]. In addition, treating children through the use of PSH also presents age-related challenges, due to physiological and surgical variability in comparison to adults [20]. For these reasons, it is imperative that the core focus of the perioperative period is the health of the patient rather than the physician or specialty supervising care [18]. Therefore, continuity of care must be maintained across specialties, subspecialties, and facilities.

This pandemic is a reminder that, as a hospital system, we are highly unequipped to deal with the unknown. In order to prepare for the unknown, a system in which patients are screened in advance for acute and chronic illnesses, hospitals or surgical centers is prepared for possible complications. Team members are all informed in advance, not only to improve patient healthcare, but it will also reduce wasteful costs, complications and cancellations. Many hospitals have yet to adapt and mandate the implementation of PSH. Studies show that the benefits of implementing the perioperative surgical home are cost saving [3,8,21]. With this knowledge, the perioperative team should work collaboratively to implement and mandate all patients that present for elective procedures receive clearance from the perioperative surgical home.

Author Contributions: A.H. conceived the paper idea, drafted the outline, wrote the initial manuscript, and read and approved the final version; R.Z. and K.G. reviewed and edited the manuscript, and read and approved the final version; R.HP.II reviewed and contributed to the initial outline, performed a literature search, wrote the abstract, derived the key words, reviewed and edited the paper, and read and approved the final version. All authors have read and agreed to the published version of the manuscript.

Funding: This research received no external funding.

Conflicts of Interest: The authors declare no conflict of interest.

References

1. COVIDSurg Collaborative; Nepogodiev, D.; Bhangu, A. Elective Surgery Cancellations Due to the COVID-19 Pandemic: Global Predictive Modelling to Inform Surgical Recovery Plans. *Br. J. Surg.* **2020**. [CrossRef]
2. Xiao, G.; van Jaarsveld, W.; Dong, M.; de Klundert, J. Stochastic programming analysis and solutions to schedule overcrowded operating rooms in China. *Comput. Oper. Res.* **2016**, *74*, 78–91. [CrossRef]
3. Desebbe, O.; Lanz, T.; Kain, Z.; Cannesson, M. The perioperative surgical home: An innovative, patient-centred and cost-effective perioperative care model. *Anaesth. Crit. Care Pain Med.* **2016**, *35*, 59–66. [CrossRef]
4. Nicolescu, T.O. Perioperative Surgical Home. Meeting Tomorrow's Challenges. *Rom. J. Anaesth. Intensiv. Care* **2016**, *23*, 141. [CrossRef]
5. Walters, T.L.; Mariano, E.R.; Clark, J.D. Perioperative Surgical Home and the Integral Role of Pain Medicine. *Pain Med.* **2015**, *16*, 1666–1672. [CrossRef] [PubMed]
6. American Society of Anesthesiologists. Perioperative Surgical Home Collaborative. Available online: https://www.perioperativesurgicalhome.org (accessed on 2 August 2020).
7. Wanderer, J.P.; Rathmell, J.P. A Brief History of the Perioperative Surgical Home. *Anesthesiology* **2015**, *123*, A23. [CrossRef] [PubMed]
8. Elhassan, A.; Elhassan, I.; Elhassan, A.; Sekar, K.D.; Cornett, E.M.; Urman, R.D.; Kaye, A.D. Perioperative surgical home models and enhanced recovery after surgery. *J. Anaesthesiol. Clin. Pharmacol.* **2019**, *35*, S46–S50. [CrossRef] [PubMed]
9. Antonelli, R.C.; McAllister, J.W.; Popp, J. Making care coordination a critical component of the pediatric health system: A multidisciplinary framework. *Commonw. Fund* **2009**, *110*, 1–26.
10. Raman, V.T. The Rise of Value-based Care in Pediatric Surgical Patients: Perioperative Surgical Home, Enhanced Recovery After Surgery, and Coordinated Care Models. *Int. Anesthesiol. Clin.* **2019**, *57*, 15–24. [CrossRef] [PubMed]
11. Kash, B.A.; Zhang, Y.; Cline, K.M.; Menser, T.; Miller, T.R. The Perioperative Surgical Home (PSH): A Comprehensive Review of US and Non-US Studies Shows Predominantly Positive Quality and Cost Outcomes. *Milbank Q.* **2014**, *92*, 796–821. [CrossRef] [PubMed]
12. American Society of Anesthesiologists. Perioperative Surgical Home. Available online: https://www.asahq.org/psh (accessed on 18 June 2020).
13. Di Gennaro, F.; Pizzol, D.; Claudia Marotta, C.; Antunes, M.; Racalbuto, V.; Veronese, N.; Smith, L. Coronavirus Diseases (COVID-19) Current Status and Future Perspectives: A Narrative Review. *Int. J. Environ. Res. Public Health* **2020**, *17*, 2690. [CrossRef] [PubMed]
14. Montemurro, N. The Emotional Impact of COVID-19: From Medical Staff to Common People. *Brain Behav. Immun.* **2020**, *87*, 23–24. [CrossRef] [PubMed]

15. Vazquez, A.O.R.; Rosenbaum, S. Anesthesia for Adults with Upper Respiratory Infection. Up-To-Date. February 2020. Available online: https://www.uptodate.com/contents/anesthesia-for-adults-with-upper-respiratory-infection (accessed on 18 June 2020).
16. Diaz, A.; Sarac, B.A.; Schoenbrunner, A.R.; Janis, J.E.; Pawlik, T.M. Elective surgery in the time of COVID-19. *Am. J. Surg.* **2020**, *219*, 900–902. [CrossRef] [PubMed]
17. American Society of Anesthesiologists. Perioperative Surgical Home: In the Spotlight. Available online: https://www.asahq.org/in-the-spotlight/perioperative-surgical-home (accessed on 18 June 2020).
18. Ferrari, L.R.; Antonelli, R.C.; Bader, A. Beyond the Preoperative Clinic: Considerations for Pediatric Care Redesign Aligning the Patient/Family-Centered Medical Home and the Perioperative Surgical Home. *Anesth. Analg.* **2015**, *120*, 1167–1170. [CrossRef] [PubMed]
19. Berry, J.G.; Ash, A.S.; Cohen, E.; Hasan, F.; Feudtner, C.; Hall, M. Contributions of children with multiple chronic conditions to pediatric hospitalizations in the United States: A retrospective cohort analysis. *Hosp. Pediatr.* **2017**, *7*, 365–372. [CrossRef] [PubMed]
20. Raman, V.T.; Tumin, D.; Uffman, J.; Thung, A.; Burrier, C.; Jatana, K.R.; Elmaraghy, C.; Tobias, J.D. Implementation of a perioperative surgical home protocol for pediatric patients presenting for adenoidectomy. *Int. J. Pediatr. Otorhinolaryngol.* **2017**, *101*, 215–222. [CrossRef] [PubMed]
21. Dexter, F.; Wachtel, R.E. Strategies for net cost reductions with the expanded role and expertise of anesthesiologists in the perioperative surgical home. *Anesth. Analg.* **2014**, *118*, 1062–1071. [CrossRef] [PubMed]

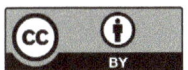

© 2020 by the authors. Licensee MDPI, Basel, Switzerland. This article is an open access article distributed under the terms and conditions of the Creative Commons Attribution (CC BY) license (http://creativecommons.org/licenses/by/4.0/).

15. Vazquez, A.O.R.; Rosenbaum, S. Anesthesia for Adults with Upper Respiratory Infection. Up-To-Date. February 2020. Available online: https://www.uptodate.com/contents/anesthesia-for-adults-with-upper-respiratory-infection (accessed on 18 June 2020).
16. Diaz, A.; Sarac, B.A.; Schoenbrunner, A.R.; Janis, J.E.; Pawlik, T.M. Elective surgery in the time of COVID-19. *Am. J. Surg.* **2020**, *219*, 900–902. [CrossRef] [PubMed]
17. American Society of Anesthesiologists. Perioperative Surgical Home: In the Spotlight. Available online: https://www.asahq.org/in-the-spotlight/perioperative-surgical-home (accessed on 18 June 2020).
18. Ferrari, L.R.; Antonelli, R.C.; Bader, A. Beyond the Preoperative Clinic: Considerations for Pediatric Care Redesign Aligning the Patient/Family-Centered Medical Home and the Perioperative Surgical Home. *Anesth. Analg.* **2015**, *120*, 1167–1170. [CrossRef] [PubMed]
19. Berry, J.G.; Ash, A.S.; Cohen, E.; Hasan, F.; Feudtner, C.; Hall, M. Contributions of children with multiple chronic conditions to pediatric hospitalizations in the United States: A retrospective cohort analysis. *Hosp. Pediatr.* **2017**, *7*, 365–372. [CrossRef] [PubMed]
20. Raman, V.T.; Tumin, D.; Uffman, J.; Thung, A.; Burrier, C.; Jatana, K.R.; Elmaraghy, C.; Tobias, J.D. Implementation of a perioperative surgical home protocol for pediatric patients presenting for adenoidectomy. *Int. J. Pediatr. Otorhinolaryngol.* **2017**, *101*, 215–222. [CrossRef] [PubMed]
21. Dexter, F.; Wachtel, R.E. Strategies for net cost reductions with the expanded role and expertise of anesthesiologists in the perioperative surgical home. *Anesth. Analg.* **2014**, *118*, 1062–1071. [CrossRef] [PubMed]

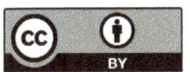

© 2020 by the authors. Licensee MDPI, Basel, Switzerland. This article is an open access article distributed under the terms and conditions of the Creative Commons Attribution (CC BY) license (http://creativecommons.org/licenses/by/4.0/).

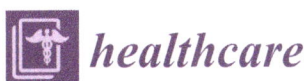 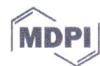

Article

Evaluation of Pediatric Surgical Site Infections Associated with Colorectal Surgeries at an Academic Children's Hospital

Kimberly Pough [1,2,*], Rima Bhakta [3], Holly Maples [1,3], Michele Honeycutt [4] and Vini Vijayan [5]

1. Department of Pharmacy Practice, Arkansas Children's Hospital, Little Rock, AR 72202, USA; MaplesHolly@uams.edu
2. Department of Pharmacy Practice, St. Christopher's Hospital for Children, Philadelphia, PA 19134, USA
3. College of Pharmacy, University of Arkansas for Medical Sciences, Little Rock, AR 72205, USA; RBhakta@uams.edu
4. Department of Infection Prevention and Hospital Epidemiology, Arkansas Children's Hospital, Little Rock, AR 72202, USA; HoneycuttMD@archildrens.org
5. Division of Infectious Diseases, Department of Pediatrics, Valley Children's Hospital, Madera, CA 93636, USA; VVijayan@valleychildrens.org
* Correspondence: Kimberly.Pough@towerhealth.org

Received: 12 March 2020; Accepted: 5 April 2020; Published: 9 April 2020

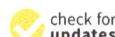

Abstract: Appropriate use of antibiotic prophylaxis (AP) is a key measure for the prevention of surgical site infections (SSI) in colorectal surgeries; however, despite the presence of national and international guidelines, compliance with AP recommendations remains low. The purpose of this study is to evaluate compliance with recommendations for the use of AP in children undergoing colorectal surgeries and to evaluate the effectiveness of antibiotics in the prevention of SSI. We collected demographic and clinical characteristics of patients who underwent colorectal surgeries, as well as microbiological and antimicrobial susceptibility data for patients who developed SSI. AP data were collected and compared with national guidelines. Antibiotic dosing and duration were most frequently in concordance with national guidelines, while antibiotic timing and selection had the lowest rates of compliance. Twelve of the 192 colorectal procedures evaluated resulted in SSI. Only 2 of the 12 children with SSI received appropriate AP for all four categories evaluated. Eight cases that resulted in SSI were due to organisms not covered by the recommended AP. We identified multiple areas for the improvement of AP in children undergoing colorectal surgery. A multidisciplinary approach to development of standardized protocols, educational interventions, and EHR-based algorithms may facilitate or improve appropriate AP use.

Keywords: colorectal surgery; pediatric; surgical prophylaxis; antibiotic prophylaxis; surgical site infections

1. Introduction

According to the Centers for Disease Control and Prevention (CDC), surgical site infections (SSI) are infections that occur at or near the surgical incision within 30 days of a procedure, or 90 days for specified procedures [1]. These infections occur in approximately 2–5% of patients undergoing inpatient surgery in the United States, and account for approximately 20% of healthcare-associated infections in adults as well as children [2]. SSI are associated with high morbidity and mortality rates, and increased durations of hospitalization and healthcare costs [2–4].

Colorectal surgeries are associated with a higher rate of SSI than for other kinds of surgeries, ranging from 5% to 45% due to exposure to the increased bacterial load in the colon and the rectum [3–7].

Current guidelines published by the CDC and the Healthcare Infection Control Practices Advisory Committee for the Prevention of Surgical Site Infection recommend appropriate utilization of systemic antibiotic prophylaxis (AP) within a surgical bundle as a key measure to prevent SSI among patients undergoing colorectal surgeries [8]. Appropriate AP in colorectal procedures is based mainly on 4 principles: (1) correct antibiotic selection; (2) correct dose; (3) timing of administration, including appropriate re-dosing for extended procedures; and (4) discontinuation of antibiotics when the procedure is completed and surgical site is closed, or no more than 24 h post-operatively. The effectiveness of AP in the prevention of SSI is well established. In 2016, the World Health Organization published evidence-based recommendations regarding the use of AP in the prevention of SSI [1,2,9–12]. However, despite the presence of international and national guidelines, compliance with AP for surgical procedures has been staggeringly low among patients undergoing colorectal procedures [13,14].

Clinical evidence in support of AP for the reduction of infectious complications following colorectal surgery is derived almost exclusively from adult literature. There are no well-controlled studies evaluating the efficacy of AP and compliance with surgical AP in children undergoing colorectal procedures. However, as children and adults have similar fecal bacterial concentration and microbiological profiles, there is little reason to suspect that current guidelines would not be adequate for children [3,15,16].

The purpose of this study is to evaluate the compliance of surgeons to national recommendations for use of AP in children undergoing colorectal surgeries with particular regard to antibiotic selection, dose, timing prior to incision and intraoperative re-dosing, and duration of postoperative antibiotic use and is to evaluate the effectiveness of antibiotics in the prevention of SSI in children undergoing colorectal surgical procedures.

2. Materials and Methods

2.1. Study Design and Setting

We performed a retrospective cohort study at Arkansas Children's Hospital (ACH) in Little Rock, Arkansas. ACH is a 336-bed academic teaching hospital and serves as the largest children's hospital in Arkansas. This project was conducted in accordance with the Declaration of Helsinki, and the institutional review board of the University of Arkansas for Medical Sciences approved this study on November 21, 2017 (Protocol number 207,026), using expedited review procedures.

2.2. Study Population

The study population included all pediatric patients <18 years of age who underwent a colorectal procedure at ACH from 1 January 2015 to 31 December 2016. We excluded surgeries that were performed as the direct result of trauma and those surgeries without anesthesia records available. A list of potentially eligible patients was provided by the hospital infection prevention team. Patients were identified through chart review of colorectal procedures and application of the standardized National Healthcare Safety Network (NHSN) definitions for SSI at the time of reporting. SSI were defined and reported to NHSN for each procedure, including all SSI types: superficial, deep, and organ space. The wound class system used in NHSN is adapted from the American College of Surgeons wound classification schema and includes Clean, Clean-Contaminated, Contaminated, and Dirty/Infected [17]. SSI were determined through prospective surveillance by four infection control practitioners who are certified in infection prevention with 4–26 years of experience. This known subset of children provided the opportunity for assessment of antibiotic prophylaxis utilization.

2.3. Data Collection/Study Procedures

We performed a comprehensive review of medical records by using a standardized data collection instrument to identify demographic information and clinical characteristics of patients who underwent colorectal surgeries at ACH. Perioperative antibiotic use, dose, timing of first administration, and duration of prophylaxis were collected and compared with the American Society of Health-System Pharmacists (ASHP) guidelines for appropriate use of antibiotics for surgical prophylaxis [9]. Microbiological and antimicrobial susceptibility data for patients who developed an SSI post-operatively were obtained from our institution's microbiology laboratory for the 2-year time period.

2.4. Definitions

Based on the ASHP guidelines, appropriate antibiotic selection for colorectal procedures was defined as those using one of the following regimens: (1) cefazolin and metronidazole, (2) ceftriaxone and metronidazole, (3) cefoxitin, (4) cefotetan, (5) ampicillin-sulbactam, or (6) ertapenem [9]. Alternative regimens for patients with a beta-lactam allergy included clindamycin or metronidazole with an aminoglycoside, aztreonam, or a fluoroquinolone [9]. Vancomycin could be used in the place of clindamycin for patients with a beta-lactam allergy [9]. Inappropriate antibiotic selection was defined as any other regimen administered preoperatively for the purposes of AP. Antibiotic dose was considered appropriate if the administered dose was within 10% of the guideline recommended dose.

Antibiotic timing was categorized as appropriate or inappropriate. Appropriate timing was defined as administration of the first dose of antibiotics within 60 min prior to surgical incision. However, given the pharmacokinetics of fluoroquinolones and vancomycin, timing of 120 min prior to incision was deemed appropriate for those antibiotics. Antibiotics not administered during these time periods were considered as inappropriate timing.

Re-dosing interval was assessed from the time of administration of the preoperative dose of the antibiotic and deemed appropriate when given within two half-lives of the agent administered, and deemed inappropriate when not administered or if there was a delay in administration. Continuation of AP for >24 h after surgery without an infectious indication was deemed as inappropriate duration.

2.5. Statistical Analysis

We performed descriptive analyses of the above variables by using SPSS version 24. Testing of proportions was performed by using a $\chi 2$ or Fisher exact test as appropriate. All reported p values are 2-tailed and were considered significant if $p < 0.05$.

3. Results

We evaluated 208 colorectal surgical procedures, of which 192 children met the inclusion criteria. Sixteen patients were excluded due to lack of anesthesia records. Of the 192 surgeries performed, 12 (6%) met the NHSN criteria for a surgical site infection; the overall SSI rate was 6.25 per 100 surgical procedures.

The median age of all patients was 4.9 months (range, 0–17.7 years), and 113 (59%) were male. Fifteen (8%) children were overweight or obese. One hundred seventy-five (91%) surgeries were categorized as scheduled or elective, and 17 (9%) were urgent or emergent. The median duration of surgery was 92 min (range, 20–579 min). The median duration of hospitalization was 13 days (range, 1–511 days). Of the 192 patients, 62 (32%) were hospitalized at least once in the previous year.

The types of surgeries most frequently performed included colorectal resection (44%), ostomy formation/revision (35%), ostomy closure (34%), exploratory laparotomy (28%), and small bowel resection (17%); most patients required multiple surgery types during their procedures. Table 1 shows the demographic, clinical, and surgical characteristics of the patients.

Table 1. Demographic and clinical characteristics of study cohort.

Variable	Patient (N = 192)	Patient (%)	SSI (N = 12)	SSI (%)	p-value
Age (range)	4.7 mo (0–17.7 yr)		3.0 yr (1.8 mo–17.1 yr)		0.009
Male	113	59	9	75	0.365
Race					0.0592
White	128	67	5	42	0.058
Black	37	19	4	34	0.251
Hispanic	18	9	2	17	0.312
Asian	2	1	1	8	0.121
Other	7	4	0	0	1.000
Co-morbidities/Exposures					
Proton Pump Inhibitor	37	19	3	25	0.704
Hyperglycemia	37	19	5	42	0.042
Immunocompromised	14	7	1	8	1.000
Steroids	19	10	2	17	0.337
Prematurity	90	47	3	25	0.143
Obese (BMI >30)	7	4	2	17	0.063
Beta-Lactam Allergy Reported	10	5	1	8	0.484
Previous hospitalizations within the year	62	32	5	42	0.473
Median Duration of Surgical Hospitalization	13 (1–511) days		19 (3–92) days		0.526
Median Surgery Duration (range)	92 (20–579) min		112.5 (76–206) min		0.037
Urgency					<0.001
Elective	175	91	7	58	<0.001
Emergent	17	9	5	42	<0.001
Surgery Type					
Appendectomy	11	6	0	0	1.000
Small Bowel Resection	33	17	5	42	0.020
Colon/Rectal resection	84	44	8	67	0.134
Chait Cecostomy	7	4	0	0	1.000
Soave	5	3	0	0	1.000
Duodenal atresia repair	16	8	0	0	0.604
Ostomy formation/revision	67	35	4	33	1.000
Ostomy closure	66	34	3	25	0.550
Exploratory laparotomy	54	28	8	67	0.005
Gastrostomy tube placement/Revision	14	7	1	8	1.000
Other	43	22	3	25	0.733
Wound Classification					0.0005
Clean-contaminated	130	68	3	25	0.002
Contaminated	33	17	2	17	1.000
Dirty	29	15	7	58	0.000016
ASA Class					0.549
I	8	4	1	8	0.409
II	80	42	5	42	1.000
III	84	44	6	50	0.652
IV	20	10	0	0	0.618

3.1. Assessment of AP Compliance

The results of compliance with antimicrobial prophylaxis are shown in Figure 1. Appropriate antibiotic dosing and duration had the highest incidence of compliance at 65% and 64% of cases, respectively. Antibiotic timing and selection had the highest rates of non-compliance at 56% and 64% of encounters being non-compliant, respectively.

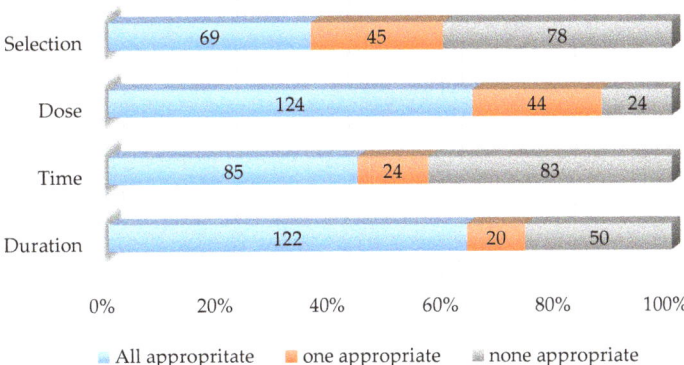

Figure 1. Appropriateness of antibiotic prophylaxis for children undergoing colorectal surgery as compared to national guideline recommendations.

Antibiotic selection was found to be in concordance with both local and national recommendations in 36% of the cases (69/192). Combination of cefazolin and metronidazole was the most common appropriately used antibiotic regimen, accounting for 26% of all surgical cases. The most common inappropriate antibiotic regimens selected included cefazolin monotherapy and a combination of vancomycin with piperacillin-tazobactam. Vancomycin alone was administered to three patients, and metronidazole alone was administered to one patient. Anaerobic coverage was not included in the antibiotic regimen in 62% of patients. Thirty-five percent of patients for whom AP was not selected appropriately were on scheduled antibiotics for an infection prior to surgery, and hence, AP was perceived to be not indicated per surgical documentation. One patient did not receive any AP, and 6% of children that did not receive appropriate AP had a documented beta-lactam allergy.

With regard to antibiotic timing, 56% (107/192) of patients received AP outside of the recommended administration time. Of the 107 inappropriately timed antibiotics, 24 (22%) were due to vancomycin administration beyond the optimal time window prior to incision (range, 97–1144 min); 9 (8%) were due to emergency procedures. We found that 24 (22%) cases of inappropriate antibiotic timing were due to delay in the administration of metronidazole following the administration of cefazolin, ceftriaxone, or a fluoroquinolone. Of the 50 patients who were already on scheduled antibiotics prior to surgery, one received antibiotics at the appropriate time prior to incision, and three were appropriately re-dosed intraoperatively.

We found that dosing of AP was inappropriate in 68/192 (35%) of our patients. Dosing errors were noted most frequently for metronidazole; 71 patients in our cohort received metronidazole preoperatively, of which 29 (41%) received a higher dose than recommended, while 13 (18%) patients received a suboptimal dose of metronidazole. Of the 23 patients that required re-dosing of antibiotics, only 8 (35%) were re-dosed appropriately. The median surgical duration for procedures that required re-dosing was 177 min (range, 52–577 min).

AP duration was inappropriate in 70/192 (36%) cases. The duration of antibiotics after surgical procedure in patients whose post-operative prophylaxis was inappropriately prolonged was a median of 48.63 h (range, 31.33–182.62 h).

Overall, noncompliance with all four elements of antimicrobial prophylaxis was 44% among the 192 cases (Table 2).

Table 2. Appropriateness of antibiotic prophylaxis in children undergoing colorectal surgery.

	Appropriate	Inappropriate	SSI Appropriate	SSI Inappropriate
	N = 192 (%)	N = 192 (%)	N = 12 (%)	N = 12(%)
Antibiotic Selection	69 (36)	123 (64)	8 (67)	4 (33)
Antibiotic Dose	124 (65)	68 (35)	6 (50)	6 (50)
Antibiotic Timing	85 (44)	107 (56)	7 (58)	5 (42)
Antibiotic Duration	122 (64)	70 (36)	10 (83)	2 (17)

Note: For dual combinations, both antibiotics had to be appropriate.

3.2. Surgical Site Infections

Twelve children (6%) in our cohort developed SSI following colorectal surgery. Of these, 5 were superficial incisional, 2 were deep incisional, and 5 were organ/space infections. The percentages of clean-contaminated, contaminated, and dirty wounds in patients who developed infection were 25%, 17%, and 58%, respectively. Of the surgical cases resulting in SSI, 42% were emergent cases. Seventeen percent of infections occurred in patients who were obese and 25% occurred in patients who were premature. The median duration of surgery in cases resulting in SSI was 112.5 min (range, 76–206 min). Cases involving bowel resections accounted for 83% of all SSI.

Of the 12 patients with SSI, only two children received the correct AP for all four categories evaluated including selection, time, dose, and duration. Antibiotics were inappropriately selected in 4/12 (33%) children who developed an SSI. AP timing, duration, and dosing were inappropriate in 6/12 (50%), 5/12 (42%), and 2/12 (17%) cases, respectively.

The organisms isolated in patients with SSI were methicillin-susceptible *Staphylococcus aureus* (MSSA), methicillin-resistant *Staphylococcus aureus* (MRSA), *Escherichia coli*, *Enterococcus faecalis*, *Pseudomonas aeruginosa*, *Klebsiella pneumoniae*, *Enterobacter cloacae*, *Candida albicans*, *Candida tropicalis*, and *Candida glabrata* (Figure 2).

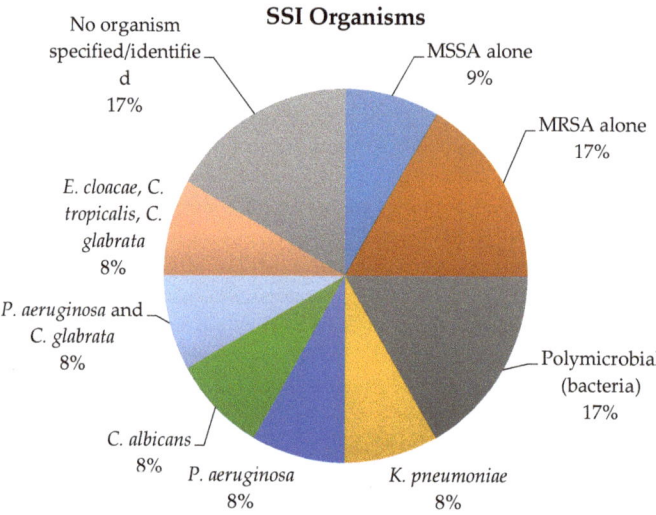

Figure 2. Organisms isolated in 12 children with a surgical site infection following colorectal surgery.

Of the 10 children with an SSI wherein an organism was identified, 8 (80%) were not covered by the recommended AP. Of these 8 cases, 3 (38%) were due to *Candida* sp., and 5 (63%) were due to organisms that were resistant to the standard AP.

4. Discussion

We found lack of compliance with national guidelines in all four facets of AP in children undergoing colorectal procedures at our institution. Appropriate antibiotic selection and timing had the highest incidence of non-compliance, but we also identified non-compliance with antibiotic dosing and duration.

Antibiotic selection had the highest rate of non-compliance in our study with the correct antibiotic being chosen in only 36% of children undergoing colorectal surgeries. At our institution, the choice of AP is at the discretion of the surgeon or anesthesiologist. Lack of familiarity with the national guidelines for AP may be a barrier to appropriate antibiotic selection. In a study published by Friedman et al., excessively broad-spectrum antibiotics were chosen for clean operations [18]. This finding was similar to that seen in our study wherein concern for serious or severe infection prompted surgeons to unnecessarily choose broader spectrum antibiotics, thereby placing patients at risk for antibiotic resistance and fungal infections. The use of clinical decision support pathways and order sets that are incorporated into the electronic medical record may help guide antibiotic selection and prevent antibiotic overuse [14,19]. These order sets should be developed with the input of pharmacists and include optimal dosing for the chosen antibiotic, thereby potentially overcoming the AP dosing issues noted in our study. A multi-disciplinary approach including pharmacy, surgeons, nursing, and anesthesia for the development of the clinical decision support pathway may help to shed light on different perspectives of patient care and hold all members of the patient care team accountable for ensuring appropriate use of AP [14,19,20].

Nearly 60% of inappropriate AP in our study was due to incorrect timing. The ASHP guidelines recommend to administer antibiotics within one hour prior to surgical incision, or within 120 min for specific antibiotics [9]. We noted that when dual antibiotics were selected for AP, the second antibiotic, most often metronidazole, was either delayed or administered at or after the time of incision. The reason for this is unclear, but lack of familiarity with the pharmacokinetics of antibiotics may be a contributing factor. Tan et al. reported that AP was perceived as a low priority when compared to the administration of anesthetics among surgeons and anesthesiologists, and that this likely influenced the timing of AP [21]. Incorporation of AP into the routine operating room workflow and administration of prophylaxis in the pre-operative area rather than in the operating room may ensure complete infusion of antibiotics prior to incision. As anesthesiologists play a critical role in postoperative infection control, the delegation of AP administration to the anesthesiology team should be considered. Nemeth et al. evaluated use of a verbal AP reminder in the surgical time-out process, but found that this intervention did not improve timeliness of administration of AP [21]. Nair et al. demonstrated the effectiveness of direct email feedback, antibiotic compliance reports, and real time alerts in improving antibiotic timing [22].

Our findings of variation in AP practices are similar to that of other studies evaluating the use of AP in pediatric surgical patients. Donà et al. noted variability in antibiotic prescribing for AP in their single-center study that evaluated the use of AP in children undergoing surgical procedures. The authors found that in the pre-intervention group, antibiotic selection was inappropriate in 51% of cases, and antibiotics were continued for a prolonged duration in 54.9% of cases [23]. Implementation of a clinical pathway proved to be a useful tool and led to a statistically significant improvement in the selection and duration of AP in pediatric patients; however, there still remained room for improvement of AP compliance in the post-intervention group [23]. Sandora et al. evaluated the national appropriateness of AP in children undergoing common surgical procedures using the Pediatric Health Information System database, and they noted significant variation in the use of AP across the 31 institutions submitting data [24]. AP was considered to be appropriate in only 64.6% of all cases in the study, with an inter-hospital variation ranging from 47.3% appropriateness to 84.4%. The authors noted that AP was commonly administered, even in cases for which AP was not indicated, revealing a significant overuse of antibiotics despite the presence of national guidelines and well described risks of antibiotic associated adverse reactions and secondary infections, such as *Clostridioides difficile* infection [24]. They also concluded that the lack of pediatric guidelines for AP may have impacted this finding of variability in AP practices between hospitals [24]. Additionally, while it is commonly inferred that the colonic composition in children is similar to that of adults, studies have demonstrated differences between the pediatric and adult gut microbiome [25,26]. Furthermore, the disproportionate differences in chronic conditions and comorbidities between children and adults may lend to different post-operative SSI risks when comparing these two populations [24]. Considering these differences, surgeons may be less inclined to extrapolate the adult guidelines to their pediatric patients.

AP was effective in the prevention of SSI in our study and only 6% developed an SSI. Of those children that developed an SSI, 80% were due to infections that were not covered by standard AP, 25% were premature infants, and 17% were in obese patients. It is well known that antibiotic overuse is frequent in neonates and significant variability exists in their use. Neonates are, therefore, at risk for antibiotic resistant organisms. Currently, there are limited data on appropriate surgical AP specific to neonates and AP in this population are based on adult guidelines [27]. Considering the unique microbiome of neonates and the morbidity associated with SSI in neonates, larger studies are warranted to determine effective AP in this particular population, as conventional AP may not be optimal. Two of the seven obese patients in this cohort developed an SSI. Patients who are obese commonly undergo longer operative times and are at risk for increased complications and prolonged hospitalizations following surgery [28]. Furthermore, the lack of data regarding antibiotic dose adjustments in obesity lends to the concern that these patients may not have adequate serum drug concentrations when standard doses of AP are utilized. Based on our small study, these special populations may benefit from a more tailored AP regimen.

This study has several limitations. This was a single-center study and, hence, the findings may not be generalizable to all pediatric surgical settings. Due to the retrospective study design, we were limited to information reported in the patients' medical records; therefore, findings may have been misclassified if the data points were not completely recorded in the chart. The application of a clinical chart review may not have captured all facets of SSI documentation. We did not evaluate the use of oral antibiotics for mechanical bowel prophylaxis prior to elective colorectal procedures, so it is unclear if those practices were impactful in preventing SSI in our cohort. Finally, SSI cases were identified using a list provided by our infection preventionists using NHSN criteria; however, cases may not have been captured if cultures were not obtained despite objective signs leading to clinical suspicion of infection, such as fever or wound drainage.

5. Conclusions

In this study, we have identified multiple areas for improvement regarding the administration of AP in children undergoing colorectal surgeries. Lack of compliance with national guidelines for AP in children undergoing colorectal surgeries was high. A multidisciplinary approach to the development of standardized protocols, educational interventions, and EHR-based algorithms may facilitate or improve appropriate AP use. Special populations, such as neonates and obese children, may benefit from a tailored regimen for AP, as these children may be at risk for SSI due to organisms not covered by conventional AP regimens. Our findings indicate the need for larger studies to investigate optimal AP choices in special populations and to determine interventions to improve the provision of AP in children.

Author Contributions: H.M. conceptualized the study. K.P. and R.B. collected and analyzed the data. K.P. and V.V. prepared the manuscript and V.V., M.H., H.M. and R.B. reviewed the manuscript. All authors have read and agreed to the published version of the manuscript.

Funding: This research received no external funding.

Conflicts of Interest: The authors declare no conflict of interest.

References

1. Berríos-Torres, S.I.; Umscheid, C.A.; Bratzle, D.W.; Leas, B.; Stone, E.C.; Kelz, R.R.; Reinke, C.E.; Morgan, S.; Solomkin, J.S.; Mazuski, J.E.; et al. Centers for Disease Control and Prevention Guideline for the Prevention of Surgical Site Infection, 2017. *JAMA Surg.* **2017**, *152*, 784.
2. Ban, K.A.; Minei, J.P.; Laronga, C.; Harbrecht, B.G.; Jensen, E.H.; Fry, D.E.; Itani, K.M.; Dellinger, E.P.; Ko, C.Y.; Duane, T.M. American College of Surgeons and Surgical Infection Society: Surgical Site Infection Guidelines, 2016 Update. *J. Am. Coll. Surg.* **2017**, *224*, 59–74. [CrossRef] [PubMed]
3. Rangel, S.J.; Islam, S.; Peter, S.D.S.; Goldin, A.B.; Abdullah, F.; Downard, C.D.; Saito, J.; Blakely, M.L.; Puligandla, P.S.; Dasgupta, R.; et al. Prevention of infectious complications after elective colorectal surgery in children: An American Pediatric Surgical Association Outcomes and Clinical Trials Committee comprehensive review. *J. Pediatr. Surg.* **2015**, *50*, 192–200. [CrossRef] [PubMed]
4. Smith, R.L.; Bohl, J.K.; Mcelearney, S.T.; Friel, C.M.; Barclay, M.M.; Sawyer, R.G.; Foley, E.F. Wound Infection After Elective Colorectal Resection. *Ann. Surg.* **2004**, *239*, 599–607. [CrossRef] [PubMed]
5. Schilling, P.L.; Dimick, J.; Birkmeyer, J.D. Prioritizing Quality Improvement in General Surgery. *J. Am. Coll. Surg.* **2008**, *207*, 698–704. [CrossRef]
6. Feng, C.; Sidhwa, F.; Cameron, D.B.; Glass, C.; Rangel, S. Rates and burden of surgical site infections associated with pediatric colorectal surgery: Insight from the National Surgery Quality Improvement Program. *J. Pediatr. Surg.* **2016**, *51*, 970–974. [CrossRef]
7. Dornfeld, M.; Lovely, J.K.; Huebner, M.; Larson, D.W. Surgical Site Infection in Colorectal Surgery. *Dis. Colon Rectum* **2017**, *60*, 971–978. [CrossRef]
8. McKibben, L.; Horan, T.; Tokars, J.I.; Fowler, G.; Cardo, D.M.; Pearson, M.L.; Brennan, P.J. Guidance on Public Reporting of Healthcare-Associated Infections: Recommendations of the Healthcare Infection Control Practices Advisory Committee. *Am. J. Infect. Control.* **2005**, *33*, 217–226. [CrossRef]
9. Bratzle, D.W.; Dellinger, E.P.; Olsen, K.M.; Perl, T.M.; Auwaerter, P.G.; Bolon, M.K.; Fish, D.N.; Napolitano, L.M.; Sawyer, R.G.; Slain, D.; et al. Clinical practice guidelines for antimicrobial prophylaxis in surgery. *Am. J. Heal. Pharm.* **2013**, *70*, 195–283. [CrossRef]
10. Anderson, D.J.; Podgorny, K.; Berríos-Torres, S.I.; Bratzle, D.W.; Dellinger, E.P.; Greene, L.; Nyquist, A.-C.; Saiman, L.; Yokoe, D.S.; Maragakis, L.L.; et al. Strategies to prevent surgical site infections in acute care hospitals: 2014 update. *Infect. Control. Hosp. Epidemiol.* **2014**, *35*, 605–627. [CrossRef]
11. Global Guidelines for the Prevention of Surgical Site Infection. Available online: http://www.who.int/iris/handle/10665/250680 (accessed on 20 July 2017).
12. Global Guidelines for the Prevention of Surgical Site Infection, 2nd ed. Available online: http://www.who.int/iris/handle/10665/277399 (accessed on 4 June 2019).
13. Tourmousoglou, C.E.; Yiannakopoulou, E.C.; Bramis, J.; Papadopoulos, J.S.; Kalapothaki, V. Adherence to guidelines for antibiotic prophylaxis in general surgery: A critical appraisal. *J. Antimicrob. Chemother.* **2007**, *61*, 214–218. [CrossRef] [PubMed]
14. Kilan, R.; Moran, D.; Eid, I.; Okeahialam, C.; Quinn, C.; Binsaddiq, W.; Williams, T.; Johnson, M.H. Improving antibiotic prophylaxis in gastrointestinal surgery patients: A quality improvement project. *Ann. Med. Surg.* **2017**, *20*, 6–12. [CrossRef] [PubMed]
15. Hopkins, M.; Macfarlane, G. Changes in predominant bacterial populations in human faeces with age and with Clostridium difficile infection. *J. Med Microbiol.* **2002**, *51*, 448–454. [CrossRef] [PubMed]
16. Hopkins, M.; Sharp, R.; Macfarlane, G.T. Age and disease related changes in intestinal bacterial populations assessed by cell culture, 16S rRNA abundance, and community cellular fatty acid profiles. *Gut* **2001**, *48*, 198–205. [CrossRef] [PubMed]
17. Centers for Disease Control and Prevention. *Costs of Intimate Partner Violence against Women in the United States*; CDC, National Center for Injury Prevention and Control: Atlanta, GA, USA, 2003.
18. Bull, A.; Russo, P.; Friedman, N.; Bennett, N.; Boardman, C.; Richards, M. Compliance with surgical antibiotic prophylaxis–reporting from a statewide surveillance programme in Victoria, Australia. *J. Hosp. Infect.* **2006**, *63*, 140–147. [CrossRef] [PubMed]
19. Putnam, L.R.; Chang, C.M.; Rogers, N.B.; Podolnick, J.M.; Sakhuja, S.; Matuszczak, M.; Austin, M.T.; Kao, L.S.; Lally, K.P.; Tsao, K. Adherence to surgical antibiotic prophylaxis remains a challenge despite multifaceted interventions. *Surgery* **2015**, *158*, 413–419. [CrossRef] [PubMed]

20. Nemeth, T.A.; Beilman, G.J.; Hamlin, C.L.; Chipman, J. Preoperative Verification of Timely Antimicrobial Prophylaxis Does Not Improve Compliance with Guidelines. *Surg. Infect.* **2010**, *11*, 387–391. [CrossRef]
21. Tan, J.A.; Naik, V.N.; Lingard, L. Exploring obstacles to proper timing of prophylactic antibiotics for surgical site infections. *Qual. Saf. Heal. Care* **2006**, *15*, 32–38. [CrossRef]
22. Nair, B.G.; Newman, S.-F.; Peterson, G.N.; Wu, W.-Y.; Schwid, H.A. Feedback Mechanisms Including Real-Time Electronic Alerts to Achieve Near 100% Timely Prophylactic Antibiotic Administration in Surgical Cases. *Anesth. Analg.* **2010**, *111*, 1293–1300. [CrossRef]
23. Donà, D.; Luise, D.; La Pergola, E.; Montemezzo, G.; Frigo, A.C.; Lundin, R.; Zaoutis, T.E.; Gamba, P.; Giaquinto, C. Effects of an antimicrobial stewardship intervention on perioperative antibiotic prophylaxis in pediatrics. *Antimicrob. Resist. Infect. Control.* **2019**, *8*, 13. [CrossRef]
24. Sandora, T.J.; Fung, M.; Melvin, P.; Graham, D.A.; Rangel, S.J. National Variability and Appropriateness of Surgical Antibiotic Prophylaxis in US Children's Hospitals. *JAMA Pediatr.* **2016**, *170*, 570. [CrossRef] [PubMed]
25. Gaufin, T.; Tobin, N.H.; Aldrovandi, G. The importance of the microbiome in pediatrics and pediatric infectious diseases. *Curr. Opin. Pediatr.* **2018**, *30*, 117–124. [CrossRef] [PubMed]
26. Hollister, E.B.; Riehle, K.; Luna, R.A.; Weidler, E.M.; Rubio-Gonzales, M.; Mistretta, T.-A.; Raza, S.; Doddapaneni, H.V.; Metcalf, G.A.; Muzny, N.M.; et al. Structure and function of the healthy pre-adolescent pediatric gut microbiome. *Microbiome* **2015**, *3*, 36. [CrossRef] [PubMed]
27. Staude, B.; Oehmke, F.; Lauer, T.; Behnke, J.; Göpel, W.; Schloter, M.; Schulz, H.; Krauss-Etschmann, S.; Ehrhardt, H. The Microbiome and Preterm Birth: A Change in Paradigm with Profound Implications for Pathophysiologic Concepts and Novel Therapeutic Strategies. *BioMed Res. Int.* **2018**, *2018*, 1–12. [CrossRef]
28. Kao, A.M.; Arnold, M.R.; Prasad, T.; Schulman, A.M. The impact of abnormal BMI on surgical complications after pediatric colorectal surgery. *J. Pediatr. Surg.* **2019**, *54*, 2300–2304. [CrossRef]

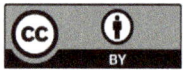

© 2020 by the authors. Licensee MDPI, Basel, Switzerland. This article is an open access article distributed under the terms and conditions of the Creative Commons Attribution (CC BY) license (http://creativecommons.org/licenses/by/4.0/).

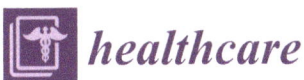

Case Report

Suspected Malignant Hyperthermia and the Application of a Multidisciplinary Response

Laura Ebbitt [1], Eric Johnson [1,*], Brooke Herndon [1], Kristina Karrick [1] and Aric Johnson [2]

1. Department of Pharmacy, University of Kentucky Medical Center, Lexington, KY 40536, USA; Laura.Means@uky.edu (L.E.); Bherndon01@uky.edu (B.H.); Kristina.Huey@uky.edu (K.K.)
2. Department of Anesthesiology, University of Kentucky Medical Center, Lexington, KY 40536, USA; Aric.Johnson@uky.edu
* Correspondence: Eric.Johnson@uky.edu

Received: 31 July 2020; Accepted: 4 September 2020; Published: 9 September 2020

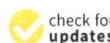

Abstract: Purpose: Malignant hyperthermia (MH) is a critical and potentially life-threatening emergency associated with inhaled anesthetic and depolarizing neuromuscular blocker administration. This is a single center's response to MH. Summary: When signs of MH are observed, a page for "anesthesia STAT-MH crisis" is called, triggering a multidisciplinary response, including the deployment of a Malignant Hyperthermia Cart. The MH cart and the delegation of duties allows nurses, physicians and pharmacists to quickly understand their role in the stabilization, transition and recovery of a suspected MH patient. Conclusion: This case highlights the importance of multi-disciplinary involvement in these rare, but potentially fatal, cases.

Keywords: malignant hyperthermia; collaborative practice; perioperative care

1. Introduction

Malignant hyperthermia (MH) is a critical and potentially life-threatening emergency associated with the administration of volatile anesthetics and depolarizing neuromuscular blockers that may occur intraoperatively, as well as during the postoperative period [1]. It is treated with dantrolene, a ryanodine receptor antagonist. Both the Malignant Hyperthermia Association of the United States (MHAUS) and American Society of Anesthesiologists (ASA) emphasize a preemptive approach to treatment, including MH supply, a medication cart and departmental training [2,3]. Furthermore, delays between the onset of MH and a coordinated response involving the administration of dantrolene have been associated with increased rates of complications [1]. Therefore, a rapid and efficient response to those with suspected MH may limit the morbidity associated with the condition. We present a case of suspected MH and illustrate the application of a multidisciplinary response in accordance with a well-rehearsed institutional protocol.

Pathophysiology

Malignant hyperthermia is an autosomal-dominant, pharmacogenetic disorder that manifests as a hypermetabolic crisis following exposure to a triggering agent. Known triggering agents include all volatile anesthetics (isoflurane, sevoflurane and desflurane), depolarizing neuromuscular blocking agents (succinylcholine) and human stressors such as vigorous exercise and heat [4]. The most common genetic mutation found to cause MH involves changes to the type 1 ryanodine receptor (RYR1), which encodes for the ryanodine receptor found on skeletal muscle [5]. The RYR1 is located on the sarcoplasmic reticulum of myocytes and is essential for regulating muscle excitation–contraction coupling. In the setting of genetic mutation and a triggering agent, rapid and uncontrolled increases in myoplasmic calcium occur, although this may not occur in the patients' initial surgeries. This is significant, as both metabolism and contraction in skeletal muscle are regulated by the concentration of intracellular calcium [6]. Manifestations of the dysregulation are indicative of a hypermetabolic state. These derangements may occur as early or late signs. Early signs may include sudden elevated end-tidal carbon dioxide, tachycardia, acidosis and muscle rigidity. Late signs may include hyperthermia and hyperkalemia [4]. If untreated, these symptoms may progress to rhabdomyolysis, myoglobinuria and acute renal failure. Life-threatening complications include disseminated intravascular coagulopathy (DIC), congestive heart failure, bowel ischemia and compartment syndrome [4]. The prompt diagnosis and treatment of MH is key to preventing the progression of symptoms and avoiding significant morbidity or death.

2. Institutional Approach/Protocol

Prior to the administration of any anesthetic, all patients should be screened for MH through a complete medical and family history analysis. This may not be possible in emergency situations. The initial signs of MH may occur at any time following the administration of a triggering agent, including immediately following the induction of general anesthesia or at any point during the maintenance phase for the anesthetic. As previously mentioned, the earliest clinical signs include an increase in the end-tidal carbon dioxide and tachycardia. As these findings are much more frequently a result of inadequate anesthesia and hypoventilation, respectively, the anesthesiologist must maintain a high level of suspicion for MH. If the anesthesiologist feels that MH is probable, or if there is no alternative diagnosis to explain the patient's clinical findings, they should immediately discontinue any triggering agents, notify the surgeon, hyperventilate with 100% inspired oxygen, increase fresh gas flow to >10 L/min, and trigger our multidisciplinary response. If available, charcoal filters should also be placed on the inspiratory and expiratory limbs of the anesthesia circuit. As MH is a potentially lethal disorder, a well-coordinated multidisciplinary approach is valuable in ensuring a timely and organized response. Figure 1 demonstrates the sequence of events initiated at our institution when MH is suspected.

An "anesthesia stat-MH crisis" is called out over the intercom to alert operating room (OR) staff including anesthesiologists, nurses and pharmacists to respond and assist in treating the patient. The anesthesiologist will serve as the primary leader for the resuscitation response and ensure that all aspects of patient care are accounted for. The primary OR nurse will retrieve the MH cart (contents shown in Table 1) from the adjoining storage area and bring it into the OR. Color-coded cards corresponding to tasks or roles are assigned to responding personnel. These roles include a registered nurse (RN) circulator, cooling nurse, medication nurse, dantrolene nurse/pharmacist and crisis management nurse. Attached to each card is a bag of supplies specific to the individual's role. The RN circulator may assign additional MH Team roles as needed. The cooling nurse procures ice and is prepared to implement advanced cooling as indicated. Cooling techniques at our institution include ice bags at the groin, axilla and neck; cooling blankets; and cold saline, as indicated. The medication nurse starts a large bore IV and works with the pharmacist to calculate the appropriate dantrolene dose. The pharmacist double-checks all drug dosing and assists with medication documentation, as well as ensuring the order of dantrolene products are utilized in the correct order to maximize efficiency and cost-effectiveness. Additionally, the pharmacists help to procure regular insulin and dextrose if needed for the treatment of hyperkalemia. Without all of these providers assessing and participating in the care of the patient, these cases would be extremely laborious. Having a multidisciplinary team attend to an MH crisis allows for the rapid control of a patient's symptoms and to potentially stabilize them quickly.

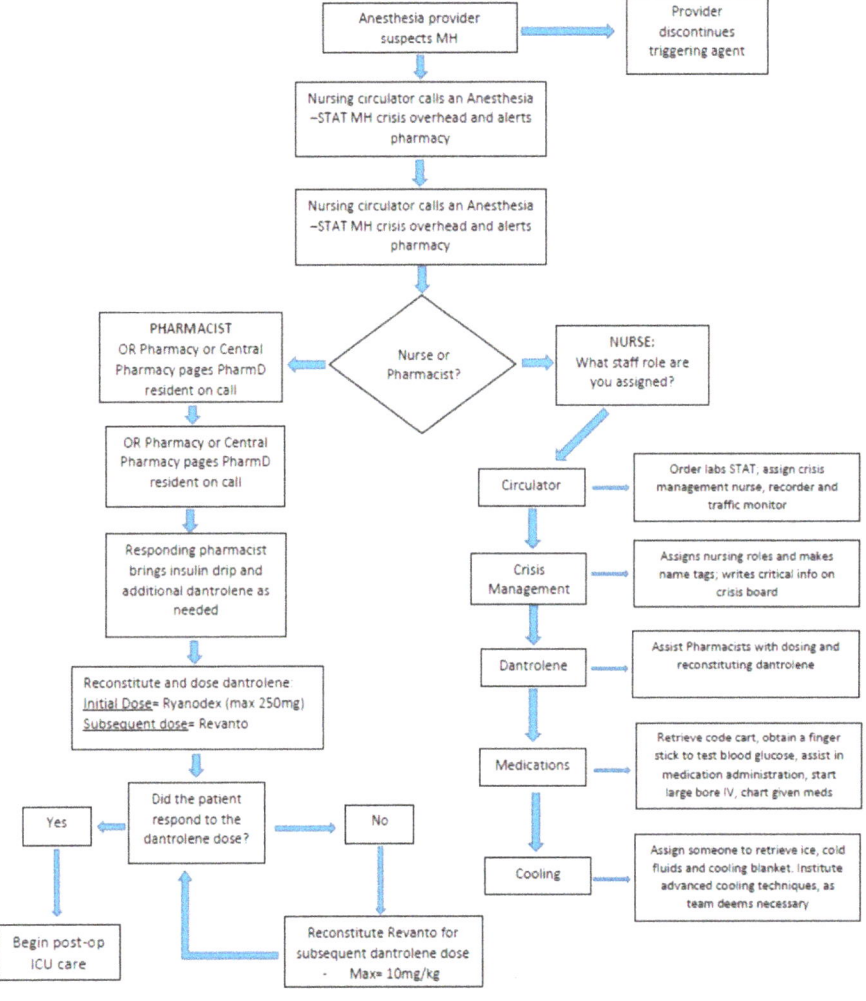

Figure 1. Sequence of events involved in Malignant Hyperthermia Response.

Table 1. Contents of Malignant Hyperthermia Cart.

Medications	Anesthesia Supply	Nursing Supplies
10% calcium chloride (1000 mg/10 mL) syringe (3)	Central line kit	Salem sump
Dextrose, 5%, syringe (1)	Arterial line kit	Rapid Infusion Catheter (RIC)
Sodium bicarbonate, 8.4% (2)	Charcoal gas machine filter	Temperature-sensing Foley
Sterile water, 50 mL (9) Revonto (dantrolene), 20 mg/60 mL (9) Ryanodex (dantrolene), 250 mg/5 mL (1)	Guidewires	Pressure bag

Two types of dantrolene are contained in our MH cart, one vial of Ryanodex and nine vials of Revonto, in addition to the 10 vials of nonbacteriostatic sterile water (nine 100 mL vials and one 20 mL vial). The Ryanodex is used for the first dose, and the nine vials of Revonto are provided for any necessary subsequent dosing. Ryanodex is a lyophilized powder form of dantrolene containing

250 mg per vial, which costs around USD 2500.00. Revonto is also a lyophilized powder but in contrast only contains 20 mg of dantrolene per vial, costing around USD 60.00 a vial. To reconstitute Ryanodex, only 5 mL of sterile water is required. When reconstituting Revonto, 60 mL is needed per vial. Ryanodex should be used for the first dose because of its ease of use and need to reconstitute fewer vials. For an average 80 kg patient, 10 vials of Revonto and 600 mL of sterile water would be required to reconstitute an initial dose. Other components of the MH cart are listed below in Table 1 and follow MHAUS recommendations [7].

Once the patient's MH symptoms and the patient are clinically stabilized, post-operative critical care and intensive care unit (ICU) admission are initiated. Patient allergies are updated to include likely triggering agents as a placeholder for future operations and hospital visits as a safety measure. When appropriate, patient and family are counseled on the importance of notifying anesthesia providers about MH history and avoiding triggering agents.

3. Case

With the consent of the patient, we present a case of a 22-year-old male admitted with an open right intercondylar fracture of the distal humerus after getting his arm caught in a steel press. In the emergency department, the patient received intravenous cefazolin, morphine, hydromorphone and a Tetanus/Diptheria/Pertussis (Tdap) vaccine. He was taken to the OR on the same day for an irrigation and debridement, as well as closed reduction of the open distal humerus fracture. General anesthesia was induced with lidocaine, fentanyl and propofol. Rocuronium was used for neuromuscular blockade. During the procedure, he was maintained on sevoflurane. No complications were noted during or after initial surgery. The following day, the patient was scheduled for a definitive internal fixation of his distal humerus fracture. General anesthesia was again induced with lidocaine, fentanyl and proprofol. Succinylcholine was administered to facilitate endotracheal intubation. The patient was maintained on isoflurane, and intermittent dosing of rocuronium was used to facilitate neuromuscular blockade. Approximately 30 min into the procedure, during the placement of an additional intravenous line, unexpected resistance was noted. Upon closer examination, his extremities were found to be rigid. A quick assessment of his vitals showed that he was tachycardic, with a heart rate of 160 bpm; hypercapnic, with an end-tidal CO_2 of 62 mmHg; and hypertensive, with systolic blood pressures >160 mmHg (baseline blood pressure was 130/82 mmHg at preoperative evaluation). A temperature-sensing catheter was placed in the bladder, and the patient was found to be normothermic at 37.4 °C. Despite the normothermia, malignant hyperthermia was suspected. The isoflurane was discontinued, and charcoal filters were placed in the circuit. Nitrous oxide was used to maintain general anesthesia, and a malignant hyperthermia response was initiated and allowed for additional responders to arrive at the patient's bedside within minutes.

The patient quickly received an initial bolus of 187.5 mg of Ryanodex (2.5 mg/kg). Additionally, 20 mg of IV push esmolol was administered to treat his tachycardia but with a negligible response. Over the next 35 min, the patient received 80 mg of Revonto via intermittent 20 mg doses. These doses were administered to treat persistent and intermittent symptoms of MH.

The non-pharmacological measures taken include ice packs applied to the axilla and the placement of cooling blankets. The patient responded to the dantrolene with marked reductions in heart rate, muscle rigidity and end-tidal carbon dioxide ($EtCO_2$). While not elevated, the patient's temperature remained normothermic. The surgical procedure was aborted, and the patient was transferred to the ICU for close monitoring, with care being assumed by the ICU intensivists.

In the ICU, the patient continued to receive Revonto 80 mg (~1 mg/kg) IV Q 6 h for 24 h. During this time period, the patient's lactate fell from 3.2 mmol/L at its peak to 0.6 mmol/L (Figure 2). His creatinine kinase (CK) peaked at 16,505 units/L and decreased to 7887 units/L prior to discharge (Figure 3). The patient's serum creatinine (SCr) was also elevated at 1.44 mg/dL and trended back down to his assumed baseline.

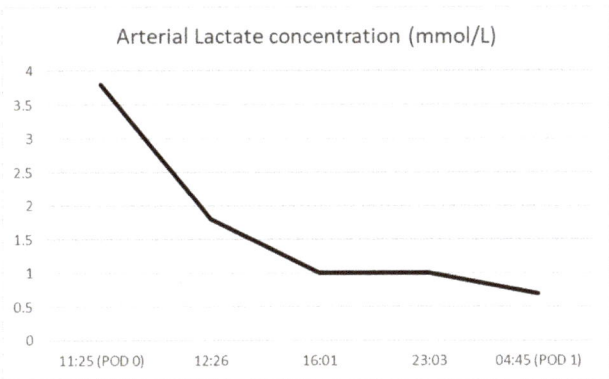

Figure 2. Arterial lactate concentration (POD = post-operative day).

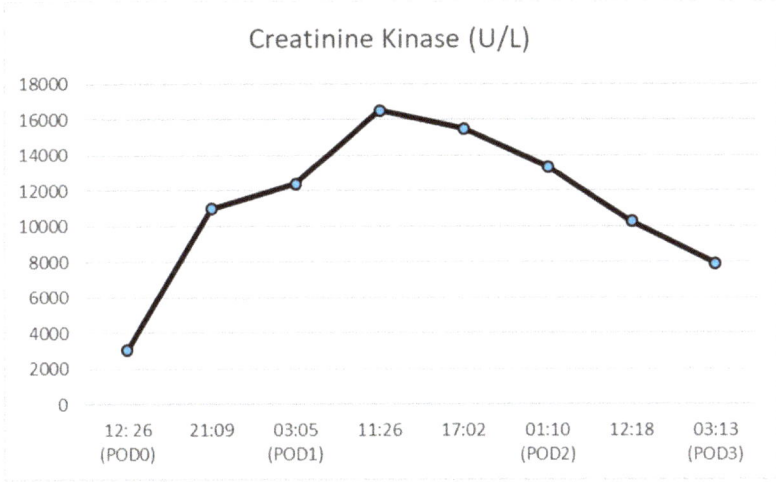

Figure 3. Creatinine kinase concentration (POD = post-operative day).

In light of the etiology and triggering factor in this case, one may incorrectly assume it was precipitated by succinylcholine alone, since the patient previously received sevoflurane without incident. However, the literature suggests that different inhaled anesthetics may trigger MH at different rates, and his initial sevoflurane exposure was not sufficient [8]. Furthermore, studies have shown that a triggering inhalation agent plus the use of succinylcholine may cause a more marked response than a single agent [9].

After the patient was stabilized, the case was discussed with the mother, who had also experienced MH in the past; however, she was not aware that this was a hereditary disease. The patient's family was educated regarding the risks of MH and the potential for genetic predisposition within the family. An allergy was also added to the patient's chart for future potential cases. The patient was extubated that evening. Four days into the patient's admission, he received an open reduction internal fixation (ORIF) of his distal humerus. Total IV anesthesia (TIVA) was used with continuous infusion of propofol and intermittent dosing of fentanyl, dexmedetomidine and rocuronium throughout the case. Aside from the CK, lactate and SCr, the patient's lab results all remained normal, and the patient progressed to his baseline function. The patient was discharged home on post-operative day 3 from the index surgery, with follow up after 2 weeks with the orthopedic service. Through the utilization of the institution's protocol, all providers were aware of their roles within the team and were able to quickly perform their assigned duties. This allowed delays to be reduced for the rapid control of the patient's MH. Without the swift initiation of an MH protocol, it is possible that patients could experience a lethal outcome.

4. Conclusions

MH is a rare but serious metabolic complication associated with the use of volatile anesthetics and depolarizing neuromuscular blocking agents. In the case of a delayed response or missed diagnosis, significant morbidity and mortality may occur. Institutions should develop, implement and train staff on how to recognize and treat this acute disorder. We present the case of a patient with an unknown family history of malignant hyperthermia. Despite proper pre-operative assessment, the family history was missed, and the patient experienced MH symptoms after receiving a triggering agent during his second surgery. Due to an extensive, multidisciplinary perioperative MH protocol, this patient was successfully treated and avoided serious complications. Providers were able to treat the patient quickly and efficiently, in great part due to the presence and utilization of the MH cart. The dosing cards and instructions readily available on the cart allowed the correct dose of Ryanodex to be verified and drawn up into a syringe by the providers while subsequent doses of Revonto were also being prepared. This case also highlights the need to ask specific questions in the pre-operative setting regarding both the patient's and the patient's family's prior history of surgeries and any events that may have occurred. We recommend that other institutions develop a similar cart, as a mechanism for providers to be able to respond to these events.

Funding: This research received no external funding.

Conflicts of Interest: All authors report no conflicts of interest, including pharmaceutical or industry support, regarding any of the information contained in this report. No relevant funding from any organization was provided to any of the authors regarding this manuscript or the ideas contained herein.

References

1. Larach, M.G.; Brandom, B.W.; Allen, G.C.; Gronert, G.A.; Lehman, E.B. Cardiac arrests and deaths associated with malignant hyperthermia in North America from 1987 to 2006: A report from the North American malignant hyperthermia registry of the malignant hyperthermia association of the United States. *Anesthesiology* **2008**, *108*, 603–611. [CrossRef] [PubMed]
2. MHAUS Website. Available online: www.MHAUS.org (accessed on 16 June 2019).
3. Litman, R.S.; Joshi, G.P. Malignant hyperthermia in the ambulatory surgery center: How should we prepare? *Anesthesiology* **2014**, *120*, 1306–1308. [CrossRef] [PubMed]
4. Rosenberg, H.; Pollock, N.; Schiemann, A.; Bulger, T.; Stowell, K.M. Malignant Hyperthermia: A Review. *Orphanet J. Rare Dis.* **2015**, *10*, 93. [CrossRef] [PubMed]
5. Brandom, B.W.; Bina, S.; Wong, C.A.; Wallace, T.; Visoiu, M.; Isackson, P.J.; Vladutiu, G.D.; Sambuughin, N.; Muldoon, S.M. Ryanodine receptor type 1 gene variants in the malignant hyperthermia-susceptible population of the United States. *Anesth. Analg.* **2013**, *116*, 1078–1086. [CrossRef] [PubMed]
6. MacLennan, D.H.; Phillips, M.S. Malignant Hyperthermia. *Science* **1992**, *256*, 789–794. [CrossRef] [PubMed]
7. Malignant Hyperthermia Association of the United States. What Should Be on an MH Cart? Available online: https://www.mhaus.org/healthcare-professionals/be-prepared/what-should-be-on-an-mh-cart/ (accessed on 16 June 2019).
8. Visoiu, M.; Young, C.M.; Wieland, K.; Brandom, B.W. Anesthetic drugs and onset of malignant hyperthermia. *Anesth. Analg.* **2014**, *118*, 388–396. [CrossRef] [PubMed]
9. Antognini, J.F. Creatine kinase alterations after acute malignant hyperthermia episodes and common surgical procedures. *Anesth. Analg.* **1995**, *81*, 1039–1042. [PubMed]

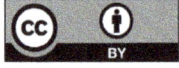

© 2020 by the authors. Licensee MDPI, Basel, Switzerland. This article is an open access article distributed under the terms and conditions of the Creative Commons Attribution (CC BY) license (http://creativecommons.org/licenses/by/4.0/).

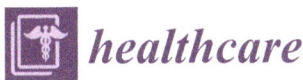

Article

Remote Monitoring of Critically-Ill Post-Surgical Patients: Lessons from a Biosensor Implementation Trial

Mariana Restrepo [1], Ann Marie Huffenberger [2], C William Hanson III [2,3], Michael Draugelis [4] and Krzysztof Laudanski [5,6,7,*]

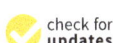

1   College of Arts and Sciences, University of Pennsylvania, Philadelphia, PA 19104, USA; rmariana@sas.upenn.edu
2   Penn Medicine Center for Connected Care, Clinical Practices of the University of Pennsylvania, PA 19104, USA; ann.huffenberger@pennmedicine.upenn.edu (A.M.H.); william.hanson@pennmedicine.upenn.edu (CW.H.III)
3   Department of Anesthesiology and Critical Care, University of Pennsylvania, Philadelphia, PA 19104, USA
4   Department of Radiology, University of Pennsylvania Health System, Philadelphia, PA 19104, USA; michael.draugelis@pennmedicine.upenn.edu
5   Department of Anesthesiology and Critical Care, Hospital of the University of Pennsylvania, Philadelphia, PA 19104, USA
6   Department of Neurology, University of Pennsylvania, Philadelphia, PA 19104, USA
7   Leonard Davis Institute of Health Economics, University of Pennsylvania, Philadelphia, PA 19104, USA
*   Correspondence: klaudanski@gmail.com

Citation: Restrepo, M.; Huffenberger, A.M.; Hanson, CW., III; Draugelis, M.; Laudanski, K. Remote Monitoring of Critically-Ill Post-Surgical Patients: Lessons from a Biosensor Implementation Trial. *Healthcare* **2021**, *9*, 343. https://doi.org/10.3390/healthcare9030343

Academic Editor: Richard H. Parrish II

Received: 13 February 2021
Accepted: 6 March 2021
Published: 18 March 2021

Publisher's Note: MDPI stays neutral with regard to jurisdictional claims in published maps and institutional affiliations.

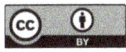

Copyright: © 2021 by the authors. Licensee MDPI, Basel, Switzerland. This article is an open access article distributed under the terms and conditions of the Creative Commons Attribution (CC BY) license (https://creativecommons.org/licenses/by/4.0/).

Abstract: Biosensors represent one of the numerous promising technologies envisioned to extend healthcare delivery. In perioperative care, the healthcare delivery system can use biosensors to remotely supervise patients who would otherwise be admitted to a hospital. This novel technology has gained a foothold in healthcare with significant acceleration due to the COVID-19 pandemic. However, few studies have attempted to narrate, or systematically analyze, the process of their implementation. We performed an observational study of biosensor implementation. The data accuracy provided by the commercially available biosensors was compared to those offered by standard clinical monitoring on patients admitted to the intensive care unit/perioperative unit. Surveys were also conducted to examine the acceptance of technology by patients and medical staff. We demonstrated a significant difference in vital signs between sensors and standard monitoring which was very dependent on the measured variables. Sensors seemed to integrate into the workflow relatively quickly, with almost no reported problems. The acceptance of the biosensors was high by patients and slightly less by nurses directly involved in the patients' care. The staff forecast a broad implementation of biosensors in approximately three to five years, yet are eager to learn more about them. Reliability considerations proved particularly troublesome in our implementation trial. Careful evaluation of sensor readiness is most likely necessary prior to system-wide implementation by each hospital to assess for data accuracy and acceptance by the staff.

Keywords: wearable biosensors; critical care; vital sign monitoring; bio-monitoring system; technology acceptance; integration; implementation

1. Introduction

The ability of biosensors to wirelessly, un-obstructively, and effortlessly monitor patients has become a fascinating prospect for healthcare [1]. They offer an opportunity to improve patient care while reducing costs and increasing patient and staff satisfaction [2,3]. At a minimum, most biosensors collect body temperature, pulse, heart rate variability, respiration rate, peripheral capillary oxygen saturation (SpO_2), sleep, and movement. Although sensors can quite often deliver additional data, it is unclear if they can increase the effectiveness of healthcare delivery.

In order to effectively integrate biosensors into healthcare workflow, several factors have to be fulfilled [4]. Foremost, the reliability of the equipment needs to be assessed. A previous study found that when comparing SpO_2 measurements between five types of biosensors and a clinical vital sign monitor, a range of 85–100% of biosensor measurements fell within three percentage points of the clinical monitor, depending on the type of biosensor [5,6]. However, the same study alternatively established that this range shifted to 93.5–100% of biosensor measurements falling within three beats per minute (BPM) of the clinical monitor [5]. It is also notable that mean skin temperature measured by biosensors can vary up to 2 °C from axillary measurements [7]. Furthermore, recordings from the research-grade biosensors proved less accurate than those intended for consumers [6,8,9]. Both the consistency and accuracy of some vital signs are much dependent on the device model [6,8,9]. Finally, the devices must take into account features specific to patients [10]. These inconsistencies across differing vital signs could introduce deceptive data trends that would undermine the feasibility of implementing biosensors in a critical care setting.

The implementation of biosensors in the workflow must be very well-planned and unit-specific [11]. The demands for perioperative care are particularly sensitive to interruption of the signal, while in other instances, accuracy may matter more. The data has to be delivered from sensors via a secure wireless network connection to provide a clear advantage over the existing infrastructure [4]. Establishing such a link securely and reliably is a complex task, especially in a hospital system with multiple entities operating off varying information system infrastructures [12]. Providing similar monitoring at home is even more complex. Acceptance of the sensor must be high across all parties involved [4,11,13,14]. Patients should value the sensor as an improvement over prior solutions. Sensors should be especially comfortable and undisruptive in perioperative settings. Providers should expect robust and reliable sets of data adding to the care being provided. Similarly, nursing staffs seek to ease the burden of continuously monitoring patients remotely, allowing biosensors to improve the quality and safety of patient care. All these requirements are particularly important for perioperative care, especially in in-home settings. A useful framework for the implementation of biosensors is provided by the ABCDEF bundle by suggesting a focus on which parameters yield most of the value [15]. Understanding potential barriers to this integration is the key to major transformations in healthcare [4,9,10,16].

This study describes the process of implementation of a multisensory biosensor platform to analyze up to 22 parameters and features in intensive care unit (ICU) patients. We aimed to describe our implementation process experiences, with special emphasis on comparing data streams from patients being monitored by biosensors versus standard hospital physiological monitoring. We also analyzed acceptance of the technology by patients, providers, and nurses. Past studies have found that while biosensors have extensive potential for real-world adaptations, functional challenges, including data validity and stability, need to be overcome first before defining practical applications [17].

2. Materials and Methods

The IRB at the University of Pennsylvania approved the study (#832633). Data were collected in 2020.

This is a pilot study testing the feasibility and robustness of the two types of wearable biosensors in anticipation of future deployment. One of the sensors is commercially available and used predominately for personal care, and it has not been previously tested in a healthcare ICU setting. The other one represented a biosensor that was developed and manufactured for healthcare use by a start-up. Both sensors collect several parameters, but we only focus on the data which are collected by the standard for medical ICU monitoring (Nihon Kohden USA; Irvine, CA, USA). The vital signs this study focuses on include heart rate, respiratory rate, and peripheral capillary oxygen saturation, as these can be collected by both types of biosensors and the Nihon Kohden monitoring system.

The study was conducted in an eight-bed medical ICU. The staff consists of an attending pulmonologist, one advanced practice provider, and four to five nurses. They were introduced to the study and hardware during a brief 10-min orientation. Patients were approached for consent while being in the ICU. Seven individuals agreed to participate, while one refused. One individual wore two sensors subsequently. The demographic characteristics of the study subjects are detailed in Table 1. After consenting, a patient was fitted with a sensor using the respective manufacturer's recommendation. The staff was instructed to keep the sensor on for a 24-h period. After the collection of data, the sensor was removed. Patients and staff members were asked to complete a quick survey in the RedCap database (Appendix A.1) [18]. In addition, we asked the staff to complete a separate survey after the trial period to explore their perception of biosensors (Appendix A.2).

Table 1. Demographic characteristics of studied cohorts.

	Patients $n = 8$	
Age (x ± SD)		59 ± 9
Sex	M	2
	F	6
Race	Caucasian	4
	Asian	1
	African American	3
How long being worn	1–4 h	0
	5–24 h	8
	1 day to 1 week	0
	Providers taking care of patients $n = 13$	
How long being worn	1–4 h	0
	5–24 h	10
	1 day to 1 week	3
Profession	MD	8
	RN	5
	Providers wearing devices $n = 16$	
How long being worn	1–4 h	8
	5–24 h	7
	1 day to 1 week	1

The data obtained from the biosensors were analyzed and compared to standard clinical monitoring provided using correlation and pathway analysis. Parametric variables were expressed as mean ± SD and compared using a Student's *t*-test. For non-parametric variables, median (Me) and interquartile ranges (IR) were computed. Mann–Whitney U statistics were employed to compare non-parametric variables. Data groups were analyzed as independent groups. A double-sided p-value of less than 0.05 was considered statistically significant for all tests. The r-Pearson statistic was calculated to determine the correlation between the studied variables. Statistical analyses were performed using Statistica 11.0 (StatSoft Inc., Tulsa, OK, USA). Graphs were generated using GraphPad Prism 8.4.2 (GraphPad Software Inc., San Diego, CA, USA).

3. Results

3.1. Data Accuracy

The biosensors' data showed varied performances with respect to different vital signs. Compared to respiratory rate and peripheral capillary oxygen saturation (SpO_2), heart rate measurements demonstrated the strongest and most consistent correlation between a biosensor and wired ICU standard recordings at rest (Figure 1A(i),(iii)) and during movement (data not shown). Although the quality of the heart rate data fluctuated throughout this specific trial, it remained above 80% for most of the measurements recorded after the application of the biosensor (Figure 1A(ii)). The difference between the biosensor's recordings and those of the Nihon Kohden system is assessed as the bias of the measurements, which is minimal and optimal for heart rate readings (Figure 1A(iv)). However, one trial demonstrated a significant lapse in the correlation during the onset of the measurements. The quality of the biosensor's measurements during this time was significantly less than once the heart rate stabilized.

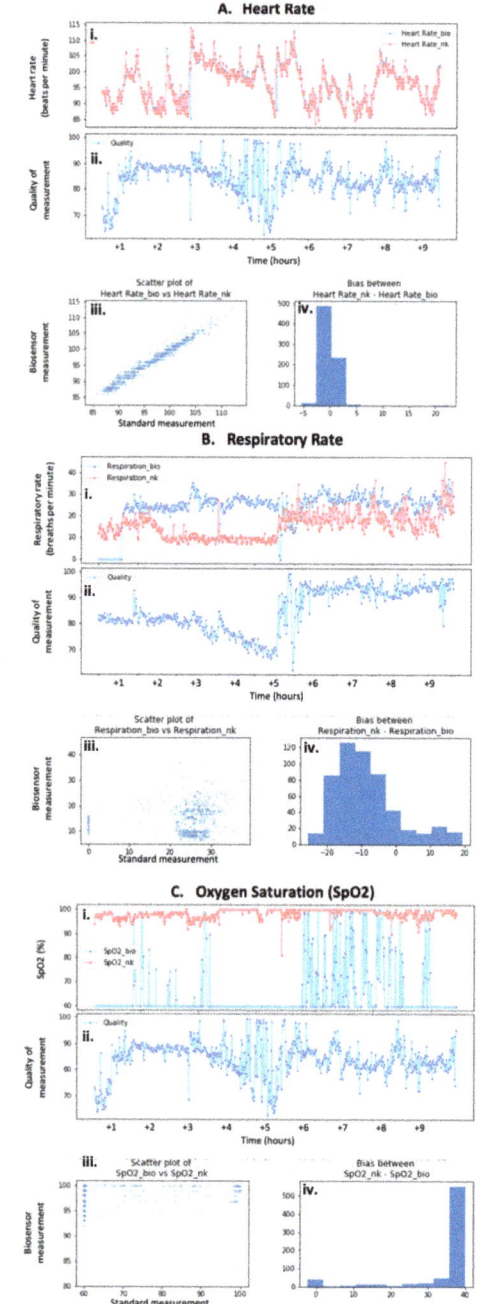

Figure 1. Correlation between data supplanted by multimodal sensor and standard ICU monitoring. Various degrees of data consistency were demonstrated by biosensors ranging from excellent for heart rate measurements (**A**), to variable for respiratory rate observations (**B**), to suboptimal SpO$_2$ recordings (**C**). In addition to the vital signs measured (**i**) and the quality of the biosensor measurements (**ii**), the correlation (**iii**), and bias (**iv**) between biosensor and Nihon Kohden recordings were also reported according to vital sign.

The correlation between biosensor and monitor-driven measurements for respiratory rate was significantly more variable than that of the heart rate recordings. One sample displayed superficially close correlations with similar results for both the biosensors and the manual measurements (Figure 1B(i)). This was confirmed by the weak positive relationship seen on the scatter plot that described the correlation between the two types of measurements (Figure 1B(iii)). Similar to the heart rate sample previously discussed, the quality of the measurements fluctuated throughout the trial, especially in the first half (Figure 1B(ii)). The bias reporting the difference between the biosensor and Nihon Kohden respiratory rates is visibly more than that seen for the heart rate data, further emphasizing the increased variability between the two forms of recording (Figure 1B(iv)).

The SpO_2 measurements showed the most variability in terms of the correlation between the biosensor and standard monitor measurements. Most samples reflected no SpO_2 measurements on the biosensors' parts (Figure 1C(i)). This lack of recording was seen in at least three different samples. Interestingly, the evaluation of the biosensors' quality did not reflect this, and instead remained at above 80% for the majority of the trial (Figure 1C(ii)). On another occasion, the biosensor only recorded periodically and at various qualities (data not shown). Similarly, the corresponding scatterplot for this sample does not reflect any correlation between the types of measurements (Figure 1C(iii)). The difference between the biosensor and standard monitor recordings seems to be greater than that of the heart rate measurements, as supported by the bias diagram (Figure 1C(iv)).

3.2. Deployment of the Sensors

The perspectives of patients wearing the biosensors, providers wearing the biosensors (providers as subject), and providers applying the biosensors on patients (provider for patients) were obtained through questionnaires to gauge the operationalization and ease of implementation of the biosensors. Determining the form factor and acceptance related to the biosensors is critical because these factors drive the discussion on implementation using the perspectives of both patients and providers. Specifically assessing the viewpoint of providers wearing the biosensors serves as an interesting comparison in relation to that of the patients they are treating.

The devices' adherence to the skin was perceived as somewhat problematic by healthy individuals. Despite small form factor, most of the users and medical staff considered sensors to interfere with daily activities (Figure 2). Medical staff included MDs (medical doctors) and RN (registered nurses). Irritation was reported by a minority of the patients, with one individual reporting skin abrasion out of a total of eight patient trials (Figure 2). Only one trial was terminated before the prescheduled time because of the irritation. The operationalization of the sensor was assessed very highly by patients wearing them when asked how much they agreed with the following: "Did you like the way the biosensor fit?", "Was it easy to apply?", "Was it easy to connect?", "Was it easy to remove?", and "How was your overall experience related to biosensor?" (Figure 2). Finally, the sensor trials were terminated on time, at the prescheduled time, in all study groups (providers as subjects = 65%, patients = 75%, providers for patients = 92%). Neither of the clinical groups discontinued the sensor because of interference with clinical care.

3.3. Perception of the Sensors

There was little difference in perception of the different domains of the sensors' usability between MDs and RNs, except for the familiarity with sensors between RNs and MDs (Figure 3A). The most common positive comments about sensors were "modern/sleek", "mobility", and "more data". The most common negative adjectives were "application", "unreliable", and "cost". The major sensor advantages were "easy application", "not-obstructive", and "portability".

The majority of MDs and RNs believed that sensors would be deployed in the next 3 to 5 years (B). The staff was feeling relatively unprepared for sensor deployment (Figure 3C).

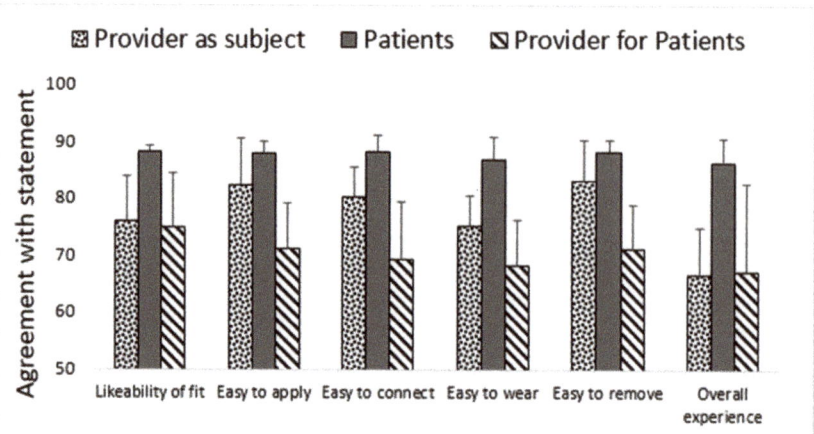

Figure 2. Experience of wearing the sensor. Experience of wearing the sensor was consistently rated higher for patient users compared to providers involved in care of patients.

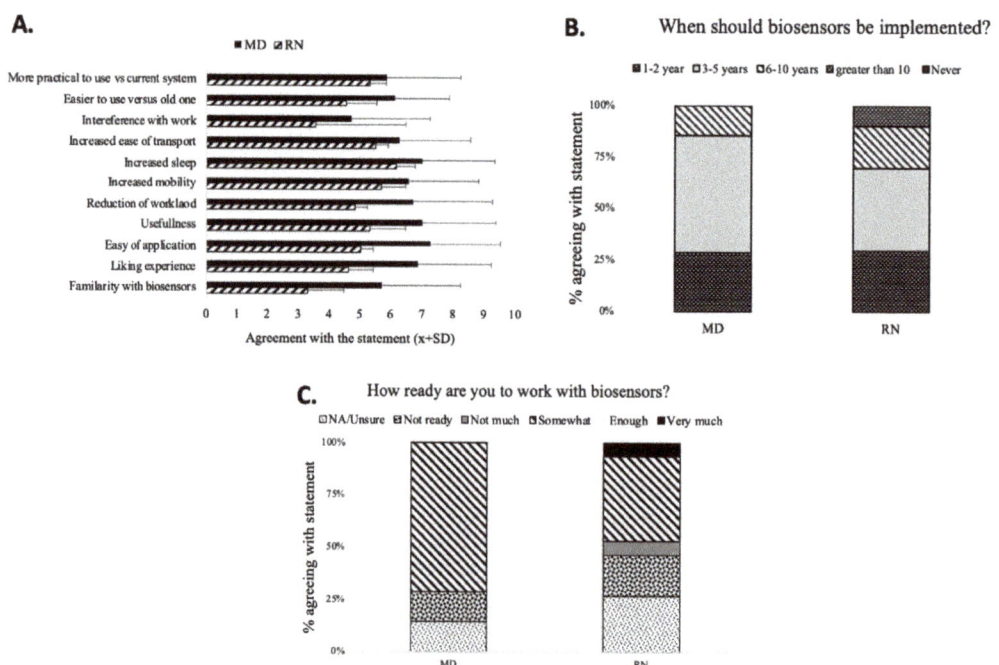

Figure 3. Readiness for implementation of biosensors. Physicians assessed the benefits of sensor deployment highly (**A**) and predicted faster implementation (**B**) than nurses. Nurses reported a more slightly unprepared perception of readiness to work with biosensors (**C**).

4. Discussion

The implementation of biosensors demonstrated several important related problems. The reliability of a sensor has to be extensively studied before the implementation. Prior reports pointed to unique problems related to the biosensors, although this was not the uniform case [12,16,19,20]. Movement, skin color, and sweating were quite often reported as the main reasons for interference [12,19]. Post-deployment interviews demonstrated that data might be lost for other reasons [14]. Sensor adherence was cited as such, but the loss of some data could not be explained exclusively. Considering that the correlations between the biosensor and clinical recordings for respiratory rate and SpO$_2$ were not significantly accurate, the variability that was introduced could negate the reliability and accuracy of the biosensors [21–24].

Overall, data correlation depended more on the data type (e.g., vital sign recorded) than on the sensor type in our study, and that was a new finding [12,16,19]. The weak correlations between readouts of the sensor and clinical standards augment the skepticism regarding integrating the biosensors with more standard critical care technology. Without a standard for accuracy, the variability will require consistent validation of the results, which will be both time sensitive and concerning if the validation fails. These problems emerged even before we could test the sensors' connection to the IT system. The unpredictability of the biosensors connecting to the appropriate downloading devices or tablets is one of the main concerns regarding this novel technology [4]. Being unable to anticipate if or where the biosensor will connect is one possible restriction that diminishes the fidelity of biosensors, given they should function to wirelessly monitor patients at all times. The stability and resiliency, among other technological obstacles, of electrochemical biosensors have proven to be focal points for barriers to their implementation, and the acceptance rate for loss signal has not being established [10]. However, our study demonstrated that multi-sensor devices might be uniquely prone to sensing errors as compared to clinical standards. This is a new and unique finding [12,16].

The adverse effects of wearing the sensors were rare. Irritation was almost not observed, while only one case of abrasion was noted in our study. The small number of enrolled subjects precluded this from being a conclusive study. Future studies should look into the incidence of adverse effects related to biosensors' application as compared to regular monitoring. However, most of the devices are fairly inert while being worn by patients [6,10,12,16].

The acceptance of the biosensor technology was particularly high for patients and slightly less so among the providers. This was the novel finding of the study, since some reported several barriers [14,16]. The reason driving the high acceptance of the biosensors was the relatively low form factor of devices [4,21,23]. A desire for non-interference of the device was frequently cited [16]. We demonstrated relatively low initial enthusiasm at the beginning of the trial that significantly increased at the completion of trials. Patients had overall positive impressions. The interference with workflow was minimal, though providers wearing the sensors reported much higher rates of premature termination of the trials secondary to adherence problems. The increased mobility of healthy individuals compared to bedridden patients may be partially responsible for this difference [14,16].

Our study has several limitations. This was not a device trial, or even a pilot study. The sample size was small, and we used two different devices. Devices were placed on few patients or staff members. However, the intention of this paper was to observe the implementation process to demonstrate potential problems. Much too often, the problems during implementation are not brought up, setting unrealistic expectations from the end-user.

5. Conclusions

We caution against an overoptimistic approach to the implementation of biosensors in a healthcare setting, as the process has several potential pitfalls. Despite being FDA-approved, biosensors need to be consistently tested against standard monitoring equipment, such as that of Nihon Kohden, in order to demonstrate readiness for implementation in high-acuity healthcare settings.

Author Contributions: M.R.—data analysis, manuscript writing, A.M.H.—design and supervision, CW.H.III—supervision, manuscript writing, M.D.—data analysis, reliability, K.L.—concept, design, data collection, analysis, manuscript writing. All authors have read and agreed to the published version of the manuscript.

Funding: This research did not receive any specific grant from funding agencies in the public, commercial, or not-for-profit sectors.

Institutional Review Board Statement: The study was approved by the Institutional Review Board at the University of Pennsylvania.

Informed Consent Statement: Informed consent was obtained from all subjects involved in the study.

Data Availability Statement: The datasets used and/or analyzed during the current study are available from the corresponding authors on reasonable request.

Acknowledgments: We would like to thank Sean Sarles for his able assistance.

Conflicts of Interest: The authors declare no conflict of interest.

Appendix A

Appendix A.1. The Questionnaire Used to Study the Attitude of the Staff towards Biosensors in Patients and Staff

1. What is your role?
    a. Attending
    b. APP
    c. RN
    d. CNA
    e. Other staff
2. Did you have contact with biosensor before
    a. Y/N
3. How familiar are you with biosensors (0—not at all; 10—extremely familiar)
    a. 0–10
4. Did you like the experience? (0—not at all; 10—extremely familiar)
5. Is the biosensor easily applied to the participants? Y/N
6. Do you think they are useful? (0—not at all; 10—extremely)
7. How much biosensor can potentially alleviate your workload? (0—not at all; 10—extremely)
8. Do you think patients like them? (0—not at all; 10—extremely)
9. How do you think it will impact the patient's experience
    a. Mobility (0—not at all; 10—extremely)
    b. sleep (0—not at all; 10—extremely)
    c. transport? (0—not at all; 10—extremely)
10. How much did they impair on the work? (0—not at all; 10—very)
11. Compared to current monitoring equipment:
    a. How esay is the biosensor to use (0—not at all; 10—very)
    b. How practical Is the biosensor to use in the healthcare setting (0—not at all; 10—very)
12. When they should be implemented?
    a. Never
    b. 1–2 years
    c. 5–6 years
    d. In 10 years
    e. Never
13. What is the main advantage of biosensor?
14. What is the major problem with biosensors?

15. List up to three adjectives describing this device?
    a. X
    b. X
    c. X
16. How familiar is the staff with devices after the trial (0—not at all; 10—very)
17. How ready is staff for their implementation? (0—not at all; 10—very)

Appendix A.2. The Questionnaire Used to Study the Attitude of the Staff towards Biosensors in Patients and Staff

1. What is your role
    a. Attending
    b. APP
    c. RN
    d. CNA
    e. Other staff
2. Did you have contact with biosensor before
    a. Y/N
3. How familiar are you with biosensors
    a. 0–10
4. Did you like the experience?
5. Do you think they are usefull
6. Do you think patients like them
7. How much did they impair on the work?
8. Do you think
9. When they should be implemented
    a. Never
    b. 1–2 years
    c. 5–6 years
    d. In 10 years
    e. Never
10. What is the main advantage for biosensor
11. What is the major problem with biosensors
12. List up to three adjective describing this device?
    a. X
    b. X
    c. X
13. How familiar is the staff with devices
14. How ready is staff for their implementation?

References

1. Bhalla, N.; Jolly, P.; Formisano, N.; Estrela, P. Introduction to biosensors. *Essays Biochem.* **2016**, *60*, 1–8. [CrossRef]
2. Ajami, S.; Teimouri, F. Features and application of wearable biosensors in medical care. *J. Res. Med. Sci.* **2015**, *20*, 1208–1215. [CrossRef]
3. Justino, C.I.; Duarte, A.C.; Rocha-Santos, T.A. Critical overview on the application of sensors and biosensors for clinical analysis. *TrAC Trends Anal. Chem.* **2016**, *85*, 36–60. [CrossRef]
4. Subramanian, S.; Pamplin, J.C.; Hravnak, M.; Hielsberg, C.; Riker, R.; Rincon, F.; Laudanski, K.; Adzhigirey, L.A.; Moughrabieh, M.A.; Winterbottom, F.A.; et al. Tele-Critical Care: An Update from the Society of Critical Care Medicine Tele-ICU Committee. *Crit. Care Med.* **2020**, *48*, 553–561. [CrossRef]
5. Li, X.; Dunn, J.; Salins, D.; Zhou, G.; Zhou, W.; Rose, S.M.S.-F.; Perelman, D.; Colbert, E.; Runge, R.; Rego, S.; et al. Digital Health: Tracking Physiomes and Activity Using Wearable Biosensors Reveals Useful Health-Related Information. *PLoS Biol.* **2017**, *15*, e2001402. [CrossRef]

6. Bent, B.; Goldstein, B.A.; Kibbe, W.A.; Dunn, J.P. Investigating sources of inaccuracy in wearable optical heart rate sensors. *NPJ Digit. Med.* **2020**, *3*, 1–9. [CrossRef] [PubMed]
7. Mony, P.K.; Thankachan, P.; Bhat, S.; Rao, S.; Washington, M.; Antony, S.; Thomas, A.; Nagarajarao, S.C.; Rao, H.; Amrutur, B. Remote biomonitoring of temperatures in mothers and newborns: Design, development and testing of a wearable sensor device in a tertiary-care hospital in southern India. *BMJ Innov.* **2018**, *4*, 60–67. [CrossRef] [PubMed]
8. Chow, H.-W.; Yang, C.-C. Accuracy of Optical Heart Rate Sensing Technology in Wearable Fitness Trackers for Young and Older Adults: Validation and Comparison Study. *JMIR mHealth uHealth* **2020**, *8*, e14707. [CrossRef] [PubMed]
9. Kaewkannate, K.; Kim, S. A comparison of wearable fitness devices. *BMC Public Health* **2016**, *16*, 1–16. [CrossRef] [PubMed]
10. Eisenhauer, C.; Arnoldussen, B.; López, D.L.; Rodríguez, S.M.; Hu, R.; Van Velthoven, M.H.; Meinert, E.; Brindley, D. Perspectives of People Who Are Overweight and Obese on Using Wearable Technology for Weight Management: Systematic Review. *JMIR mHealth uHealth* **2020**, *8*, e12651. [CrossRef]
11. Malhotra, S.; Jordan, D.; Shortliffe, E.; Patel, V.L. Workflow modeling in critical care: Piecing together your own puzzle. *J. Biomed. Inform.* **2007**, *40*, 81–92. [CrossRef]
12. Breteler, M.J.M.; KleinJan, E.J.; Dohmen, D.A.J.; Leenen, L.P.H.; van Hillegersberg, R.; Ruurda, J.P.; van Loon, K.; Blokhuis, T.J.; Kalkman, C.J. Vital Signs Monitoring with Wearable Sensors in High-risk Surgical Patients. *Anesthesiology* **2020**, *132*, 424–439. [CrossRef] [PubMed]
13. Birchley, G.; Huxtable, R.; Murtagh, M.; Ter Meulen, R.; Flach, P.; Gooberman-Hill, R. Smart homes, private homes? An empirical study of technology researchers' perceptions of ethical issues in developing smart-home health technologies. *BMC Med. Ethics* **2017**, *18*, 23. [CrossRef] [PubMed]
14. Mackintosh, K.A.; Chappel, S.E.; Salmon, J.; Timperio, A.; Ball, K.; Brown, H.; Macfarlane, S.; Ridgers, N.D. Parental Perspectives of a Wearable Activity Tracker for Children Younger Than 13 Years: Acceptability and Usability Study. *JMIR mHealth uHealth* **2019**, *7*, e13858. [CrossRef]
15. Marra, A.; Ely, E.W.; Pandharipande, P.P.; Patel, M.B. The ABCDEF Bundle in Critical Care. *Crit. Care Clin.* **2017**, *33*, 225–243. [CrossRef] [PubMed]
16. Keogh, A.; Dorn, J.F.; Walsh, L.; Calvo, F.; Caulfield, B. Comparing the Usability and Acceptability of Wearable Sensors among Older Irish Adults in a Real-World Context: Observational Study. *JMIR mHealth uHealth* **2020**, *8*, e15704. [CrossRef]
17. Kim, J.; Campbell, A.S.; De Ávila, B.E.-F.; Wang, J. Wearable biosensors for healthcare monitoring. *Nat. Biotechnol.* **2019**, *37*, 389–406. [CrossRef]
18. Harris, P.A.; Taylor, R.; Minor, B.L.; Elliott, V.; Fernandez, M.; O'Neal, L.; McLeod, L.; Delacqua, G.; Delacqua, F.; Kirby, J.; et al. The REDCap consortium: Building an international community of software platform partners. *J. Biomed. Inform.* **2019**, *95*, 103208. [CrossRef]
19. Msc, M.J.M.B.; Huizinga, E.; Van Loon, K.; Leenen, L.P.H.; Dohmen, D.A.J.; Kalkman, C.J.; Blokhuis, T.J. Reliability of wireless monitoring using a wearable patch sensor in high-risk surgical patients at a step-down unit in the Netherlands: A clinical validation study. *BMJ Open* **2018**, *8*, e020162. [CrossRef]
20. Nasseri, M.; Nurse, E.; Glasstetter, M.; Böttcher, S.; Gregg, N.M.; Nandakumar, A.L.; Joseph, B.; Attia, T.P.; Viana, P.F.; Bruno, E.; et al. Signal quality and patient experience with wearable devices for epilepsy management. *Epilepsia* **2020**, *61*. [CrossRef]
21. Kim, J.; Campbell, A.S.; Wang, J. Wearable non-invasive epidermal glucose sensors: A review. *Talanta* **2018**, *177*, 163–170. [CrossRef] [PubMed]
22. Cheung, C.C.; Krahn, A.D.; Andrade, J.G. The Emerging Role of Wearable Technologies in Detection of Arrhythmia. *Can. J. Cardiol.* **2018**, *34*, 1083–1087. [CrossRef] [PubMed]
23. Sawka, M.N.; Friedl, K.E. Emerging Wearable Physiological Monitoring Technologies and Decision Aids for Health and Performance. *J. Appl. Physiol.* **2018**, *124*, 430–431. [CrossRef] [PubMed]
24. Topfer, L.-A. Wearable Artificial Kidneys for End-Stage Kidney Disease. In *CADTH Issues in Emerging Health Technologies*; Canadian Agency for Drugs and Technologies in Health: Ottawa, ON, Canada, 2016.

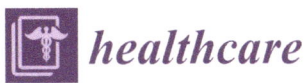

Review

A Meta-Analysis on Prophylactic Donor Heart Tricuspid Annuloplasty in Orthotopic Heart Transplantation: High Hopes from a Small Intervention

Alberto Emanuel Bacusca [1,2,†], **Andrei Tarus** [1,2,†], **Alexandru Burlacu** [2,3,*], **Mihail Enache** [1,2] **and Grigore Tinica** [1,2]

1. Department of Cardiovascular Surgery, Cardiovascular Diseases Institute, 700503 Iasi, Romania; alberto-bacusca@email.umfiasi.ro (A.E.B.); andrei.tarus@umfiasi.ro (A.T.); mihail.enache@umfiasi.ro (M.E.); grigore.tinica@umfiasi.ro (G.T.)
2. Faculty of Medicine, University of Medicine and Pharmacy "Grigore T Popa", 700115 Iasi, Romania
3. Department of Interventional Cardiology, Cardiovascular Diseases Institute, 700503 Iasi, Romania
* Correspondence: alexandru.burlacu@umfiasi.ro; Tel.: +40-7-4448-8580
† Both authors contributed equally.

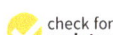

Citation: Bacusca, A.E.; Tarus, A.; Burlacu, A.; Enache, M.; Tinica, G. A Meta-Analysis on Prophylactic Donor Heart Tricuspid Annuloplasty in Orthotopic Heart Transplantation: High Hopes from a Small Intervention. *Healthcare* **2021**, *9*, 306. https://doi.org/10.3390/healthcare9030306

Academic Editor: Richard H. Parrish II

Received: 18 February 2021
Accepted: 8 March 2021
Published: 10 March 2021

Publisher's Note: MDPI stays neutral with regard to jurisdictional claims in published maps and institutional affiliations.

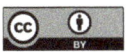

Copyright: © 2021 by the authors. Licensee MDPI, Basel, Switzerland. This article is an open access article distributed under the terms and conditions of the Creative Commons Attribution (CC BY) license (https://creativecommons.org/licenses/by/4.0/).

Abstract: (1) Background: Tricuspid regurgitation (TR) is the most frequent valvulopathy in heart transplant recipients (HTX). We aimed to assess the influence of prophylactic donor heart tricuspid annuloplasty (TA) in orthotopic HTX (HTX-A), comparing the outcomes with those of HTX patients. (2) Methods: Electronic databases of PubMed, EMBASE, and SCOPUS were searched. The endpoints were as follows: the overall rate of postprocedural TR (immediate, one week, six months, and one year after the procedure), postoperative complications (permanent pacemaker implantation rate, bleeding), redo surgery for TR, and mortality. (3) Results: This meta-analysis included seven studies. Immediate postprocedural, one-week, six-month and one-year tricuspid insufficiency rates were significantly lower in the HTX-A group. There was no difference in permanent pacemaker implantation rate between the groups. The incidence of postoperative bleeding was similar in both arms. The rate of redo surgery for severe TR was reported only by two authors. In both publications, the total number of events was higher in the HTX cohort, meanwhile pooled effect analysis showed no difference among the intervention and control groups. Mortality at one year was similar in both arms. (4) Conclusion: Our study showed that donor heart TA reduces TR incidence in the first year after orthotopic heart transplantation without increasing the surgical complexity. This is a potentially important issue, given the demand for heart transplants and the need to optimize outcomes when this resource is scarce.

Keywords: heart transplant; tricuspid annuloplasty; tricuspid regurgitation; prophylactic; meta-analysis

1. Introduction

Tricuspid regurgitation (TR) is the most frequent valvulopathy in heart transplant recipients (HTX), with a reported incidence ranging between 19% to 84% [1,2]. The tricuspid valve (TV) integrity manifests a significant impact on the long-term clinical progress and survival of orthotopic HTX. Although most of the patients present a small degree of tricuspid insufficiency, moderate or greater grades were associated with significantly worse survival and higher post-transplant complications [3]. TR etiology is multifactorial, with several viable hypotheses still debatable: biatrial transplantation technique, allograft dysfunction or rejection, donor-recipient size mismatch, or structural damage during endomyocardial biopsy [4–8].

Postoperative moderate or severe TR negatively affects the overall survival rates after HTX [9]. Despite the fact there is a reported improvement of the degree of tricuspid regurgitation six months after the transplantation, the nature of this valvulopathy is progressive. Studies with more extended follow-up periods reported an increase in severe TR incidence from 7.8% at five years to 14.2% at ten years [10].

The most frequently reported indication for heart surgery after HTX was the atrioventricular valve reconstructions or replacement. 62.5% of these cases were related to the tricuspid valve [11]. Surgical repair or replacement is required when right heart failure becomes refractory to conservative medical treatment [10,12]. The mean duration from transplantation to severe TR diagnosis is reported to be 43 +/- 6.38 months [10]. The cardiac mechanics portending right ventricular failure can be accurately predicted using either right cardiac catheterization or by noninvasive methods computational modeling of hemodynamic and cardiac mechanics using lumped-parameter and biventricular finite element analysis [13,14].

To improve the TV function and avoid the risks associated with redo heart surgery, prophylactic tricuspid annuloplasty (TA) on the donor's heart was proposed as a simple solution to a problem that triggered an increasing concern. Already an established and widely performed surgery, primarily in functional TR treatment, TA accomplished either by DeVega's technique or by a ring is associated with excellent long-term results [15,16]. TA was envisioned to enhance posttransplant hemodynamics and prevent late moderate/severe TR. Moreover, the importance of TV repair was emphasized not only in heart transplanted patients but also in those receiving left ventricular assist devices either as a bridge therapy or as destination therapy, in which concomitant TV repair may reduce postoperative right ventricular failure [17].

Although a significant reduction in TR after this procedure was reported by most of the authors, actual data are controversial, and opinions regarding its impact on overall survival are heterogeneous. To date, there is no consensus on the concomitant management of the TV during heart transplant [18].

The purpose of this study is to assess the influence of prophylactic donor heart tricuspid annuloplasty (in terms of postoperative complications, effects on hemodynamic parameters, short- and long-term tricuspid regurgitation, and mortality) in orthotopic heart transplant recipients.

2. Materials and Methods

The preferred reporting items for systematic reviews and meta-analysis (PRISMA) checklist was applied in each step of the meta-analysis conduction (Supplementary Table S1).

2.1. Search and Eligibility

We performed an extensive search for studies comparing heart transplantation with and without prophylactic tricuspid annuloplasty in three electronic databases: PubMed, EMBASE, and SCOPUS from inception to 20th December 2020. We used the following interrogation terms: "heart transplantation," "tricuspid regurgitation," "tricuspid valvuloplasty," "de Vega." Two independent authors (A.E.B. and A.T.) checked titles and abstracts for eligibility. Fulltext was retrieved for selected papers and verified for fulfilling the following inclusion criteria: (1) study design—randomized control trials, observational studies, propensity score match studies; (2) population—patients with orthotopic heart transplantation; (3) intervention—donor heart tricuspid annuloplasty; (4) comparators—heart transplanted patients without prophylactic tricuspid annuloplasty; (5) outcomes—reported at least post-transplantation tricuspid regurgitation. Both authors scanned the references in relevant articles. The third reviewer (G.T.) mediated the situations when consensus regarding a manuscript's inclusion was not achieved.

2.2. Intraoperative Timing and Outcomes

We compared intraoperative timing between two cohorts (ischemic time, cardiopulmonary bypass time, and cross-clamp time). The endpoints were as follows: the overall rate of postprocedural TR (immediate, one week, six months, and one year after the procedure), postoperative complications (permanent pacemaker implantation rate, bleeding), redo surgery for TR, and mortality.

2.3. Data Collection and Synthesis

The same reviewers extracted data only from retrieved published manuscripts and registered them in standard tables. When the ratio of events and not raw data were available, we calculated the event number from the described ratio and total cohort.

Review Manager (RevMan) Version 5.3 (Nordic Cochrane Centre, The Cochrane Collaboration, 2012, Copenhagen, Denmark) software was used to generate the pooled effect size with odds ratio (OR) and 95% confidence intervals (CI) by Mantel–Haenszel method and random effect model for dichotomous data. A p-value of less than 0.05 was considered significant. Conversion to mean and standard deviation (SD), when median and IQR were available, was performed following the methods published by Luo et al. and Wan et al. [10,11]. The pooled sample mean and pooled standard deviation for selected studies were calculated according to the Cochrane Handbook's recommendation for Systematic Reviews. We used MedCalc Statistical Software version 14.8.1 (MedCalc Software bvba, Ostend, Belgium; http://www.medcalc.org (accessed on 20 December 2020); 2014) for comparative statistics. Chi-squared and t-Student's tests were used to compare dichotomous and continuous data.

2.4. Studies Quality Assessment

The risk of publication bias was assessed with the Newcastle–Ottawa quality assessment scale (NOS) for cohort studies and the Cochrane risk of bias tool for randomized controlled trials.

3. Results

3.1. Literature Search and Study Selection

The digital search identified a total of 1506 titles. After duplicates removal, a total of 1068 references were screened by title and abstract. There were 26 articles selected for full-text analysis (Figure 1).

Seven full-text articles that compared the incidence of moderate or severe tricuspid regurgitation, postoperative complications, and late mortality in heart transplant patients with donor tricuspid annuloplasty with cohorts with no prophylactic tricuspid valve repair during OHT were retrieved [2,19–24]. Two of the studies had the same cohort of patients and reported the same outcomes at different periods [22,23]. Two other studies have been conducted by the same authors in the same center [2,20]. The criteria for patient selection and the reported outcomes were the same. We have considered the data presented in the most recent study that also included the more representative cohorts of patients.

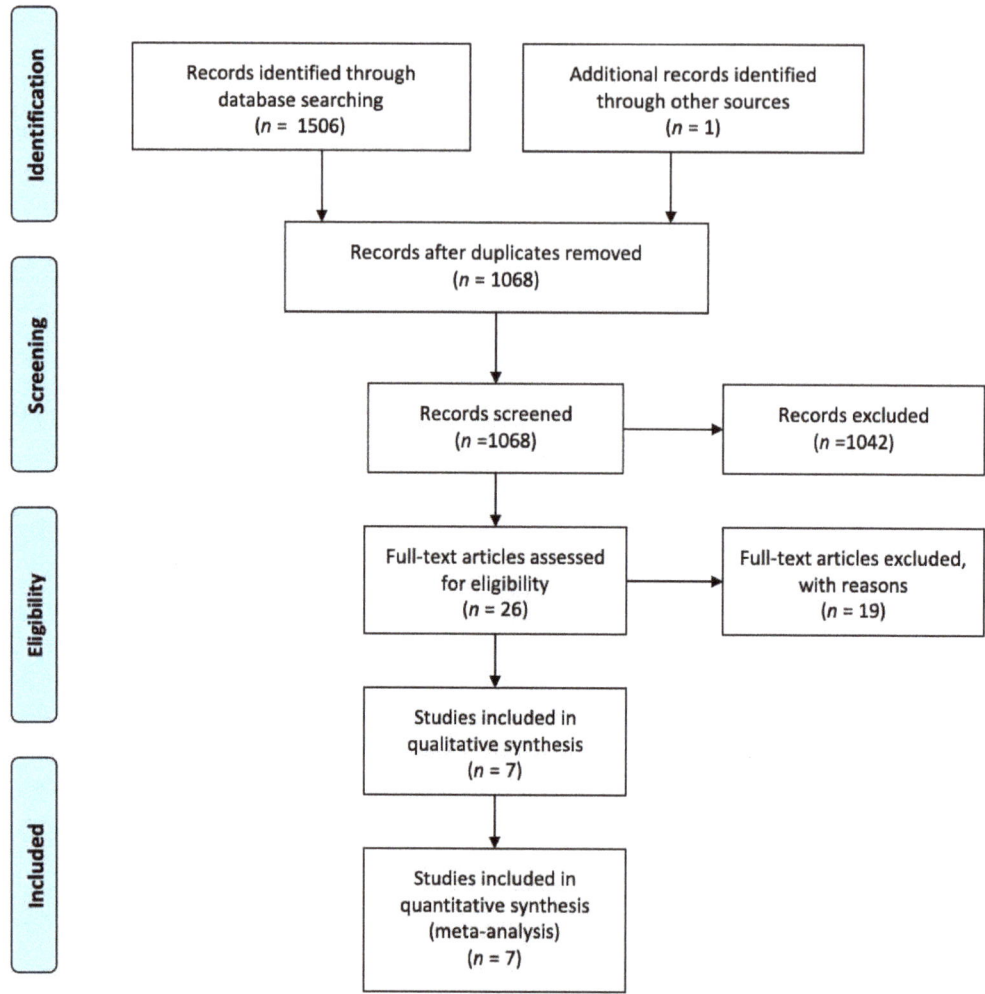

Figure 1. Preferred reporting items for systematic reviews and meta-analysis (PRISMA) flow diagram for study selection.

3.2. Study Characteristics and Risk of Bias

The characteristics of the selected studies are presented in Table 1. All studies were appreciated to have a good quality design (Supplementary Table S2).

3.3. Patient and Periprocedural Characteristics

The final analysis included 730 patients, of which 359 heart transplant recipients with prophylactic donor tricuspid annuloplasty (HTX-A) and 371 patients without tricuspid valve repair (HTX group). Both bicaval and biatrial heart transplantation techniques were taken into account. De Vega and Ring tricuspid valve annuloplasty procedures were analyzed.

Baseline characteristics and periprocedural data distinguishing each group are summarized in Table 2. Patients in both groups predominantly male and had similar ages.

Table 1. Summary of included studies.

Author	Year	Country	No. of Centers	Type of Study	Time Period	Type of Surgery	Patient Group	No. of Patients Per Group	Follow-Up
Jeevanandam	2004	USA	1	RCT	April 1997–March 1998	Bicaval orthotopic heart transplantation with DeVega TVA	HTX HTX-A	30 30	1 year
Jeevanandam	2006	USA	1	RCT	April 1997–December 2003	Bicaval orthotopic heart transplantation with DeVega TVA	HTX HTX-A	30 30	5.7 to 6.7 years
Rubin, G	2018	USA	1	Retrospective observational	2013–2017	Orthotopic heart transplantation with DeVega TVA	HTX HTX-A	104 76	32 months
Greenberg J	2017	USA	18	Retrospective observational-Propensity score-matched	January 2002–December 2016	Bicaval orthotopic heart transplantation with DeVega TVA	HTX HTX-A	117 130	7.9 ± 4.3 years 5.2 ± 2.9 years
Fiorelli	2007	Brazil	1	Prospective Observational- nonrandomized	March 1985–December 2005	Bicaval orthotopic heart transplantation with DeVega TVA	HTX HTX-A	10 10	14.6 ± 4.3 months
Fiorelli	2010	Brazil	1	Prospective Observational- nonrandomized	2002–2010	Bicaval orthotopic heart transplantation with DeVega TVA	HTX HTX-A	15 15	26.9 ± 5.4 months
Brown	2004	USA	1	Retrospective Observational	November 1999–July 2001	Biatrial cardiac transplantation with a Cabrol modification with either a DeVega (n = 10) or Ring (n = 15) TVA	HTX HTX-A	25 25	6 months

HTX—heart transplantation; HTX-A—heart transplantation with tricuspid annuloplasty; TVA—tricuspid valve annuloplasty.

Table 2. Baseline characteristics and periprocedural data.

Parameters	No. of Studies	No. of HTX Patients	No. of HTX-A Patients	HTX Mean ± SD or (%)	HTX-A Mean ± SD or (%)	p-Value
Demographics						
Age	5	331	319	51.48 ± 10.20	51.92 ± 11.32	0.6
Male	5	331	319	72.2%	73.3%	0.8
Preoperative data						
Ischemic etiology of the end-stage heart failure	4	132	148	88.63%	67.57%	0.0001
Inotropic medication	2	172	188	30.23%	37.76%	0.2
Preoperative renal function						
Creatinine	2	187	203	1.26 ± 0.93	1.22 ± 0.46	0.6
BUN	2	187	203	23.73 ± 11.90	23.56 ± 11.82	0.9
Hemodynamic parameters						
Pulmonary capillary wedge pressure	2	187	203	17.16 ± 8.55	19.71 ± 9.14	0.005
Pulmonary vascular resistance woods units	5	298	300	2.29 ± 1.00	2.17 ± 1.02	0.15
Mechanical circulatory support	4	306	304	55.88%	52.63%	0.5
Intraoperative times						
CPB duration	3	144	116	173.33 ± 27.75	154.15 ± 25.89	<0.0001
Ischemic time	5	326	314	181.75 ± 40.83	165.32 ± 41.72	<0.0001
Aortic cross-clamp	4	169	141	88.02 ± 20.50	86.89 ± 13.86	0.6

Ischemic etiology of the end-stage heart failure was more frequent in the HTX group (88.63% vs. 67.57%, $p = 0.0001$). There was no difference in preoperative renal status, mechanical circulatory support, or inotropic drug use. The pulmonary capillary wedge pressure was higher in the HTX-A group (19.70 ± 9.13 vs. 17.15 ± 8.54, $p = 0.0047$), but pulmonary vascular resistance was similar.

3.4. Intraoperative Times

Intraoperative data analysis revealed longer cardiopulmonary bypass time (173.32 ± 27.75 vs. 154.14 ± 25.88, $p < 0.0001$) and ischemic time (181.75 ± 40.82 vs. 165.31 ± 41.72, $p < 0.0001$) in the HTX group, but no difference in the aortic cross-clamp time.

3.5. Outcomes

3.5.1. Tricuspid Regurgitation

Forest plots for postoperative TR in different periods are shown in Figure 2a–d. Immediate postprocedural, one week, six months and one year tricuspid insufficiency rate was significantly lower in HTX-A group (HTX-A vs. HTX: OR: 0.04, 95% CI, 0.01 to 0.34, $I^2 = 0\%$); (HTX-A vs. HTX: OR: 0.25, 95% CI, 0.06 to 1.03, $I^2 = 8\%$); (HTX-A vs. HTX: OR: 0.18, 95% CI, 0.05 to 0.66, $I^2 = 0\%$); (HTX-A vs. HTX: OR: 0.17, 95% CI, 0.04 to 0.77, $I^2 = 0\%$).

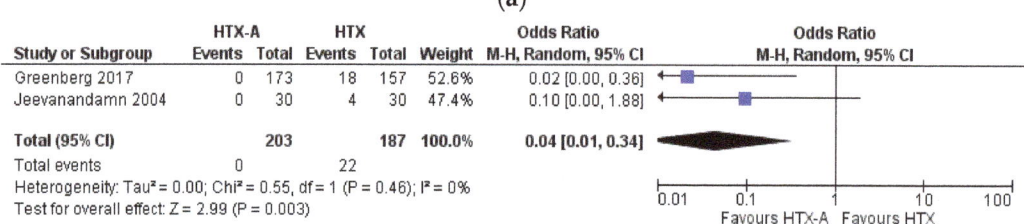

Figure 2. Cont.

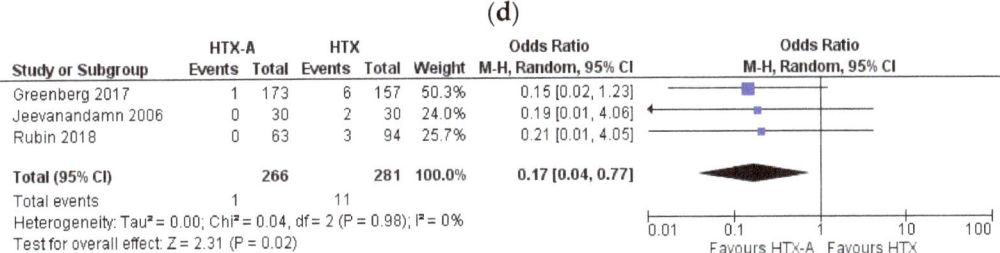

Figure 2. Forest plot depicting post-transplantation TR: (**a**) immediate; (**b**) after 1 week; (**c**) after 6 months; (**d**) after 1 year.

3.5.2. Periprocedural Complications

There were no difference in permanent pacemaker implantation rate between the goups (HTX-A vs. HTX: OR: 2.19, 95% CI, 0.50 to 9.64, $I^2 = 0$%) (Figure 3a). Incidence of postoperative bleeding was similar in both arms (HTX-A vs. HTX: OR: 1.00, 95% CI, 0.23 to 4.28, $I^2 = 0$%) (Figure 3b).

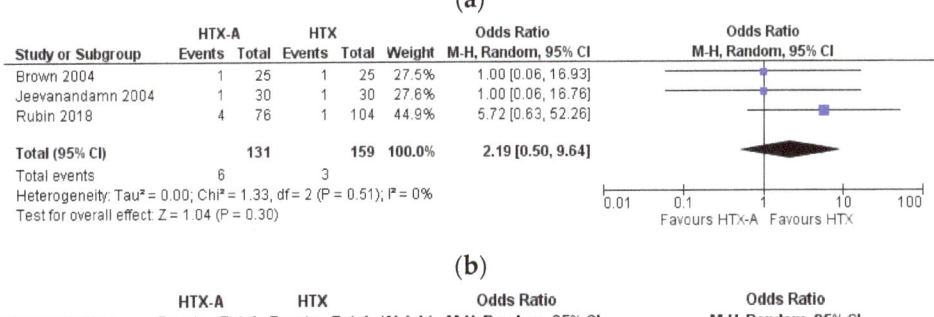

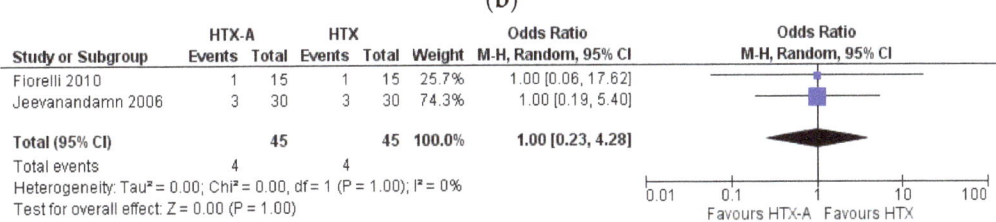

Figure 3. Forest plot depicting periprocedural complications: (**a**) permanent pacemaker implantation rate; (**b**) postoperative severe bleeding rate.

3.5.3. Reoperation and Survival

The rate of redo surgery for severe TR was reported only by two authors. In both publications, the total number of events was higher in the HTX cohort, meanwhile pooled effect analysis showed no difference among the intervention and control groups (HTX-A vs. HTX: OR: 0.13, 95% CI, 0.02 to 1.11, $I^2 = 0$%) (Figure 4a). Mortality at 1 year was similar in both arms (HTX-A vs. HTX: OR: 1.01, 95% CI, 0.41 to 2.49, $I^2 = 0$%) (Figure 4b).

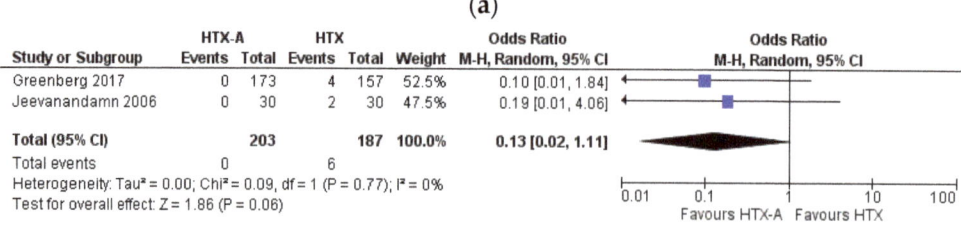

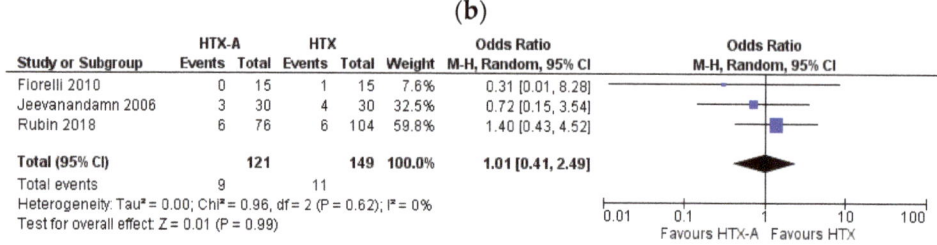

Figure 4. Forest plot depicting: (**a**) reoperation rate on tricuspid valve after transplantation; (**b**) 1-year survival.

4. Discussion

Our meta-analysis shows that donor heart tricuspid annuloplasty reduces tricuspid regurgitation incidence in the first year after orthotopic heart transplantation without increasing the surgical complexity. No significant benefit or harm was revealed on long-term mortality. Performed in high-experienced centers, prophylactic donor tricuspid annuloplasty could be routinely considered during orthotopic heart transplantation as it tends to incline the balance to a more favorable evolution.

Tricuspid regurgitation is a common problem after heart transplantation. There are two main types of tricuspid insufficiency. Type I dysfunction is more common and occurs earlier, with a reported average time from the procedure to the onset of severe TR of 13 months [25]. In this scenario, the regurgitation is due to the alteration in the TV geometry and right atrium, followed by annular/ventricular dilation. The tricuspid valve leaflet motion is normal. Evolution under medical therapy is usually mild but may become severe and require surgical correction [25,26].

Type II dysfunction has a reported average time to onset of severe TR of 28 months and is characterized by an excessive leaflet motion mostly due to chordal disruption after right ventricular endomyocardial biopsy [25]. Mild to moderate TR may be well-tolerated, but recurrent injury or spontaneous rupture of the chordae tendineae could also lead to severe symptomatic TR that may require surgical repair [27,28].

The etiology of the disease is multifactorial. In a multivariate analysis, the standard biatrial transplantation technique is considered the most independent predictor for early and late TR in heart transplant recipients [5]. Due to a higher distortion and dilatation of the tricuspid annulus, biatrial transplantation can lead to a more frequent and severe type I tricuspid regurgitation in all time scales following transplantation. After a one-year follow-up, the patients who underwent transplantation by the biatrial technique showed higher right-sided pressures and thus added another risk factor in developing the TR [5].

Despite these findings, some authors disagree with this hypothesis. Kim and colleagues found that the occurrence of TR was not related to the anastomosis technique [29], and Kalra et al. revealed in an echocardiographic study comparing bi-caval versus atrial anastomosis technique, no effect of the technique on tricuspid regurgitation [30]. Another study identified that the strongest predictor of moderate to severe TR would rather be the presence of intraoperative RV dysfunction [3]. Other risk factors associated with the development of type I TR are the donor age, the preoperative pulmonary hemodynamics, pre-transplant dilated cardiomyopathy weight mismatch, and more than two cellular rejection episodes [5,9,29].

The development of long-term significant type II TR after transplantation was correlated with the number of endomyocardial biopsies performed (EMB) [5]. (*A significant correlation between the occurrence of tricuspid valve injury and EMB number performed per patient was observed* [12].) Percutaneous transvenous EMB remains the most suitable method for the early identification of histopathologic alterations; thus, the gold standard in the diagnose of cardiac rejection [31]. The reported TR caused by iatrogenic injury during EMB was 6–32% of cases [3,32,33], and almost half of all myocardial fragments recovered from patients with significant TR revealing the presence of chordae tendineae [12]. The risk factors of developing tricuspid injury are EMB technique, bioptome type, method of bioptome guidance, and access route and team experience [12,32,34]. Noninvasive methods sought to replace the EMB yet did not prove able to overcome histological analysis's advantages [35,36]. Gallium-67 scintigraphy used as a screening method has resulted in favorable outcomes, with an approximately 10-fold reduction of EMB per patient [37]. Although TV annuloplasty is performed to maintain the annulus's standard size, minor structural damage caused by EMB could also be attenuated due to the annulus reduction [23].

The impact of TR on transplantation outcomes is unquestionable. Anderson and colleagues report a 38% operative mortality in patients with mild or greater severity TR versus 7% in patients with no or trace TR. In the absence of RV dysfunction, one-year survival rates were 92% for those with no or trace TR vs. 57% with mild or greater severity TR. A vital survival gap was also noticed in the patients with RV failure (83% vs. 63%) [3]. After ten years, follow-up in Algharni et al. reported 90% survival rates in patients with less than moderate tricuspid regurgitation compared to 43% for moderate and severe TR [9]. Individuals with higher grades of TR also had more extended hospital stays and higher renal dysfunction rates and dialysis [18]. They were also more prone to need mechanical circulatory support and required more often redo open chest procedures [3].

Although prompt surgical repair of severe TR that develops early after transplantation is regarded as a safe procedure in selected patients, with an improvement in the overall survival after 1, 5 and 10 years due to better cardiac performance and alleviation of associated organ dysfunction, this redo surgery is not risk-free [11,38]. The postoperative evolution was marked by high rates of prolonged ventilation (33%), new-onset requirement of hemodialysis treatment (36.8%), and infectious complications (11.1%). The reported early mortality was 11.1% [11].

Tricuspid valve annuloplasty had been proven already as a simple, safe, effective, and reliable surgical procedure [39]. Moreover, because it is the least expensive way to treat functional TR, De Vega's TVA established itself as the treatment of choice for functional TR [39]. The procedure adds little additional time of 5 to 10 min to the operation, the fact that it is also suggested by similar aortic cross-clamp times between the HTX and HTX-A groups [40]. Instead, our results show that TVA contributed to a shorter cardiopulmonary bypass and ischemic time fact attributed to improved right ventricular performance and hemodynamic parameters [23].

TVA has been hypothesized to exert its significant benefits in the early postoperative period [23]. Our meta-analysis of immediate postprocedural, one-week, six-month, and one-year tricuspid insufficiency rates showed significantly lower values in the HTX-A group. This finding would explain the rationale behind establishing the prophylactic donor tricuspid annuloplasty procedure as standard practice. On the other hand, contrary to expected, there was no other significant improvement in the postoperative outcomes. Even though multiple authors have brought strong arguments about the TR's impact on morbidity and mortality rates, our results revealed no difference in one-year mortality between groups. Unfortunately, the fact that survival data were very heterogenous reported could be why these inexplicable results.

One of the most significant drawbacks of the procedure revolves around the complications involving the conduction system. Rubin and colleagues conducted the most edifying study that focuses on the electrophysiologic consequences associated with tricuspid annuloplasty in heart transplantation. The conduction disturbances reported as significantly more common in the experimental group were the right bundle branch block, left anterior fascicular block, and complete heart block. Permanent pacemaker (PPM) implantation was also more frequent in patients receiving DVA. The authors advise that annuloplasty should be integrated within the context of an equitable tradeoff between the possible risk of conduction abnormalities that occur in the immediate postoperative period and the benefit of preventing late moderate/severe TR [24].

The reported incidence of PPM implantation in heart transplanted patients varies between 5.3% and 10.9% [24,41,42]. Older patients undergoing a biatrial surgical technique with a previous history of amiodarone use are already more susceptible to necessitate pacing without tricuspid intervention [43,44]. Our results showed no difference in the PPM between the groups. However, the negative effect of tissue-damaging during annuloplasty may have been counterbalanced by a shorter ischemic time in the HTX-A group previously reported to contribute to the occurrence of the conduction disturbances [44].

All in one, TA is a simple technique that is worth considering when it comes to orthotopic heart transplantation. The procedure's aim is clear: to reduce the annulus dilatation development and thus the long-term tricuspid regurgitation. If the results are according to what was initially expected when they were first introduced is still debatable. Correctly performed, it could reduce the risk of severe regurgitation and thus, improve the survival rates and postoperative outcomes while carrying no additional risk for the patient. Some surgeons have discontinued this procedure two years after its implementation, some have assimilated it into the transplantation protocol on the presumption that it has its advantages. However, in the lack of precise data regarding long-term benefits, the basic principle is that TA could be performed as a routine adjunct to orthotopic heart transplantation by experienced surgeons.

Limitations

This meta-analysis has some significant limitations. First, it includes three observational retrospective studies: a matched case–control study, two prospective nonrandomized studies, and two RCTs. Second, two of the studies authored by the same team of researchers included the same cohort of patients and reported mostly the same outcomes at different periods, the first after a follow-up of 1 year and the second after a follow-up of 5.7 to 6.7 years. Another group of studies authored by the same authors was conducted respecting identical patient selection criteria and the reported outcomes. To avoid biased results, we have considered the meta-analysis of the data presented in the most recent and representative of them. Third, TR was not uniformly graded in all of the studies. Jeevandaman described four degrees of regurgitation, while the authors used a three-stage classification. Fourthly, there were significant discrepancies regarding the surgical technique. Rubin did not report the technique of heart transplantation at all. The patients included in the study conducted by Brown had undergone biatrial heart transplantation, while the other authors used the bicaval technique. TA was performed by De Vega's technique in all of the studies, except for Brown, who also included the annuloplasties performed using rings.

5. Conclusions

Our study showed that donor heart tricuspid annuloplasty reduces tricuspid regurgitation incidence in the first year after orthotopic heart transplantation without increasing the surgical complexity. Further large randomized clinical trials are necessary to evaluate the impact of this procedure on long-term insufficiency and outcome benefits. Regarding one-year and long-term mortality, no significant benefit or harm was revealed. Thus, we emphasize the importance of extending the follow-up period on larger cohorts. In conclusion, if performed in high-experienced centers, prophylactic donor tricuspid annuloplasty could be routinely considered during orthotopic heart transplantation as it tends to incline the balance to a more favorable evolution without adding any additional risks.

Supplementary Materials: The following are available online at https://www.mdpi.com/2227-9032/9/3/306/s1, Table S1: preferred reporting items for systematic reviews and meta-analysis (PRISMA) checklist, Table S2: Risk of publication bias assessment.

Author Contributions: Conceptualization, A.E.B. and A.T.; methodology, A.B.; software, A.E.B.; validation, G.T., A.B. and M.E.; writing—original draft preparation, A.E.B., A.T.; writing—review and editing, A.B.; visualization, M.E.; supervision, G.T.; project administration, A.B. All authors have read and agreed to the published version of the manuscript.

Funding: This research received no external funding.

Institutional Review Board Statement: Not applicable.

Informed Consent Statement: Not applicable.

Data Availability Statement: The data presented in this study are available on request from the corresponding author.

Conflicts of Interest: The authors declare no conflict of interest.

References

1. Wong, R.C.C.; Abrahams, Z.; Hanna, M.; Pangrace, J.; Gonzalez-Stawinski, G.; Starling, R.; Taylor, D. Tricuspid Regurgitation After Cardiac Transplantation: An Old Problem Revisited. *J. Heart Lung Transplant.* **2008**, *27*, 247–252. [CrossRef]
2. Fiorelli, A.I.; Oliveira, J.L.; Santos, R.H.; Coelho, G.B.; Oliveira, A.S.; Lourenço-Filho, D.D.; Lapenna, G.; Dias, R.R.; Bacal, F.; Bocchi, E.A.; et al. Can tricuspid annuloplasty of the donor heart reduce valve insufficiency following cardiac transplantation with bicaval anastomosis? *Heart Surg. Forum* **2010**, *13*, E168–E171. [CrossRef] [PubMed]
3. Anderson, C.A.; Shernan, S.K.; Leacche, M.; Rawn, J.D.; Paul, S.; Mihaljevic, T.; Jarcho, J.A.; Stevenson, L.W.; Fang, J.C.; Lewis, E.F.; et al. Severity of intraoperative tricuspid regurgitation predicts poor late survival following cardiac transplantation. *Ann. Thorac. Surg.* **2004**, *78*, 1635–1642. [CrossRef]
4. Bainbridge, A.D.; Cave, M.; Roberts, M.; Casula, R.; Mist, B.A.; Parameshwar, J.; Wallwork, J.; Large, S.R. A prospective randomized trial of complete atrioventricular transplantation versus ventricular transplantation with atrioplasty. *J. Heart Lung Transpl.* **1999**, *18*, 407–413. [CrossRef]
5. Aziz, T.M.; Burgess, M.I.; Rahman, A.N.; Campbell, C.S.; Deiraniya, A.K.; Yonan, N.A. Risk factors for tricuspid valve regurgitation after orthotopic heart transplantation. *Ann. Thorac. Surg.* **1999**, *68*, 1247–1251. [CrossRef]
6. De Simone, R.; Lange, R.; Sack, F.U.; Mehmanesh, H.; Hagl, S. Atrioventricular valve insufficiency and atrial geometry in orthotopic heart transplantation. *Cardiologia* **1994**, *39*, 325–334. [CrossRef]
7. Leyh, R.G.; Jahnke, A.W.; Kraatz, E.G.; Sievers, H.H. Cardiovascular dynamics and dimensions after bicaval and standard cardiac transplantation. *Ann. Thorac. Surg.* **1995**, *59*, 1495–1500. [CrossRef]
8. Deleuze, P.; Benvenuti, C.; Mazzucotelli, J.P.; Perdrix, C.; Le Besnerais, P.; Mourtada, A.; Hillion, M.L.; Patrat, J.F.; Loisance, D.Y. Orthotopic cardiac transplantation with caval anastomoses: A comparative randomised study with the standard procedure in 81 cases. *Arch. Des Mal. Du Coeur Et Des Vaiss.* **1996**, *89*, 43–48.
9. Algarni, K.D.; Arafat, A.A.; Pragliola, C.; Alhebaishi, Y.S.; AlFayez, L.A.; AlOtaibi, K.; Bakhsh, A.M.; Amro, A.A.; Adam, A.I. Tricuspid Valve Regurgitation After Heart Transplantation: A Single-Center 10-year Experience. *J. Saudi Heart Assoc.* **2020**, *32*, 213–218. [CrossRef] [PubMed]
10. Chan, M.C.; Giannetti, N.; Kato, T.; Kornbluth, M.; Oyer, P.; Valantine, H.A.; Robbins, R.C.; Hunt, S.A. Severe tricuspid regurgitation after heart transplantation. *J. Heart Lung Transplant.* **2001**, *20*, 709–717. [CrossRef]
11. Farag, M.; Arif, R.; Raake, P.; Kreusser, M.; Karck, M.; Ruhparwar, A.; Schmack, B. Cardiac surgery in the heart transplant recipient: Outcome analysis and long-term results. *Clin. Transplant.* **2019**, *33*, e13709. [CrossRef] [PubMed]
12. Mielniczuk, L.; Haddad, H.; Davies, R.A.; Veinot, J.P. Tricuspid valve chordal tissue in endomyocardial biopsy specimens of patients with significant tricuspid regurgitation. *J. Heart Lung Transplant.* **2005**, *24*, 1586–1590. [CrossRef] [PubMed]
13. Bellavia, D.; Iacovoni, A.; Agnese, V.; Falletta, C.; Coronnello, C.; Pasta, S.; Novo, G.; di Gesaro, G.; Senni, M.; Maalouf, J.; et al. Usefulness of regional right ventricular and right atrial strain for prediction of early and late right ventricular failure following a left ventricular assist device implant: A machine learning approach. *Int. J. Artif. Organs* **2020**, *43*, 297–314. [CrossRef]
14. Scardulla, F.; Agnese, V.; Romano, G.; Di Gesaro, G.; Sciacca, S.; Bellavia, D.; Clemenza, F.; Pilato, M.; Pasta, S. Modeling Right Ventricle Failure After Continuous Flow Left Ventricular Assist Device: A Biventricular Finite-Element and Lumped-Parameter Analysis. *Cardiovasc. Eng. Technol.* **2018**, *9*, 427–437. [CrossRef] [PubMed]
15. Morishita, A.; Kitamura, M.; Noji, S.; Aomi, S.; Endo, M.; Koyanagi, H. Long-term results after De Vega's tricuspid annuloplasty. *J. Cardiovasc. Surg.* **2002**, *43*, 773–777.
16. Kuwaki, K.; Morishita, K.; Tsukamoto, M.; Abe, T. Tricuspid valve surgery for functional tricuspid valve regurgitation associated with left-sided valvular disease. *Eur. J. Cardiothorac. Surg.* **2001**, *20*, 577–582. [CrossRef]
17. Lee, C.H.; Wei, J. Successful continuous-flow left ventricular assist device implantation with adjuvant tricuspid valve repair for advanced heart failure. *Cardiovasc. J. Afr.* **2016**, *27*, e14–e16. [CrossRef]

18. Bishawi, M.; Zanotti, G.; Shaw, L.; MacKenzie, M.; Castleberry, A.; Bartels, K.; Schroder, J.; Velazquez, E.; Swaminathan, M.; Rogers, J.; et al. Tricuspid Valve Regurgitation Immediately After Heart Transplant and Long-Term Outcomes. *Ann. Thorac. Surg.* **2019**, *107*, 1348–1355. [CrossRef] [PubMed]
19. Brown, N.E.; Muehlebach, G.F.; Jones, P.; Gorton, M.E.; Stuart, R.S.; Borkon, A.M. Tricuspid annuloplasty significantly reduces early tricuspid regurgitation after biatrial heart transplantation. *J. Heart Lung Transplant.* **2004**, *23*, 1160–1162. [CrossRef]
20. Fiorelli, A.I.; Stolf, N.A.; Abreu Filho, C.A.; Santos, R.H.; Buco, F.H.; Fiorelli, L.R.; Issa, V.; Bacal, F.; Bocchi, E.A. Prophylactic donor tricuspid annuloplasty in orthotopic bicaval heart transplantation. *Transplant. Proc.* **2007**, *39*, 2527–2530. [CrossRef]
21. Greenberg, J.; Teman, N.R.; Haft, J.W.; Romano, M.A.; Pagani, F.D.; Aaronson, K.D.; Wu, A.H. Association of Donor Tricuspid Valve Repair With Outcomes After Cardiac Transplantation. *Ann. Thorac. Surg.* **2018**, *105*, 542–547. [CrossRef] [PubMed]
22. Jeevanandam, V.; Russell, H.; Mather, P.; Furukawa, S.; Anderson, A.; Grzywacz, F.; Raman, J. A one-year comparison of prophylactic donor tricuspid annuloplasty in heart transplantation. *Ann. Thorac. Surg.* **2004**, *78*, 759–766. [CrossRef] [PubMed]
23. Jeevanandam, V.; Russell, H.; Mather, P.; Furukawa, S.; Anderson, A.; Raman, J. Donor Tricuspid Annuloplasty During Orthotopic Heart Transplantation: Long-Term Results of a Prospective Controlled Study. *Ann. Thorac. Surg.* **2006**, *82*, 2089–2095. [CrossRef] [PubMed]
24. Rubin, G.A.; Sanchez, J.; Bayne, J.; Avula, U.M.R.; Takayama, H.; Takeda, K.; Naka, Y.; Garan, H.; Farr, M.A.; Wan, E.Y. Conduction Abnormalities Associated with Tricuspid Annuloplasty in Cardiac Transplantation. *ASAIO J.* **2019**, *65*, 707–711. [CrossRef] [PubMed]
25. Filsoufi, F.; Salzberg, S.P.; Anderson, C.A.; Couper, G.S.; Cohn, L.H.; Adams, D.H. Optimal surgical management of severe tricuspid regurgitation in cardiac transplant patients. *J. Heart Lung Transplant.* **2006**, *25*, 289–293. [CrossRef] [PubMed]
26. Cladellas, M.; Abadal, M.L.; Pons-Lladó, G.; Ballester, M.; Carreras, F.; Obrador, D.; Garcia-Moll, M.; Padró, J.M.; Aris, A.; Caralps, J.M. Early transient multivalvular regurgitation detected by pulsed Doppler in cardiac transplantation. *Am. J. Cardiol.* **1986**, *58*, 1122–1124. [CrossRef]
27. Yankah, A.C.; Musci, M.; Weng, Y.; Loebe, M.; Zurbruegg, H.R.; Siniawski, H.; Mueller, J.; Hetzer, R. Tricuspid valve dysfunction and surgery after orthotopic cardiac transplantation. *Eur. J. Cardiothorac. Surg.* **2000**, *17*, 343–348. [CrossRef]
28. Braverman, A.C.; Coplen, S.E.; Mudge, G.H.; Lee, R.T. Ruptured chordae tendineae of the tricuspid valve as a complication of endomyocardial biopsy in heart transplant patients. *Am. J. Cardiol.* **1990**, *66*, 111–113. [CrossRef]
29. Kim, G.S.; Kim, J.J.; Kim, J.B.; Kim, D.H.; Song, J.M.; Yun, T.J.; Choo, S.J.; Kang, D.H.; Chung, C.H.; Song, J.K.; et al. Fate of atrioventricular valve function of the transplanted heart. *Circ. J.* **2014**, *78*, 1654–1660. [CrossRef]
30. Kalra, N.; Copeland, J.G.; Sorrell, V.L. Tricuspid regurgitation after orthotopic heart transplantation. *Echocardiography* **2010**, *27*, 1–4. [CrossRef]
31. Stewart, S.; Winters, G.L.; Fishbein, M.C.; Tazelaar, H.D.; Kobashigawa, J.; Abrams, J.; Andersen, C.B.; Angelini, A.; Berry, G.J.; Burke, M.M.; et al. Revision of the 1990 working formulation for the standardization of nomenclature in the diagnosis of heart rejection. *J. Heart Lung Transplant.* **2005**, *24*, 1710–1720. [CrossRef] [PubMed]
32. Saraiva, F.; Matos, V.; Gonçalves, L.; Antunes, M.; Providência, L.A. Complications of endomyocardial biopsy in heart transplant patients: A retrospective study of 2117 consecutive procedures. *Transplant. Proc.* **2011**, *43*, 1908–1912. [CrossRef] [PubMed]
33. Mügge, A.; Daniel, W.G.; Herrmann, G.; Simon, R.; Lichtlen, P.R. Quantification of tricuspid regurgitation by Doppler color flow mapping after cardiac transplantation. *Am. J. Cardiol.* **1990**, *66*, 884–887. [CrossRef]
34. Fiorelli, A.I.; Coelho, G.H.B.; Oliveira, J.L., Jr.; Aiello, V.D.; Benvenuti, L.A.; Santos, A.; Chi, A.; Tallans, A.; Igushi, M.L.; Bacal, F.; et al. Endomyocardial Biopsy as Risk Factor in the Development of Tricuspid Insufficiency After Heart Transplantation. *Transplant. Proc.* **2009**, *41*, 935–937. [CrossRef] [PubMed]
35. Warnecke, H.; Müller, J.; Cohnert, T.; Hummel, M.; Spiegelsberger, S.; Siniawski, H.K.; Lieback, E.; Hetzer, R. Clinical heart transplantation without routine endomyocardial biopsy. *J. Heart Lung Transplant.* **1992**, *11*, 1093–1102.
36. Camargo, P.R.; Mazzieri, R.; Snitcowsky, R.; Higuchi, M.L.; Meneghetti, J.C.; Soares Júnior, J.; Fiorelli, A.; Ebaid, M.; Pileggi, F. Correlation between gallium-67 imaging and endomyocardial biopsy in children with severe dilated cardiomyopathy. *Int. J. Cardiol.* **1990**, *28*, 293–297. [CrossRef]
37. Fiorelli, A.I.; Coelho, G.H.; Aiello, V.D.; Benvenuti, L.A.; Palazzo, J.F.; Santos Júnior, V.P.; Canizares, B.; Dias, R.R.; Stolf, N.A. Tricuspid valve injury after heart transplantation due to endomyocardial biopsy: An analysis of 3550 biopsies. *Transplant. Proc.* **2012**, *44*, 2479–2482. [CrossRef]
38. Bollano, E.; Karason, K.; Lidén, H.; Dellgren, G. How should we manage early tricuspid valve regurgitation after heart transplantation? *Int. J. Cardiol.* **2016**, *214*, 191–193. [CrossRef]
39. Wei, J.; Chang, C.Y.; Lee, F.Y.; Lai, W.Y. De Vega's semicircular annuloplasty for tricuspid valve regurgitation. *Ann. Thorac. Surg.* **1993**, *55*, 482–485. [CrossRef]
40. Kanter, K.R.; Doelling, N.R.; Fyfe, D.A.; Sharma, S.; Tam, V.K.H. De Vega tricuspid annuloplasty for tricuspid regurgitation in children. *Ann. Thorac. Surg.* **2001**, *72*, 1344–1348. [CrossRef]
41. Cantillon, D.J.; Tarakji, K.G.; Hu, T.; Hsu, A.; Smedira, N.G.; Starling, R.C.; Wilkoff, B.L.; Saliba, W.I. Long-term outcomes and clinical predictors for pacemaker-requiring bradyarrhythmias after cardiac transplantation: Analysis of the UNOS/OPTN cardiac transplant database. *Heart Rhythm* **2010**, *7*, 1567–1571. [CrossRef] [PubMed]
42. Mallidi, H.R.; Bates, M. Pacemaker Use Following Heart Transplantation. *Ochsner J.* **2017**, *17*, 20–24. [PubMed]

43. Hamon, D.; Taleski, J.; Vaseghi, M.; Shivkumar, K.; Boyle, N.G. Arrhythmias in the Heart Transplant Patient. *Arrhythmia Electrophysiol. Rev.* **2014**, *3*, 149–155. [CrossRef] [PubMed]
44. Cui, G.; Kobashigawa, J.; Margarian, A.; Sen, L. Cause of atrioventricular block in patients after heart transplantation. *Transplantation* **2003**, *76*, 137–142. [CrossRef] [PubMed]

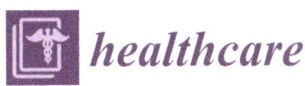

Book Review

Book Review: Cohn, S.L. (Ed.). Decision Making in Perioperative Medicine: Clinical Pearls. (New York: McGraw-Hill), 2021. ISBN: 978-1-260-46810-6

Richard H. Parrish II

Department of Biomedical Sciences, Mercer University School of Medicine, Columbus, GA 31902, USA; parrish_rh@mercer.edu; Tel.: +1-(706)-321-7218

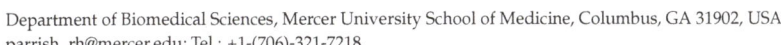

Citation: Parrish II, R.H. Book Review: Cohn, S.L. (Ed.). Decision Making in Perioperative Medicine: Clinical Pearls. (New York: McGraw-Hill), 2021. ISBN: 978-1-260-46810-6. *Healthcare* **2021**, *9*, 687. https://doi.org/10.3390/healthcare9060687

Academic Editor: Andreas G. Nerlich

Received: 6 May 2021
Accepted: 3 June 2021
Published: 7 June 2021

Publisher's Note: MDPI stays neutral with regard to jurisdictional claims in published maps and institutional affiliations.

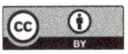

Copyright: © 2021 by the author. Licensee MDPI, Basel, Switzerland. This article is an open access article distributed under the terms and conditions of the Creative Commons Attribution (CC BY) license (https://creativecommons.org/licenses/by/4.0/).

Cohn's work fills a void in the perioperative care literature by providing a concise, comprehensive, practical, and authoritative guide to the medical management of common periprocedural issues and scenarios. The book is organized logically according to the typical flow of patient management, beginning with an introduction to perioperative patient care, prevention of common complications, treatment of co-existing diseases and special populations (such as the cancer patient and surgery in the older patient), and finishing with the management of common post-operative problems.

The book has a number of strengths, and could be easily converted into a computer app to aid utilization for practice enhancement and teaching at the bedside. It contains many helpful tables and figures (algorithms) that assist the reader to form a complete picture of the topic. The importance of conducting a careful risk assessment to avoid exacerbation of co-morbidities or prevention of various post-operative complications is well highlighted. The 'clinical pearls' found at the end of each chapter provide the reader with high yield and pertinent information on important treatment decision making aspects. The chapters in the section on common post-operative problems are well-written and succinct.

There are also a number of areas where the book could be improved, perhaps in subsequent editions. Because there are 26 co-authors of the various chapters, the scope, depth, and detail of each chapter seems to vary considerably. Some chapters have guideline or clinical trial citations; some important statements were uncited. For example, in the prevention of surgical site infections (SSI) with antimicrobials, the current workhorse antibiotic and dosing for prophylaxis of SSIs, cefazolin, is not mentioned by name; not all cephalosporins are indicated for prophylaxis [1]. This variation is also true of the 'clinical pearls' bullet points, and the source or attribution of the pearl often varies. Some of the pearls are summative statements discussed in-depth in the chapter; others are based on the author's experience or expertise. Moreover, several citations are not the most up to date, such as the management of post-operative nausea and vomiting (PONV) [2]. In this regard, while PONV is a major reason for delayed discharge from the hospital or outpatient surgery center, its assessment and management are scattered among several chapters. It would have been more helpful to the reader if PONV had its own chapter, placed either in the prophylaxis or common problems section. There are several redundancies and omissions regarding medication management. For example, both the chapter on medication management and ischemic heart disease identify cardiac medications that need to be withheld or continued during the perioperative period. Medications to treat myasthenia gravis (pyridostigmine and azathioprine) are omitted in the robust table (chapter 4, page 34), and importance of avoiding general anesthesia and neostigmine reversal in these patients is paramount to safe emergence by using newer agents, perhaps sugammadex (which is not mentioned in the text at all) [3–5]. At times, use of medication names, either brand or generic, is not consistent. There is no chapter on the pediatric patient, which would be another excellent addition to the next edition placed in the special populations section. Considering the recent major paradigm shift in perioperative care culture, the treatment of enhanced recovery programs is somewhat cursory [6–8].

On balance, while the book has some minor limitations, it is an excellent collection of tips and wisdom proven to be very helpful in the management of the perioperative patient. It is recommended as required reading for any surgery, general medicine, or pharmacy resident or fellow in training or on rotation, as well as a comprehensive reference for experienced practitioners and allied health professionals working in the periprocedural space. It might also serve as the basis of a shared mental model for collaborative practice development among surgeons, anesthesiologists, hospitalists, clinical pharmacists, nurses, dietitians, and other therapists managing the care of the periprocedural patient.

Funding: This research received no external funding.

Institutional Review Board Statement: Not applicable.

Informed Consent Statement: Not applicable.

Data Availability Statement: Not applicable.

Conflicts of Interest: The authors declare no conflict of interest.

References

1. Bratzler, D.W.; Dellinger, E.P.; Olsen, K.M.; Perl, T.M.; Auwaerter, P.G.; Bolon, M.K.; Fish, D.N.; Napolitano, L.M.; Sawyer, R.G.; Slain, D.; et al. Clinical practice guidelines for antimicrobial prophylaxis in surgery. *Am. J. Health Syst. Pharm.* **2013**, *70*, 195–283. [CrossRef] [PubMed]
2. Gan, T.J.; Belani, K.G.; Bergese, S.; Chung, F.; Diemunsch, P.; Habib, A.S.; Jin, Z.; Kovac, A.L.; Meyer, T.A.; Urman, R.D.; et al. Fourth Consensus Guidelines for the Management of Postoperative Nausea and Vomiting. *Anesth. Analg.* **2020**, *131*, 411–448. [CrossRef] [PubMed]
3. Sanders, D.B.; Wolfe, G.I.; Narayanaswami, P.; MGFA Task Force on MG Treatment Guidance. Developing treatment guidelines for myasthenia gravis. *Ann. N. Y. Acad. Sci.* **2018**, *1412*, 95–101. [CrossRef] [PubMed]
4. Collins, S.; Roberts, H.; Hewer, I. Anesthesia and Perioperative Considerations for Patients With Myasthenia Gravis. *AANA J.* **2020**, *88*, 485–491. [PubMed]
5. Fernandes, H.D.S.; Ximenes, J.L.S.; Nunes, D.I.; Ashmawi, H.A.; Vieira, J.E. Failure of reversion of neuromuscular block with sugammadex in patient with myasthenia gravis: Case report and brief review of literature. *BMC Anesthesiol.* **2019**, *19*, 160. [CrossRef] [PubMed]
6. Smith, T.W.J.; Wang, X.; Singer, M.A.; Godellas, C.V.; Vaince, F.T. Enhanced recovery after surgery: A clinical review of implementation across multiple surgical subspecialties. *Am. J. Surg.* **2020**, *219*, 530–534. [CrossRef] [PubMed]
7. Arrick, L.; Mayson, K.; Hong, T.; Warnock, G. Enhanced recovery after surgery in colorectal surgery: Impact of protocol adherence on patient outcomes. *J. Clin. Anesth.* **2019**, *55*, 7–12. [CrossRef] [PubMed]
8. Currie, A.; Soop, M.; Demartines, N.; Fearon, K.; Kennedy, R.; Ljungqvist, O. Enhanced Recovery After Surgery Interactive Audit System: 10 Years' Experience with an International Web-Based Clinical and Research Perioperative Care Database. *Clin. Colon. Rectal. Surg.* **2019**, *32*, 75–81. [CrossRef] [PubMed]

MDPI
St. Alban-Anlage 66
4052 Basel
Switzerland
Tel. +41 61 683 77 34
Fax +41 61 302 89 18
www.mdpi.com

Healthcare Editorial Office
E-mail: healthcare@mdpi.com
www.mdpi.com/journal/healthcare

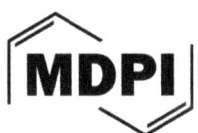

www.ingramcontent.com/pod-product-compliance
Lightning Source LLC
LaVergne TN
LVHW070559100526
838202LV00012B/516